Essential Geriatrics

Henry Woodford

BSc, MRCP
Consultant in Elderly Medicine
Cumberland Infirmary, Carlisle

Foreword by
James George

Hon. Clinical Senior Lecturer, University of Newcastle
Consultant Physician and Clinical Director, North Cumbria Acute Trust

Radcliffe Publishing
Oxford • New York

Radcliffe Publishing Ltd
18 Marcham Road
Abingdon
Oxon OX14 1AA
United Kingdom

www.radcliffe-oxford.com
Electronic catalogue and worldwide online ordering facility.

British Library Cataloguing in Publication Data

A catalogue record for this book is available from the British Library.

ISBN-13: 978 1 84619 170 1

Typeset by Advance Typesetting Ltd, Oxford
Printed and bound by TJI Digital, Padstow, Cornwall

Contents

To my wife, Leanne

Foreword

Geriatric medicine, with over a thousand consultants, is now the largest medical specialty in the UK. With the ageing population, the development of subspecialties in geriatrics and the increasing acute workload, the specialty is expected to expand rapidly over the next decade. Dr Woodford has highlighted a gap in the market which this book fills. Although there are now numerous large textbooks on geriatric medicine, there is no concise practical evidence-based guide for the beginner in the specialty. Geriatrics is both an 'old' and a 'new' specialty. 'Old' in the sense that it dates from the 1940s when Marjory Warren, in her seminal work, recognised that older people benefit from proper assessment and rehabilitation, and a new specialty was born. 'New' in that much of the evidence base is relatively new and comprehensive geriatric assessment, for example, was not confirmed as a beneficial intervention by a meta-analysis until the 1990s. Geriatric medicine has long had a passionate beating 'heart', attracting doctors, nurses and therapists with tremendous enthusiasm to improve the care for older people, but only relatively recently has the specialty developed a definite 'soul' of a sound evidence base to ensure this enthusiasm is targeted to achieve better outcomes for older people. This book eloquently describes the knowledge and evidence base essential for practitioners of geriatric medicine.

Although the book is written primarily for doctors starting in the specialty, it will also be valuable for all members of the multidisciplinary team and also established geriatricians who wish to update themselves. Hopefully, it will encourage research into the many areas in which our evidence base is still uncertain. There are four sections covering the 'geriatric giants' (falls, confusion, immobility and incontinence) and three sections on therapeutics, cardiovascular topics and end of life issues. Each section can be read in under an hour, but also can be dipped into when particular queries arise, for example during and after ward rounds. The evidence base for treatment and intervention in older people is clearly described, evaluated and referenced. Older people are particularly vulnerable in two ways. Firstly, they may sometimes be denied treatment that is clearly of benefit to them simply because of their age. Secondly, and no less importantly, they may sometimes be offered treatment simply because it is feasible rather than being necessarily beneficial, especially as older people are likely to have multiple symptoms and diseases. Fortunately, older patients are often wiser than their doctors and when given the alternative options for their individual situation will make the right decision for themselves. The book gives geriatricians the information to inform and to share difficult decisions with our older patients.

Dr Woodford is to be congratulated for his practical approach and critical review of the literature. Enthusiasm and passion for the specialty are important but no longer enough as we enter a new era for geriatrics. Hopefully this book will inspire the new generation of geriatricians to improve their clinical care of older patients and improve clinical outcomes. I look forward to multiple further editions as our evidence base expands. Read, learn and enjoy.

James George
Consultant Geriatrician, Carlisle
January 2007

About the author

Henry Woodford was born in York and went to school in Yorkshire. He then went to medical school at King's College London. During this time he did an intercalated degree incorporating physiology. His elective period was spent in British Columbia, Canada. He did his house jobs in the south-east of England but then moved to the north-east for further training. He did his specialist registrar rotation based around Newcastle upon Tyne. One year was taken out of the programme to work at the Westmead Hospital in Sydney, Australia. He has recently taken a consultant post in elderly medicine with a special interest in stroke at Cumberland Infirmary, Carlisle, UK. He is married and, so far, has one daughter.

Introduction

The population is getting older. Over the next 30 years the number of people aged over 90 years within the UK is set to double from the value recorded in 1999.[1] Thus, those who specialise in the treatment of older people will be needed more than ever. Coupled to this rising demand, the specialty is becoming more evidence-based with increasing research into the care of this important section of the community.

When I first became a specialist registrar in geriatric medicine I looked for a suitable textbook to introduce me to the finer points of the specialty. Those available seemed to be either extremely long or short, but above all not meeting the criteria of being both evidence-based and practical. As I progressed through my training I found that I was searching through textbooks, journal articles and web resources to cover the key subjects. I came to the conclusion that I may be able to prevent other people doing the same – this idea forms the basis for this book.

This text specifically focuses on the key aspects of elderly care, aiming to be a bridge between general medicine and the particular problems that are encountered in geriatrics (targeted at the 'geriatric giants'[2]). It is envisaged that it will help the reader have a stepping-stone into this peculiar specialty. The subjects covered are chosen because they are not traditionally covered well in medical texts. At the end of each section there is often an attempt to convert the available evidence into a practical guide for the management of the covered conditions. Trying to practise evidence-based elderly medicine can be a frustrating thing as there are so many gaps in the evidence. Some of the guidance in this book reflects this – it tries to represent a reasonable approach, but not everyone will agree.

This book is designed to be of high practical value to the busy clinician. For the more theoretical subspecialty of gerontology (the study of the process of ageing), the interested reader is advised to start with an excellent book by Tom Kirkwood.[3] Within his book the 'disposable soma' theory of ageing is discussed in plain English.

The geriatrician should never forget that our aim is not simply to prolong life or extend the dying process. We are charged with reducing illness and suffering in older people. It appears to be possible that we may achieve the apparent paradox of increased lifespan with reduced lifetime morbidity.[4] We should consider this as one of humanity's greatest successes.

References

1 Khaw KT. How many, how old, how soon? *BMJ*, 1999; **319**: 1350–2.
2 Isaacs B. *The Challenge of Geriatric Medicine*. Oxford: Oxford University Press, 1992.
3 Kirkwood T. *Time of Our Lives*. London: Phoenix, 2000.
4 Tallis R. *Hippocratic Oaths: medicine and its discontents*. London: Atlantic Books, 2004.

Brain

Chapter 1

Dementia

Definition

Dementia is a syndrome attributed to disease of the brain, usually of a chronic or progressive nature, in which there is disturbance of multiple brain functions. These impairments may include calculation, learning capacity, language and judgement. It is usually only considered present when there is resultant impact on social or occupational function, or both. Consciousness is usually unaltered. There may also be deterioration in emotional control, social behaviour or motivation. In other words, it is not simply memory loss but a complex condition that affects more than one cognitive aspect.

Epidemiology

Approximately 8–10% of people over the age of 65 years in the Western world have dementia. The prevalence rises from around 2% of those aged 65 to more than 35% of those over 85 years (Figure 1.1).[1–3] This figure represents, roughly, a doubling in prevalence for every five-year increase in age. A more positive thought is that around two-thirds of the very old do not have dementia. The number of people worldwide with dementia is predicted to double every 20 years.[4]

In addition, there is a significant population of individuals with some clinical evidence of cognitive impairment that is not severe enough to meet the criteria for a diagnosis of dementia. This also appears to increase with advancing age – perhaps affecting around 17% of people over the age of 65 years.[5] This figure may have some impact on functional status and the need for care-home placement.

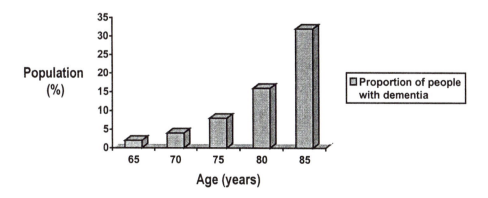

Figure 1.1   The rising prevalence of dementia with age.

Memory

Loss of memory is not always a feature of dementia but it is a common finding. Traditionally it has been loosely divided into short-term and long-term components. More recently, memory has been classified into four categories,[6] which are outlined below.

- **Episodic memory**: The memory of specific personal events and experiences, for example what you did on holiday last year. Predominantly mediated by the medial temporal lobes (including the hippocampus). Insults to this system tend to affect more recently learned memories more than older ones (i.e. short-term memory is more affected than long-term memory).
- **Semantic memory**: Knowledge of the world not related to personal experiences. This includes the names of objects, for example the names of animals. This is predominantly mediated by the inferolateral temporal lobes.
- **Procedural memory**: The memory of how to perform tasks, such as riding a bike. The basal ganglia and cerebellum predominantly mediate this. It occurs at a subconscious level. It may be particularly affected in movement disorders (*see* Chapter 4).
- **Working memory**: Short-term (seconds to minutes) 'keeping it in your head'. It can be phonologic (e.g. a phone number) or spatial (e.g. manipulating an object in your mind). The prefrontal cortex is important in this process along with other brain areas depending on the nature of the task. For an effective working memory, it is also necessary to be able to maintain attention/concentration.

Memories may be conscious (declarative) or non-conscious (non-declarative). Confabulation is the making-up of new 'memories' to replace those that have been lost.

Assessment

History

The history is usually best taken with the help of a carer. It should incorporate all the features of a thorough medical history in other situations, for example past medical problems, current medication, and so on. The following is a guide to the specific features required in cognitive assessment.

Onset and progression

The rate and nature of cognitive decline are helpful in distinguishing between different types of dementia. For example: Alzheimer's disease (AD) has an insidious, progressive nature; vascular dementia (VaD) may be stepwise; and a more rapid decline is seen in Creutzfeldt–Jakob disease (CJD). A fluctuating course may be associated with delirium (*see* Chapter 2) or dementia with Lewy bodies (DLB) (*see* p 76). This is represented graphically in Figure 1.2. The initial presenting problem may be helpful in distinguishing subtypes when the presentation is late and deficits in multiple cognitive domains have developed.

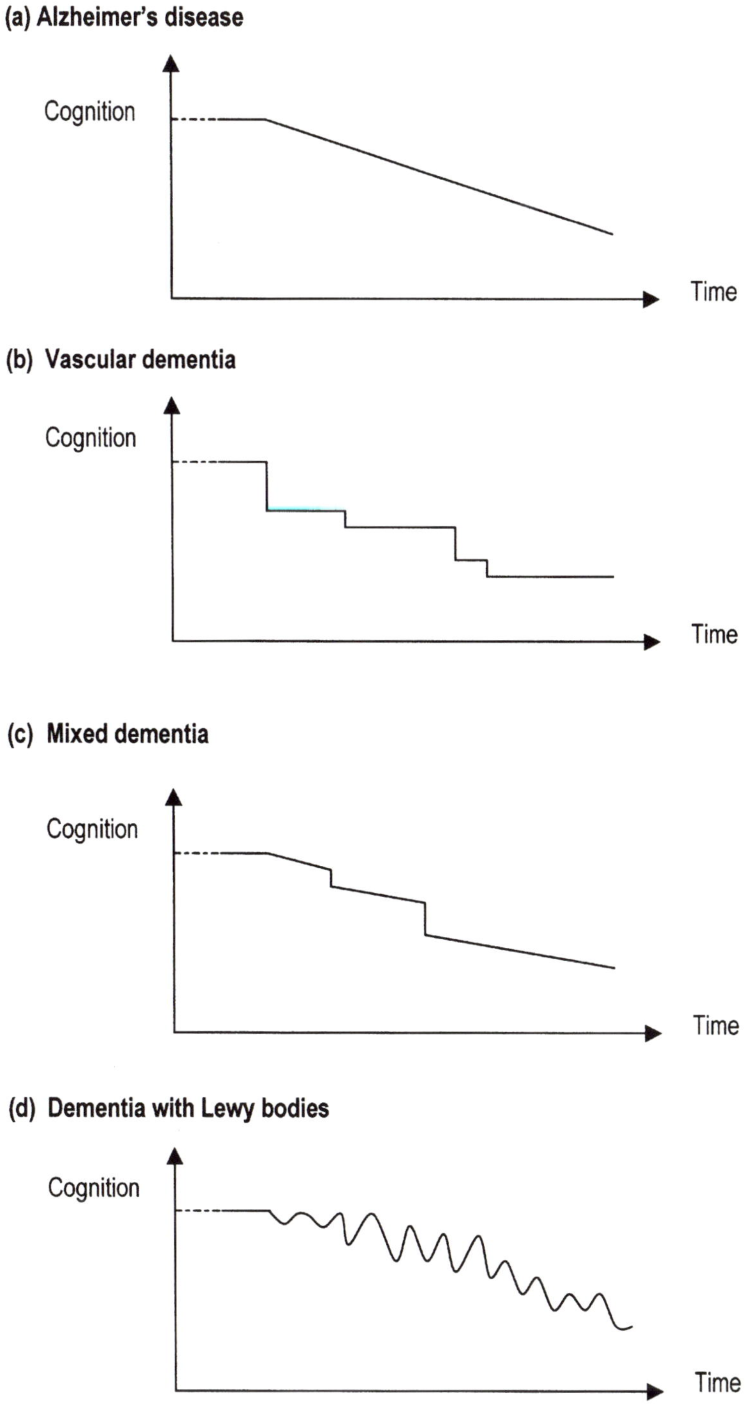

(a) Alzheimer's disease

(b) Vascular dementia

(c) Mixed dementia

(d) Dementia with Lewy bodies

Figure 1.2 Change in cognitive function over time with different types of dementia: (a) Alzheimer's disease; (b) vascular dementia; (c) mixed dementia; (d) dementia with Lewy bodies.

Cognitive deficits

It is important to explore different cognitive areas during the questioning in order to fully identify all the deficits. These functions will then be more formally tested during the mental state examination.

- *Memory loss*: both short and long-term aspects.
- *Language impairment*: problems including word-finding difficulties (dysphasia) and the use of inappropriate words (paraphrasias).
- *Calculation impairment*: may manifest as difficulty with financial matters.
- *Visuospatial problems*: such as getting lost in familiar environments.
- *Praxia*: the inability to perform learned movements despite intact motor function. This may present as difficulty with tasks, such as opening cans or turning on taps.
- *Executive functions*: complex tasks, goal-directed behaviour and insight.
- *Agnosia*: the inability to recognise objects despite intact sensory function.

Behavioural changes

- *Personality*: changes in social interaction and inappropriateness are common in frontotemporal dementia (FTD).
- *Sleep*: changes in diurnal variation. Early morning waking is associated with depression, which may co-exist with, or mimic dementia (*see* Chapter 3). REM disorders (vivid dreams, jerking or thrashing movements during sleep) are associated with DLB.
- *Food preferences*: a change in dietary preferences, especially a tendency to like more sweet foods, is associated with FTD.
- *Sexuality*: sexual drive may be increased or reduced.
- *Delusions and hallucinations*: early visual hallucinations are a feature of DLB, but may occur in other conditions, especially delirium.
- *Continence*: if urinary incontinence is an early feature then VaD or normal pressure hydrocephalus (NPH) (*see* p 84) should be considered. Incontinence is important as a predictor of nursing home placement and survival.

Past medical history

A history of depression makes current depression more likely. Previous vascular disease or vascular risk factors may add weight to a diagnosis of vascular dementia.

Medication

Anticholinergic medication use is frequently associated with impaired cognition in the elderly (but not an increased risk of developing dementia).[7] (*See* Table 2.1, Table 3.2 and p 148.)

Social and functional

A number of example questions to explore social and functional background are listed below.

- Who else is at home and what kind of residence is it?
- What help is required for mobility, self-care, cooking, cleaning, laundry, finances, etc? Are they still driving? If so how safe does the carer feel to be in the car with the patient?
- Do they have any external help – friends, family, Social Services? Are there any hazards and has there been an occupational therapist involved in home assessment?
- Are there any issues regarding carer well-being?
- Does the patient smoke or drink (important as risk factors for VaD and alcohol-related dementias)? If alcoholism is suspected, then explore the patient's prior drinking habits and ask about specific problems, such as withdrawal seizures.

Sociocultural background

Neuropsychological assessment is interpreted in light of previous education. What age did the patient leave school and with what qualifications? What was their employment?

Familial history

Although not the norm, some dementing illnesses have a familial component. This is more likely with FTD when there is a history of onset before the age of 60 years.

Examination

This is divided into mental state and physical examinations.

Mental state

In clinical practice, time usually limits the depth and complexity of testing of the mental state. The 10-point Abbreviated Mental Test (AMT) may suffice for an 'on the ward' screening tool (*see* Appendix A). However, the 30-point Mini Mental State Examination (MMSE) should be considered the minimum for cognitive assessment. Here, the higher the score the better, with a score of 25 or below suggesting significant impairment (*see* Appendix A). In the clock-drawing test the patient is asked to draw a circle, add numbers as though drawing a clock face and then place on the hands to indicate a specific time (e.g. 10 past 11). There are differing scoring systems, but in the simplest of these one point is allocated for correctly completing each of the three elements just listed. It has been found to be a reasonable screening test for dementia.[8]

Formal neuropsychological testing usually involves a series of tests that assess specific aspects of brain function. This process often takes far longer (typically two to three hours) than practical for a medical assessment, plus the results can only accurately be interpreted by a specialist with comparison to data on normal populations. A reasonable intermediate step between the MMSE and formal neuropsychology is the Addenbrookes Cognitive Examination (ACE).[9] This series of questions incorporates the MMSE and the clock-drawing test along with more elaborate tests of specific cognitive domains to give a score out of 100. The higher the score, the better the cognition, with a cut-off point suggesting significant impairment of below 87. Subtle deficits will only be detected with more complex testing. In late dementia all areas of cognition will become impaired and the discriminatory ability to diagnose specific dementia syndromes will become diminished.

Domains tested include attention, memory, language, visuospatial skills and executive function. These are discussed in turn below. The process attempts to localise deficits within the brain. A simplified overview of the function of cortical regions is shown in Figure 1.3.

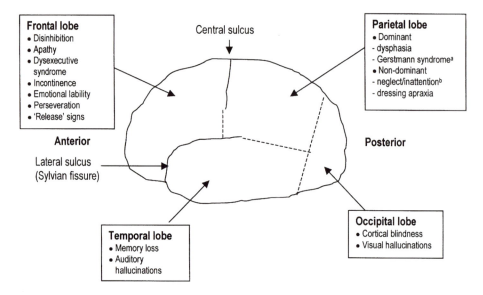

Figure 1.3 Cognitive functional neuro-anatomy of the brain: the basic features of damage to specific brain regions (*see also* Figure 5.5): [a]Gerstmann syndrome: difficulty with writing (dysgraphia) and calculation (dyscalculia), left–right indistinction and inability to identify fingers (finger agnosia); [b]dominant parietal lesions may also cause neglect and inattention, but they tend to be less severe.

Attention

Attention is the ability to focus on a task and is determined by both concentration and arousal. Patients with reduced attention are easily distracted. Simple tests of attention include digit span (the patient is asked to recall series of numbers), reverse sequences (e.g. recite the months of the year backwards or count down from 20 to 1), and 'serial sevens' (subtract sevens from 100). It requires an intact reticular activating system as well as cortical components. When attention is impaired the rest of the neuropsychological examination may be hard to interpret.

Memory

Giving the patient a series of words to remember is a simple test of memory. A person who is able to recall words after clues are given is more likely to have a subcortical deficit that impairs memory retrieval rather than memory formation.

Orientation questions (day, month, year, etc.) also test the ability to form new memories. The non-dominant lobe predominantly determines visuospatial memory. Asking the patient to remember and then reproduce images can test this. Remote memory (e.g. recalling the dates of World War II) is more dependent on cortical processes than the limbic system (*see* Figure 1.6).

Language

The dominant hemisphere encodes language. Spontaneous speech during the history may have given some clues to linguistic function. The assessment of speech is discussed in Chapter 5. 'Prosody' is a term for the melodic and rhythmic qualities of speech. 'Paraphrasia' is the insertion of incorrect words into sentences. There may be semantic errors (using an incorrect but related word, for example saying 'apple' instead of 'orange'). Language disturbance is a common component of AD but rarely features in subcortical dementias.

Visuospatial skills

Asking patients to copy figures can test visuospatial skills. This function is commonly impaired in dementia or delirium but rarely involved with primary psychiatric disorders. Deficits are more common and more severe when the non-dominant rather than the dominant lobe is affected.

Executive function

Executive skills enable the performance of complex tasks or behaviours. The frontal lobes are important for their generation. They can be tested by asking patients to continue sequences, which can be alpha-numeric (e.g. 1A, 2B, 3C ...) or drawn repetitive patterns. Alternative methods include verbal fluency (e.g. ask the patient to list as many names of animals as they can in one minute), describe similarities between words (e.g. shirt and trousers) or to interpret the meanings of proverbs (e.g. people who live in glass houses shouldn't throw stones).

Gerstmann syndrome is caused by a lesion of the dominant lobe's angular gyrus (within the parietal lobe), which results in dyscalculia, dysgraphia, left–right disorientation and finger agnosia.

Physical

The physical examination should incorporate the features of a good general medical assessment, in particular looking for signs of neurological and vascular disease. Speech will have been assessed as part of the mental state examination. Cranial nerves may show reduced up and down gaze with progressive supranuclear palsy (PSP) (*see* p 77). Impaired saccadic eye movements may provide more subtle signs of an underlying movement disorder (*see* Figure 4.5). Pyramidal tract or cerebellar signs may indicate VaD. Increased tone with cogwheeling and bradykinesia suggests an underlying movement disorder (*see* Chapter 4).

Frontal release signs

- *Grasp reflex*: the patient grasps an object that is stroked across the palm.
- *Pout (snout) reflex*: a pouting facial expression is produced when the area lateral to the upper lip is stroked.
- *Glabellar tap*: the area between the eyebrows is gently tapped (with the examiner's arm approaching from above/behind to prevent blinking to a threatening stimulus). A positive result is achieved when the patient continues to blink beyond the first three taps.

The frontal release signs are neurological phenomena that originate from the brainstem or below.[10] These signs are present in newborn children until subcortical myelination is completed. They may recur in later life in normal individuals or in association with cerebral damage.[11] They are then termed 'release' signs due to the loss of the cortical inhibition of the brainstem-mediated mechanisms. They have been detected in 55% of patients with AD (mean age 68 years) compared to 9% of normal control subjects (mean age 62).[12] In general their occurrence does not correlate well with cognitive function. The presence of grasp and pout reflexes appears to be the most suggestive of cognitive impairment.[10,13]

Test for dyspraxia by asking the patient to mime tasks with both hands individually and together, and to mime some tasks involving the face, such as combing hair, cutting bread, whistling. The Luria task is a test of executive function. It is a three-step hand sequence that the patient is asked to copy (*see* Figure 1.4). Hemiplegic or 'marche à petits pas' (small-stepping) gaits are associated with VaD. Parkinsonian gaits may signify an underlying movement disorder. The gait of NPH is broad-based with a 'foot stuck to the floor' appearance.

'Cut'   'Fist'   'Slap'

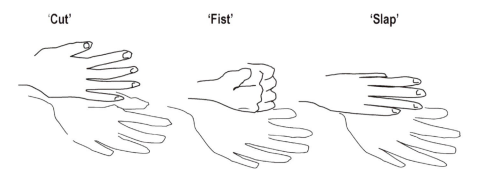

Figure 1.4 The Luria task. The patient is asked to copy the three-stage hand sequence shown above. A normal individual can correctly repeat this within several attempts.

Investigations

There are no laboratory tests to diagnose the common forms of dementia. Investigations may help to exclude potentially reversible causes. The standard 'dementia screen' bloods: ESR, vitamin B_{12} and TSH should be performed (to exclude vasculitis, combined degeneration and hypothyroidism). Syphilis serological testing (venereal disease research laboratory test; VDRL) may be considered – *see* Box 1.1. Brain imaging (CT or MRI) can exclude NPH or space-occupying lesions. Focal cerebral atrophy is rarely seen in early disease. Global cerebral atrophy is often seen in normal ageing and does not correlate with cognitive function. Vascular disease may be seen, lending weight to a diagnosis of VaD. Areas of leukoaraiosis (white matter lesions) are found in a third of those aged over 65 and have questionable clinical significance (*see* p 16). Definitive diagnosis can only be achieved by correlation of clinical features with pathological specimens, usually post-mortem. Rarely a brain biopsy is undertaken. This typically involves obtaining a full-thickness frontal cortical section. One retrospective analysis found that diagnostic information was obtained in 57% of biopsies, and treatment decisions were affected in 11%.[14] Complications are seen in around 10% and include seizures, haemorrhage and infection. Biopsy should be considered when a reversible condition, such as an inflammatory process, is suspected clinically but cannot be confirmed by an alternative method. More specific tests may be indicated in some individuals according to their clinical history, for example HIV serology.

Box 1.1   Note on syphilis

Syphilis serology is often performed as part of a dementia 'work-up'. It should be remembered that a VDRL stays positive after exposure to syphilis. There are also a number of conditions causing false positives (e.g. systemic lupus erythematosus; SLE). A *Treponema pallidum* haemaggultinin antibody (TPHA) test is only positive at the time of acute infection. Neurosyphilis is a form of tertiary syphilis that occurs in about 10% of people who are untreated. The median age of onset has now fallen to 39 years and is mostly seen in relation to HIV infection.[15] The form of neurosyphilis associated with cognitive impairment is called 'general paresis'. This occurs between three and 40 years after exposure. The clinical features are reduced attention, memory and executive abilities. There may be associated delusions (classically grandiose), hallucinations and confabulation. Physical examination may reveal upper motor neuron signs in the limbs and possibly associated tabes dorsalis (demyelination of the dorsal columns). With adequate penicillin treatment 50% will improve.

   In summary, neurosyphilis is an extremely rare presentation of cognitive impairment in the elderly. VDRL testing may well give a positive result in the absence of active syphilis. It should be considered when clinical suspicion is present, but its value as a routine screening test in dementia is questionable.

Differential diagnosis of dementia

Normal ageing and cognition

A number of cognitive changes are commonly found in healthy older adults. These include slowing of cognition (bradyphrenia), a reduced capacity to form novel solutions to problems, becoming more cautious in behaviour and having reduced memory recall. These subtle changes need to be distinguished from an abnormal dementia process.

Delirium and depression

Delirium and depression are the most important differential diagnoses of dementia in the elderly. These are discussed in chapters 2 and 3, respectively. Core features that may help to distinguish them are outlined in Table 1.1.

Table 1.1 A comparison of the distinguishing features of dementia, delirium and depression[a]

	Dementia	Delirium	Depression
Onset	Insidious	Acute/subacute	Rapid
Course	Progressive	Fluctuating	Stable
Impaired consciousness	−	+	−
Reduced attention span	−	+	−
Impaired visuospatial skills	+	+	−
Hallucinations	−	+	−
Delusions	−	+	−
Psychomotor retardation	−	+	+
Psychomotor activation	−	+	−
Personal or family history of depression	−	−	+
Low mood	−	−	+
Poor appetite	−	−	+
Weight loss	−	−	+
Sleep disturbance	−	+	+
Insight preserved	−	−	+
Improves during the day	−	−	+
Response to antidepressants	−	−	+

[a] Its purpose is to act as a guide rather than a rigid scheme. For example, hallucinations are most commonly seen with delirium, but may be associated with either dementia with Lewy bodies or psychotic depression. + = a characteristic feature; − = not usually a feature.

Distinguishing dementia subtypes

A broad division of the subtypes of dementia into cortical and subcortical has been proposed. This is not a perfect divide as much overlap exists[16] but it probably has some role as a simplistic model.

- *Cortical* (e.g. AD, FTD, asymmetric cortical atrophies): These dementias are characterised by deficits in specific cortical domains: memory problems, aphasia, apraxia, visuospatial impairment, reduced calculation and agnosia (perceptual difficulty).
- *Subcortical* (e.g. VaD, movement disorders (e.g. PSP), NPH, infections, toxins): These dementias are thought to affect circuits of the basal ganglia and thalamus (*see* Figure 4.1). There is reduced speed of thought (bradyphrenia) and delayed access to information. There tend to be frontal-executive features, such as perseveration, sequencing problems and reduced verbal fluency (rather than aphasia). The use of clues may aid memory retrieval, whereas this is less likely to benefit those with a cortical deficit. There may be more prominent apathy and associated reduced speech quality, for example dysarthria and hypophonia (reduced volume).

Table 1.2 outlines some of the distinguishing features of these two categories.

Table 1.2 Properties that may help to distinguish between cortical and subcortical patterns of dementia

	Cortical	Subcortical
Psychomotor speed	Normal	↓
Speech	Dysphasia or paraphrasia	Hypophonia or dysarthria
Executive function	Normal or ↓	↓↓
Verbal fluency	Normal or ↓	↓↓
Memory	Amnesia	↓ retrieval speed

Personality change

A change in personality suggests frontal lobe involvement and makes a diagnosis of FTD, VaD or CJD more likely.

Hallucinations and delusions

Visual hallucinations and cognitive impairment are suggestive of DLB. Alternative diagnoses include delirium, VaD and psychotic depression. Auditory hallucinations are more compatible with schizophrenia. Delusions are common in advanced AD but may be an early feature of DLB.

Neurological signs

Focal neurological signs may help to diagnose VaD. Alternatively, a small-stepping gait (marche à petits pas) may be detected. Movement disorders with associated dementia usually have characteristic physical signs; however, the cognitive features may predate the motor features by up to one year.

Specific conditions causing dementia

In the Western world the most common cause of dementia is AD (50–60%).[17] The other common causes of dementia in the elderly are VaD, mixed dementia (VaD–AD) and DLB (together accounting for around 30–40% in total). Alternative diagnoses represent less than 10% of cases in older people (*see* Figure 1.5). The estimates of actual prevalence vary quite widely between studies, in part due to differing diagnostic definitions and differing age groups studied. For example, FTD is a more common cause of dementia in younger people (<65 years), where it may represent as many as 20% of cases.

Alzheimer's disease

- Percentage of all dementia: 50–60.

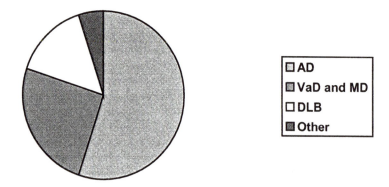

Figure 1.5 The approximate contribution of subtypes of dementia in the elderly.

- Prevalence: 6% of people over 65 years.
- Survival: approximately 10 years.
- Key early features: memory loss, language deficits, visuospatial problems.

Alzheimer's disease most commonly presents as an initial loss of short-term memory. Usually procedural memory is retained in the early stages. Language problems present as word-finding difficulties and paraphrasias (using the wrong words). Verbal fluency may be reduced – particularly the generation of semantic lists (e.g. the names of animals). Visuospatial problems are prominent (e.g. a history of getting lost or difficulty with copying objects or clock drawing). Later in the disease comprehension is also reduced and there may also be repetition of other peoples' words (echolalia) or their own words (palilalia). Also, apraxia, agnosia and reduced executive functioning become more apparent. Patients usually continue to perform activities of daily living well until late in the disease.

Behavioural symptoms are not a significant presenting feature but may develop later. The most common early change is to become apathetic with reduced social interaction and participation in activities. Late changes may include disinhibition, wandering, psychosis and aggression. Delusions commonly develop in later disease and are often persecutory in nature. A study of 50 patients with AD of varying severity found that 80% had some form of behavioural change.[18] The most common were apathy (72%), agitation (60%), and anxiety (48%). The emergence of agitation, dysphoria, apathy and aberrant motor behaviour was significantly correlated with cognitive decline. Visual hallucinations may occur. They are more common in people with underlying visual impairment.[19] Neurovegetative changes (sleep, appetite and sexuality) are common. Neurological features, including extrapyramidal signs, gait disturbance and seizures, can occur in the late stages.

Familial forms also exist, which show an autosomal dominant pattern of inheritance.[20] These tend to have a younger age of onset. There are a number of implicated genes: apolipoprotein E4 allele (APOE4) on chromosome 19, presenilin 1 (chromosome 14), presenilin 2 (chromosome 1), amyloid precursor protein (APP) (chromosome 21), plus others. As yet the role of genetic analysis in clinical practice is not well established.

The accumulation of beta-amyloid plaques (also called neuritic plaques) within the brain appears to be the key mechanism in the pathogenesis of AD.[21] It has been termed the 'amyloid cascade'. The genetic links listed above all seem to enhance the accumulation of amyloid proteins. Secondary pathological changes include tau protein hyperphosphorylation (to form neurofibrillary tangles), inflammation, lipid peroxidation and excitotoxicity. The net result is neuronal cell death in specific brain areas. The parietal and temporal lobes are most frequently affected, although variants involving other brain areas have been described. The limbic system, which lies predominantly within the temporal lobes, is thought to play a crucial role in the processing of memories (*see* Figure 1.6). Acetylcholine, norepinephrine and serotonin pathways are affected. The cholinergic neuronal projections of the nucleus basilis of Meynert within the limbic system to the cortex are particularly impaired.

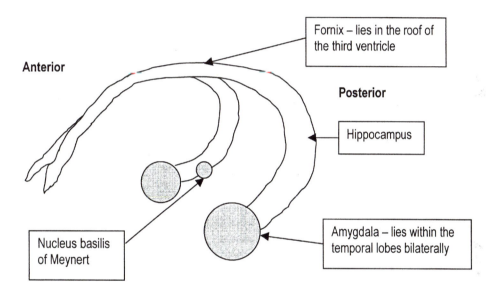

Figure 1.6   A three-dimensional representation of the limbic system.

The diagnosis is classified as definite only when confirmatory pathology is available (usually post-mortem). Probable AD is based on a clinical diagnosis alone (possible AD is when it is considered the most likely diagnosis but there are atypical features).

The rate of cognitive decline is around 3 points on the MMSE scale (out of 30) or 6–7 points on the ADAS-cog scale (out of 70) (*see* Appendix A) per year. The mean survival period is around 10 years.

Vascular dementia

The prevalence of vascular dementia is hard to accurately establish due to a large proportion of patients with mixed pathology (*see below*). Estimates range from approximately 1% to 4% of people over the age of 65 years.

VaD encompasses a variety of clinical presentations. It can result from a range of vascular lesions, including a single cortical stroke, a number of subcortical events, cerebral haemorrhage or episodes of hypoperfusion. 'Binswanger disease' is a term for dementia in association with extensive peri-ventricular white matter lesions (leukoaraiosis) usually caused by atherosclerosis of deep penetrating end-arterioles. Diagnostic criteria for VaD usually require three factors:[17]

- dementia
- clinical and imaging evidence of cerebrovascular disease
- a temporal link between the above two components.

The nature of the cognitive impairment can be quite diverse. Small-vessel ischaemia appears to be the most common cause and this characteristically tends to result in a subcortical pattern of dementia. A clinical picture similar to that of either Parkinson's disease (PD) or NPH can occur. The onset is often abrupt and tends to deteriorate in a stepwise fashion. However, a gradually progressive dementia can occur. The history will usually reveal vascular risk factors. CT scanning may help to demonstrate vascular lesions but it is not, alone, diagnostic.

Patches of leukoaraiosis tend to be peri-ventricular in distribution and are seen as lucencies on CT scanning and areas of increased signal intensity on T2-weighted MRI scans. They are seen more commonly in patients with VaD, but are also seen in normal elderly people. Their role, if any, in the pathogenesis of dementia is unclear. They appear to be related to vascular insufficiency in the white matter, either through infarction or chronic hypoperfusion.[16] Pathological changes seen include loss of myelin and neurons. Identified risk factors for these lesions include hypertension, hypotension and having a labile blood pressure. Other conditions may mimic their MRI appearance (e.g. multiple sclerosis).

Around 20–30% of patients who have sustained an acute stroke will develop dementia in the following three-year period and about 10% will have dementia prior to the onset of this stroke.[22,23] Of those who develop post-stroke dementia, two-thirds seem to meet diagnostic criteria for VaD and one-third for AD.[22,24] These findings further suggest a large overlap between VaD and neurodegenerative changes. Features that make the development of dementia more likely include older age, pre-existing cognitive impairment, atrial fibrillation (AF) and severity of stroke.[23]

Treatment includes addressing vascular risk factors such as blood pressure control, cholesterol and antiplatelet agents where indicated (*see* Chapter 5).

Mixed aetiology

As already mentioned, there is a great deal of overlap between the dementia disorders. Many of the neurodegenerative diseases share common pathologic findings. Also, there is an association of AD with vascular lesions. So, it is not unexpected to find that some dementias are classified as being of mixed aetiology. The most common variant is a mixed AD–VaD condition, and most studies have defined mixed dementia as this combination of pathologies. Estimates of prevalence have varied considerably depending on diagnostic criteria. It is estimated that it accounts for around 20–40% of dementia.[25] Neuropathologic studies have found that pure vascular dementia in the elderly is rare and is almost always associated with some AD-type changes.[17]

In patients with AD, the presence of vascular lesions appears to make the degree of dementia worse.[26] The neuropsychological deficits appear to resemble VaD more closely than AD.[25] A pattern of stepwise deterioration in combination with a progressive decline suggests a mixed aetiology (*see* Figure 1.2).[17]

Frontotemporal dementia

- Percentage of all dementias: 2–5%.
- Mean age of onset: 56–61 years.[27,28]
- Survival: approximately 10 years.

Key early features: personality change, altered personal and interpersonal conduct, emotional blunting, loss of insight, behavioural disorder.

Frontotemporal dementia has several variants, including Pick disease. This latter condition is distinguished pathologically by the presence of Pick bodies, which are argentophilic intracellular inclusions. Tau protein is a normal cellular component of microtubules. FTD is associated with abnormal processing of this protein, often with hyperphosphorylation. Other conditions associated with tau abnormalities include AD, PSP and corticobasal degeneration (CBD) (*see* pp 77 and 79) – together termed 'tauopathies'. As suggested by the name, FTD predominantly affects the frontal and anterior temporal lobes. Overall it represents around 2–5% of dementia but it is a more common cause of younger-onset dementia. It uncommonly occurs after the age of 65.[28]

FTD has an insidious onset and slow progression. Memory and visuospatial ability are relatively spared in the early stages. Patients tend to score adequately on the MMSE. There may be economy or stereotypy (patterns of repetition) of speech. Behavioural features may include reduced personal hygiene, dietary change and disinhibition.[29] Compulsive-like repetitive or stereotyped actions may occur. There may be perseveration of responses and utilisation behaviour. Some individuals become more impulsive and hyperactive; others become apathetic and less active. Urinary incontinence may occur early in the condition. Neurological examination may reveal primitive reflexes.

Obtaining a family history is important as around 40% will have an affected first-degree relative.[27,28] The majority of familial forms show an autosomal dominant pattern of inheritance.[28] Individuals with an affected first-degree relative have a 3.5 times increased risk of dementia before the age of 80 years compared to matched control subjects.[27]

Klüver–Bucy syndrome is a pattern of clinical features that results from bilateral anterior temporal lobe dysfunction. These features include dietary changes (e.g. eating only sweet things), emotional blunting, altered sexual behaviour, sensory agnosia and oral exploratory behaviour (e.g. putting inedible objects into the mouth). Neuroimaging may reveal focal atrophy of frontal and temporal lobes but this is usually only detectable late in the disease course.

Involvement of the left frontotemporal region alone can lead to a presentation with progressive non-fluent aphasia. Semantic dementia is a variant where fluent speech is preserved but there are problems with naming and word comprehension. Other variants of FTD include overlap syndromes with features of PD, motor neuron disease or CBD. A familial form of FTD with PD features is linked to chromosome 17 (FTDP-17). It has a younger age of onset and more rapid progression.

Dementia in movement disorders

The majority of movement disorders affecting older people are neurodegenerative in aetiology. It is not surprising to find that there is a great deal of overlap with the neurodegenerative dementias. Movement disorders presenting in the elderly and with associated cognitive changes include:

- Parkinson's disease
- progressive supranuclear palsy
- dementia with Lewy bodies
- corticobasal degeneration
- normal pressure hydrocephalus.

These are discussed in Chapter 4. The pattern of dementia is generally of a subcortical type, as discussed earlier.

Other causes of dementia

Many causes of dementia have been identified, most of which are very rare in the elderly. These include HIV-associated dementia, Huntington disease, Wilson disease and neurosyphilis (*see* Box 1.1). Selected conditions are discussed below.

Alcohol-related dementia

Although mild to moderate alcohol intake may be protective against dementia (*see* p 20), heavy intake appears to confer an increased risk. A study of 2873 people over the age of 65 found that 8.9% had a definite history of alcohol abuse (DSM criteria).[30] Of this subgroup (mean age 78 years) 48% had evidence of dementia compared to 35% of those with no history of abuse (mean age 82 years).

There is more than one alcohol-related mechanism causing dementia. The first is simple alcohol dementia, which appears to be induced by more than 10 years of excessive alcohol intake. It may be more common in binge drinkers and those with a low thiamine level. It presents with a subcortical pattern of cognitive impairment.

Wernicke–Korsacoff syndrome is caused by thiamine (B_1) deficiency. The Wernicke stage is usually the precursor and has the clinical characteristics of ophthalmoplegia, ataxia and delirium. The Korsacoff stage usually, but not always, follows one or more episodes of Wernicke syndrome. This is a prolonged amnesic disorder affecting the ability to form new memories. It often causes the patient to confabulate. The pathological finding is of haemorrhagic necrosis of the mamillary bodies.

Marchiafava–Bignami disease is caused by acute demyelination of the corpus callosum. It was first described in middle-aged Italian men who drank excessive quantities of red wine. Associated with the dementia are seizures and inter-hemispheric disconnection.

Cognition may improve with thiamine replacement and abstinence.

Hypothyroidism

Profound hypothyroidism has been associated with memory impairment, psychomotor slowing and visuospatial impairments.[31] Impairments such as these are probably only partially reversed by adequate treatment.

B₁₂ deficiency

The common cause of B_{12} deficiency is pernicious anaemia that is attributed to reduced absorption secondary to insufficient gastric secretion of intrinsic factor.[32] It has been estimated to be present, yet undiagnosed, in around 2% of the population over the age of 60 and is more common in women than men (2:1).[33] Neuronal lesions may cause demyelination or even cell death. Rarely, cerebral involvement can present as progressive personality change or memory loss.[32] Advanced neurological complications may not be reversed by replacement therapy.

Creutzfeldt–Jakob disease

Creutzfeldt–Jakob disease (CJD) is mediated by a prion. In such disorders, a cellular prion protein (PrP^C) becomes pathogenic by misfolding into a harmful form (PrP^{SC}).[20] This is then capable of inducing change in other prion proteins with a resultant cascade and accumulation of protein aggregates (*see* Figure 1.7).[34] Pathological changes include spongiform degeneration and astrogliosis.[20] It is most commonly sporadic in nature (85%) but familial (10–15%) and infectious forms (<5%) also exist.[35] The infectious forms include new variant (nvCJD) that is related to the ingestion of infected animal products. The sporadic form has a mean age of onset of 62 years and runs a short course (mean survival five months).[35,36] Overall it has an incidence of around one per million per year but this figure rises to around five per million in those over the age of 60 years.[20] Key clinical features are listed below:

- a rapidly progressive subcortical dementia
- myoclonus
- ataxia
- pyramidal or extrapyramidal signs.

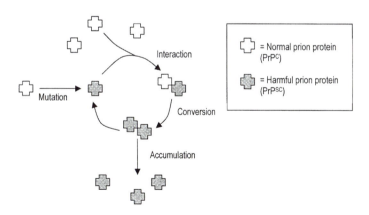

Figure 1.7 The proposed actions of harmful prion proteins.

In the sporadic form, around 60% will have periodic sharp wave complexes in their EEG (compared to 30% of people with AD),[37] around 90% will have 14–3–3 protein in their cerebrospinal fluid (CSF).[37–39] However, 14–3–3 protein is a normal cellular component and its presence in the CSF is merely a marker of cell turnover.[39]

It may be present following cerebral insults such as a stroke. It has been detected in 10% of people with non-CJD dementia.[37–39] MRI scanning has demonstrated signal hyperintensity in the basal ganglia of 67% of patients with CJD compared to just 7% of non-CJD dementia control subjects.[40] The use of diffusion-weighted MRI may further increase diagnostic accuracy.[41] Autopsy studies have found the commonest misdiagnosis in older people is rapidly progressive AD.[42] The combination of clinical criteria and a CSF positive for 14–3–3 protein or a suggestive EEG has a high diagnostic sensitivity and specificity.[38,39]

There is no effective treatment for this condition.

Motor neuron disease

Motor neuron disease (MND) is a disorder related to degeneration of anterior horn cell motor neurons. Onset is between the ages of 40 and 80 years. It is marginally more common in men than women. Ten per cent of cases are familial. There tends to be a mixed pattern of upper and lower motor lesions. There are no sensory signs or bladder or bowel neurological involvement. There is usually weakness with associated stiffness and fasciculations. The voice may become hoarse. Cognition is significantly affected in only one-third of patients.[43] A pattern of deficits similar to FTD is most commonly seen.

Preventing the development of dementia

Non-modifiable risk factors for the development of dementia include age, family history and Down syndrome. A wide range of strategies has been proposed to protect against the development of dementia. Some of these are discussed below.

Alcohol intake

The Rotterdam study is a prospective population-based cohort study of patients over the age of 55 years in a suburb of Rotterdam. Over a mean follow-up period of six years, dementia was diagnosed in 197 of 5395 participants (74% AD, 15% VaD, 11% other dementia).[44] There was a lower associated risk of dementia in those who consumed, on average, up to three alcoholic drinks per day compared to those who did not drink alcohol. The hazard ratio (HR) for people drinking one to three drinks per day for all types of dementia was 0.58 (95% confidence interval (CI) 0.38–0.90). All subtypes of dementia appeared to be reduced with alcohol intake and all types of alcohol (beer, wine and spirits) appeared to offer a similar benefit. Similarly, a comparison of 373 individuals (mean age 78 years) who developed dementia with matched controls within the Cardiovascular Health Study ($n = 5888$) found that mild to moderate alcohol intake appears to confer a lower risk of dementia.[45] The odds ratio (OR) compared to non-drinkers was lowest for those who reported drinking between one and six drinks per week (OR 0.46, 95% CI 0.27–0.77). Other studies seem to support these findings.[46–48] In terms of cardiovascular risk reduction, the benefit of alcohol appears to be mediated by changes in LDL and HDL cholesterol levels.[49] A similar mechanism may protect against cerebral small-vessel ischaemia.

Conversely, alcohol abuse is associated with an increased risk of dementia (*see* p 18).

Prevention of obesity

Over 10 000 men and women who were aged between 40 and 45 years when they were enrolled in the Kaiser Permanente program between the years 1964 and 1973 have been assessed for the development of dementia on average 27 years later.[50] Some 713 people developed dementia at a mean age of onset of 74.5 years. The investigators found that increased weight in middle age was associated with an increased risk of developing dementia. Obese people (body mass index (BMI) $\geq$30 kg/m^2) had a 74% increased risk (HR 1.74, 95% CI 1.34–2.26) and overweight people (BMI 25.0–29.9) had a 35% increased risk (HR 1.35, 95% CI 1.14–1.60) compared to people of normal weight. These differences were not explained by the presence of co-morbid conditions. The mechanism of this apparent effect is not understood. It could be related to changes in vascular risk factors. One study has found that obesity is correlated with brain atrophy.[51] The onset of the clinical phase of dementia is usually accompanied by weight loss.

Vascular risk factors

Smoking, hypertension, high cholesterol and diabetes have all been found to be associated with an increased risk of dementia in later life.[52] This finding is clearly logical for VaD. The degree to which vascular factors are important in the genesis of AD is not known but they do appear to play some role.[53] The Syst-Eur trial randomised 2418 patients with hypertension but without dementia (mean age 70 years, mean blood pressure (BP) 173/86 mmHg) to placebo or BP control with a combination of agents.[54] BP fell in both groups, but significantly more in the treatment group. Mean values achieved were 160/83 mmHg for the placebo group compared to 152/80 mmHg in the treatment arm. After a median follow-up of two years, the incidence of dementia was significantly lower in the treatment group: 3.8 cases per 1000 patient-years vs 7.7 per 1000 patient-years in the placebo arm. Having a higher BP in middle age is also associated with an increased risk of cognitive impairment in later life.[55]

Vitamin E

It had been believed that the antioxidant properties of vitamin E might have a protective role against the development of dementia. A recent study of 769 people with mild cognitive impairment failed to demonstrate any benefit.[56] Further to this, there is some evidence that vitamin E may be harmful in high doses. A meta-analysis of studies comparing vitamin E supplementation to placebo in 136 000 people found an increase in all-cause mortality in the treatment arm.[57]

Oestrogens

A series of small studies and meta-analyses had suggested a benefit of oestrogens in protecting against the development of dementia. The Women's Health Initiative Memory Study involved over 7000 women aged 65–79 years receiving either oestrogen alone or in combination with progesterone (depending on womb status) vs placebo.[58] Not only did these agents not protect against dementia but also there was a trend towards an increased incidence. Therefore, they should not be used to try to prevent dementia.

Exercise

Regular exercise has been associated with a delay in the age of onset of dementia.[59] The mechanism of this apparent effect has not been defined.

Treatment

Education, support and respite care can be helpful for caregivers and can delay nursing home placement.[60] A study of 206 people with dementia who lived at home and had a carer found that a series of six sessions (lasting around $1\frac{1}{2}$ hours each) of individual and family counselling plus support group involvement was able to delay the time of admission to a nursing home by, on average, 329 days compared to a control group.[61] The sessions included education on AD and strategies to cope with problem behaviours. Patients with mild to moderate AD had more benefit from the intervention than those with advanced disease.

General management issues

Some simple measures such as installing safety devices, including smoke alarms and gas detectors, within the home may improve an individual's ability to live independently. Day centre visits and respite periods within residential care facilities can be useful for carers' well-being. Longer-term issues such as nursing home placement should be discussed. Advance directives, wills and power of attorney orders should be considered prior to cognitive decline to the point of mental incapacity (*see* p 32).

Driving

In patients who currently drive, consideration needs to be given to stopping. Patients with early dementia of the Alzheimer type and VaD with mean MMSE scores of 23 and 25, respectively, have been found to perform significantly less well in driving test scores compared to age-matched control subjects.[62] This observed decline in function correlated with the degree of MMSE reduction. However, important factors such as impairments in judgement and visuospatial skills may not be detected if MMSE screening is used alone. It can be useful to ask relatives how they feel when in the car with the patient driving to help gauge the risk. For example, would they allow their mother or father to pick up the grandchildren from school? A formal driving assessment can also be arranged. Further details regarding regulations within the UK are available at the DVLA website (www.dvla.gov.uk/at_a_glance/ch4_psychiatric.htm). Links to information relating to countries outside the UK are given in Box 1.2.

Box 1.2 International driving regulations

Useful web resources for driving regulations related to medical illnesses in some selected countries are given below.

Australia

Austroads has produced a guide 'Assessing Fitness to Drive' available from their website (www.austroads.com.au/upload_files/docs/AFTD%202003-F_A-WEBREV1.pdf). The Road and Traffic Authority of New South Wales has produced a booklet for older drivers (www.rta.nsw.gov.au/licensing/downloads/2005_03_gfod.pdf).

Canada

The Canadian Council of Motor Transport Administrators has produced a guide of medical standards for drivers (www.ccmta.ca/english/pdf/medical_standards_july04.pdf).

USA

The physician's guide to assessing and counselling older drivers is available from the American Medical Association website (www.ama-assn.org/ama/pub/category/10791.html).

Cognition

Functioning can be maximised by maintaining daily routines and providing written down to-do lists. Orientation may be improved by providing readily visible clocks and calendars.[63]

Cholinesterase inhibitors

The development of a treatment for dementia would be a major achievement and it is understandable why great excitement was initially expressed in relation to cholinesterase inhibitors. Early trials suggested a significant benefit in cognition in AD and possibly also VaD and DLB. Unfortunately more recent studies have been less favourable. Side effects from this type of medication include nausea, vomiting, diarrhoea, weight loss and somnolence.

The AD2000 study randomised 565 patients with mild to moderate AD (mean age 76, range 46–93 years; mean MMSE score 19, range 10–27) to receive either donepezil (5 mg or 10 mg daily) or placebo over a three-year period.[64] There was a mean better MMSE score of 0.8 (out of 30) and a mean better Bristol Activities of Daily Living Scale (BADLS) score of 1.0 (out of 60) over the first two years in the donepezil group ($p<0.0001$ for both values). These suggest a minor cognitive and functional benefit with treatment; however, the clinical significance of such a minor change is questionable. Coupled to this, there were no significant differences in either the rate of institutionalisation or the progression of disability after three years. Also, no benefits in terms of behavioural symptoms or carer stress were demonstrated. The study concluded that the benefits were clinically insignificant and did not justify the high associated costs.

Some people have argued that a subset of patients responds well to these medications. The AD2000 study found a normally distributed response-to-treatment curve (rather than a bimodal distribution), which would not favour this idea. Further, those patients who responded best initially were the ones who were more likely to score badly at the subsequent evaluation (i.e. demonstrating the phenomenon of regression to the mean[65]). Therefore, the practice of using a three-month MMSE score to predict those who will benefit from continued treatment is flawed.

Cholinesterase inhibitors have also been proposed for the slowing or prevention of development of AD. A trial of 769 patients with mild cognitive impairment (mean age 73 years, mean MMSE score 27/30) did not demonstrate a difference in rate of progression to AD over a three-year period compared to placebo.[56]

A meta-analysis of 22 trials looking at the use of the cholinesterase inhibitors donepezil, galantamine and rivastigmine in AD has been published.[66] The majority of trials used the Alzheimer's Disease Assessment Scale – cognitive subscale (ADAS-cog) as a primary outcome measure (*see* Appendix A). Values obtained showed a net improvement of between 1.5 and 3.9 points on this scale (out of 70). The trial lengths were variable, ranging from six weeks to three years. A number of methodological deficiencies were noted within most of the trials. These included incomplete or inaccurate data for patients who did not complete the trial, which, given that dementia is associated with a progressive cognitive decline, could artificially exaggerate the treatment effect. The small benefit derived coupled with the trial deficiencies further questions the use of these agents.

In conclusion, sadly, the cholinesterase inhibitors are not a solution for AD. They may have a small benefit in cognition but this is of questionable clinical significance and appears to be short-lived (less than three years). Their main benefit has perhaps been the provocation of a new interest in dementia and the establishment of memory clinics.

Memantine

Memantine is a glutamate antagonist that acts at N-methyl-D-aspartate (NMDA) receptors. It has been proposed that it may reduce excitatory neurotoxicity in dementia. A series of small trials of short duration (six months) have shown a possible mild benefit on cognition, function and behaviour in moderate to severe AD, but benefits are unclear in mild to moderate AD or VaD.[67] Larger, longer-term studies are required before memantine can be recommended for use in dementia.

Non-cognitive symptoms

Agitation

The term 'agitation' is used to cover a number of behavioural disturbances in dementia. An alternative term 'behavioural and psychological symptoms of dementia' is also used (BPSD). It ranges from the more mild problems of apathy, fidgeting and wandering to the more alarming difficulties of verbal and physical aggression. Some such symptoms occur in the majority of people with advanced dementia. Agitation can be a sign of unhappiness and associated reversible factors should be sought (e.g. pain or depression). A significant number of problem behaviours will spontaneously resolve and so, unless very severe, a policy of watching to see if it persists over a one-month period may be adopted.[68]

Non-pharmacological management

Evidence for the efficacy of non-pharmacological interventions is, at best, minimal. However, in the absence of a good alternative and given the lack of adverse effects, their implementation seems reasonable. In general, people with dementia respond better when they are in familiar, calm and quiet environments and in stable daily routines. Behavioural problems may become worse later in the day ('sun downing'). Confrontation of patients with problem behaviours may lead to escalation.

Identifying the trigger factors that are associated with problem behaviours can lead to being able to avoid their occurrence. One approach is for the carer to complete a diary, recording the antecedent, behaviour and consequences (ABC) each time a problem arises.[69] Typical data would include the people present and the activity being undertaken before the problem. Also, the outcome of the event should be noted to see if any reinforcement of negative behaviours is taking place.

Brief educational programmes and support groups for carers may have a small benefit but do not affect patient outcomes.[60] In episodes of aggression, the carer should be advised to remain clam and try to avoid contradicting, arguing or confrontation. The agitated patient should be approached from the front and addressed at eye level. Questions may be used to distract the person's attention and aim to refocus on something more pleasurable.[69] In patients who are resistant to their caregivers, setting more limited goals can be effective. For example, if showering is a particular problem, less frequent showering may help to reduce conflict.

In people who wander, increased daytime activity and exercise, preferably outdoors, can limit this tendency. Rooms might be labelled to reduce the chance of getting lost. Patients who wander at night may be less likely to become lost if night-lights are fitted. Caffeine, alcohol and daytime naps may all affect sleep patterns and should be avoided. Alarms that are activated when a wandering person leaves a building or opens a door can be useful. Environmental adaptations such as putting stop signs or mirrors on doors can prevent persons from exiting through them. Alternatively, concealed or childproof locks may be fitted to external doors. A patient may be allowed to wander within a safe environment. Medications are usually ineffective for this problem.

A study that recruited 81 people with dementia who resided in a nursing home (mean age 82 years, mean MMSE score 9/30) compared an intervention consisting of an activity program, medication review and educational sessions for staff to a control group over a six-month period.[70] It was found that behavioural disorders and antipsychotic drug use reduced in both groups but the sizes of the reductions were greater in the treatment group (by 23% and 9%, respectively). However, this was achieved with additional staff usage and so financial costs were greater.

Aromatherapy has been suggested as an effective treatment to reduce behavioural symptoms in dementia. A study compared the use of an essential oil (lemon balm) mixed with a base lotion and applied to patients' arms and faces to a placebo lotion in 72 patients with dementia plus agitation over a four-week period.[71] Sixty per cent of the treatment group compared to 14% of the placebo group were judged to have had a significant improvement with this therapy. Sensory stimulation such as soft background music may cause a small reduction in problem behaviours.[60]

Light therapy has been advocated to try and correct abnormal circadian rhythms in the institutionalised elderly with reduced sunlight exposure. Patients sit in front of a box that emits strong light for around two hours per day. Small initial studies suggest it may provide a minor benefit in behavioural control.[72] Pet therapy may also be tried.

Pharmacological management

Medications used to control problem behaviours may worsen a patient's cognitive function leading to increased confusion and, paradoxically, worsened behaviour.

Antipsychotic medications

Antipsychotic drugs (also termed 'neuroleptics') are roughly divided into two categories: the older 'typical' and newer 'atypical' agents. Haloperidol is the most commonly used typical agent. Atypical agents include clozapine, risperidone, olanzapine and quetiapine. Comparing the groups, atypical agents tend to have lesser antagonism of dopamine receptors, but more anticholinergic, serotinergic and alpha-adrenergic effects.[73]

Adverse effects

Adverse events with all of these medications are considerable. Among these are drug-induced movement disorders (*see* p 80) and an increased risk of falls (*see* p 185). They have also been found to be associated with an increased rate of cognitive decline in patients with dementia compared to those not taking such medications.[74–76] This finding may be mediated by the anticholinergic properties of these drugs (*see* Table 3.2). Some of the atypical agents (olanzapine and clozapine) have been associated with increased weight gain and new onset of type 2 diabetes.[77] These problems may be mediated by serotinergic or histaminergic receptor actions.[78]

More recently, concerns have been generated that atypical antipsychotic medications may be associated with an increased risk of stroke.[79,80] This is based on results from trials comparing these agents to placebo where a two to three times increased relative risk for cerebrovascular events was observed. This has led to the Committee on Safety of Medicines recommending that olanzapine and risperidone are no longer appropriate for use in elderly people with dementia. A retrospective review of the records of 32 710 people prescribed either typical (17 845) or atypical antipsychotic agents (14 865) failed to demonstrate a difference in hospitalisation rates for stroke between the medication groups (HR 1.01, 95% CI 0.81–1.26).[81] This suggests that either the association with stroke is artefactual or, perhaps more likely, that both subgroups of antipsychotic agent are associated with an increased stroke risk. However, studies of this nature cannot account for prescriber bias.

A meta-analysis of trials comparing atypical antipsychotic drug use to placebo in patients with dementia found an increased risk of death with these agents (OR 1.54, 95% CI 1.06–2.23, $p = 0.02$).[82] It is not known whether this also applies to conventional antipsychotic agents as similar safety data in dementia are not available. However, a recent retrospective analysis of mortality in elderly patients (mean age 83 years) found a higher risk of death with typical compared to atypical agents (within 180 days of commencement risk ratio (RR) 1.37, 95% CI 1.27–1.49).[83] Of course, caution must be used when interpreting such data as there are significant differences between the medication groups, the subjects did not all have dementia (less than half), and prescriber bias cannot be analysed.

Efficacy

Risperidone and haloperidol have been compared to placebo in 344 people with advanced dementia and agitation within institutional care facilities (median age 81, range 56–97 years; mean MMSE score 8/30) over a 12-week period.[84] After dose titration, mean doses of 1.1 mg/day and 1.2 mg/day were attained for the risperidone and haloperidol groups, respectively. At the end of the trial there were no significant differences in total behavioural scores for the three groups. A subgroup analysis suggested that both risperidone and haloperidol were better than placebo for control of aggression. There was a 35% drop-out rate for this study (similar amounts of patients from each group). The majority of participants discontinued due to either adverse events (50%) or lack of efficacy (44%). Twenty-two per cent of patients on haloperidol had extrapyramidal side effects compared to 15% on risperidone and 11% on placebo. Somnolence was more common in both treatment arms compared to placebo. Similarly, when other neuroleptics have been compared, they all appear to have a similar, mild efficacy.[85]

Haloperidol, trazadone, behavioural management techniques (BMT), and placebo have been compared in 149 community-dwelling people with AD and agitation (mean age 75 years, mean MMSE score 13/30) over a 16-week period.[86] Doses of the medications were gradually titrated up, achieving mean doses of 1.8 mg/day for haloperidol and 200 mg/day for trazadone. The BMT consisted of 11 sessions, including education and strategies to reduce agitation. There were no significant differences between the groups in primary outcome measures. There was a 38% discontinuation rate overall, with no significant differences between the groups. Extrapyramidal side effects occurred more commonly in the haloperidol arm.

A dose of 2–3 mg per day of haloperidol has been found to be more effective than 0.5–0.75 mg per day in controlling disruptive behaviours (mainly psychosis and/or aggression) in 71 outpatients with dementia (mean age 72 years).[87] However, there was a 20% incidence of extrapyramidal side effects rated as 'moderate to severe' at this higher dose.

Quetiapine has been compared to placebo and rivastigmine treatment for the management of agitation in 93 demented individuals over the age of 60 years who live in institutional care over a 26-week period.[75] Not only did quetiapine not improve agitation but it also was associated with a significant cognitive decline compared to the other groups.

A trial randomised 345 people with dementia (mean age 83 years, mean MMSE score 5/30) plus aggressive behaviour, who lived in nursing homes, to receive either risperidone (mean dose 0.95 mg per day) or placebo over a 12-week period.[88] There was a significant reduction in aggression in the risperidone arm. Adverse effects occurring more commonly in the risperidone group included somnolence (37% vs 25%), cerebrovascular events (9% (including two deaths due to stroke) vs 2%) and extrapyramidal disorders (6% vs 3%). Similarly, another trial of 625 patients with dementia plus psychotic and behavioural symptoms (mean age 83 years, mean

MMSE score 7/30) comparing risperidone to placebo over a 12-week period found a significantly lower rate of aggression and psychosis with risperidone.[89]

A recent study compared olanzepine, quetiapine or risperidone to placebo in patients with AD plus aggression, psychosis or agitation over a 36-week period.[90] Overall they found similar discontinuation rates between the groups, with discontinuation due to inefficacy more common with placebo, but this was offset by higher discontinuation due to adverse effects with the active drugs (including Parkinsonism, sedation and cognitive changes).

A study of 206 demented people (most of whom displayed aggression) (mean age 83 years, mean MMSE score 7/30) over a six-week period found that olanzapine (5–10 mg per day) was superior to placebo in the control of psychosis and behavioural disturbance.[91] Patients in the treatment arm had a significantly higher incidence of somnolence and abnormal gait.

A Cochrane review of the use of haloperidol for agitation in dementia concluded that there was evidence to support the use of haloperidol to reduce aggression but not for any other behavioural problems.[92]

When a programme of reduction of antipsychotic use in nursing homes was implemented, no worsening of behavioural features was encountered compared to a matched group of patients without a reduction in their medication.[93] Such a technique may be even more effective if coupled to nursing education programmes to teach alternative management strategies to medication use.[94]

These studies emphasise the point that many nursing home residents are on medication that is either unjustified or ineffective. Investigators have found that 17–24% of nursing home residents are on antipsychotic medication.[95–97] Yet the majority of these prescriptions (up to 88%) are inappropriate according to expert guidelines.[98] The trigger to prescribe many of these medications appears to be nursing home admission and is associated with little, if any, specialist input.[96]

Summary

In summary, antipsychotic agents may have a role in controlling aggression in dementia but not other forms of agitation. They are generally overprescribed, especially within nursing home environments. Atypical antipsychotics are more expensive and no more effective. They have only been studied in a small number of trials with short durations.[98] They appear to cause fewer extrapyramidal side effects but this may be at the expense of an increased risk of stroke and death. The clinical relevance of reduced extrapyramidal effects is unclear as all of the agents are associated with a similarly increased risk of falls (*see* p 185). They are likely to result in cognitive decline if taken over a prolonged time period. When indicated, haloperidol should be used at the lowest possible dose for the shortest possible duration. When unacceptable extrapyramidal side effects occur or for aggression in DLB, atypical antipsychotics may be considered. Regular review with attempts to withdraw antipsychotic agents should be undertaken at least six-monthly.[99]

Cholinesterase inhibitors

Most studies assessing the effect of cholinesterase inhibitors were not primarily designed to assess non-cognitive symptoms. The AD2000 study did not demonstrate an improvement in behavioural symptoms in patients with mild to moderate AD on donepezil.[64]

A study of 134 patients with AD (mean age 81 years, mean MMSE score 20/30) and neuropsychiatric symptoms (Neuropsychiatric Inventory (NPI) score >11) (*see* Appendix A) compared the effect of continued donepezil therapy (10 mg/day) to medication replacement with placebo over a 12-week period.[100] The mean NPI score for both groups was 15.2 at randomisation, this fell to 12.3 in the continued donepezil group and rose to 18.5 in the placebo group (*p* = 0.02). However, only 60% of the participants completed the study. Most withdrawals were due to adverse events or inefficacy of the medication. It cannot be excluded that the difference between the groups is due to drug withdrawal effects rather than a true benefit of continued donepezil.

A trial of 120 people with DLB (mean age 74 years, mean MMSE score 17/30) compared rivastigmine to placebo in the control of behavioural features of the condition over 23 weeks.[101] NPI scores were used as the main outcome measure. A benefit was found with rivastigmine in the symptom domains of apathy, anxiety, delusions and hallucinations but overall differences failed to reach statistical sig-nificance. Side effects occurring more commonly in the treatment group included nausea (37%), vomiting (25%), anorexia (19%) and somnolence (9%). A worsen-ing of parkinsonian features with pro-cholinergic medication was not found in this study but there have been a few case reports of this occurring.[102] Similarly, rivastigmine was not found to improve agitation in individuals with AD.[75]

In summary, there is little evidence to support the use of cholinesterase inhibitors for the control of non-cognitive symptoms in dementia. Available studies recruited only small numbers of patients and used short time periods. When a difference has been found, the magnitude has been small and of doubtful clinical significance.[103]

Anti-epileptic agents

Carbamazepine and valproate have been suggested as treatments for agitation in dementia. Carbamazepine (mean dose 304 mg/day) has been compared to placebo in 51 patients with dementia plus agitation (mean age 86 years, mean MMSE score 6/30) over a six-week period.[104] Previously used psychotropic agents were with-drawn prior to the study. Carbamazepine was started at 100 mg/day and increased by 50 mg every 3–4 days if no side effects occurred. A significant reduction in behavioural scores was noted in the treatment group. Side effects were significantly more common in the carbamazepine group (59% vs 29%). These included increased incidences of drowsiness, ataxia and disorientation. However, the behav-ioural efficacy of carbamazepine was not demonstrated in a subsequent study.[103]

A number of small, short-duration studies have evaluated the use of valproate for agitation in dementia. A Cochrane review concluded that lower doses of valproate (from 480 mg per day) were ineffective and higher doses (up to 1 g per day) were associated with an unacceptably high rate of adverse effects, including sedation.[105]

Benzodiazepines

Benzodiazepines have also been tried in the management of behavioural disturbance in dementia. Alprazolam (a short to intermediate half-life benzodiazepine given at a dose of 0.5 mg bd) has been compared to haloperidol (mean dose 0.64 mg) in the management of disruptive behaviours in 68 elderly people (mean age 83, range 65–98 years) with cognitive impairment, in a crossover design, over a 12-week period.[106] There were no significant differences between the groups for outcome measures. Alarmingly, there was a trend for a worsening of behaviour following commencement of either agent after the placebo pre-treatment phase. It seems fair to assume that benzodiazepines are equally ineffective as neuroleptics in the control of agitation and are associated with their own range of significant adverse effects (e.g. sedation, confusion and falls).

Antidepressants

Various antidepressant drugs have been proposed for the management of agitation in dementia. Trazadone is a sedating antidepressant agent with serotinergic agonist and antagonist properties. It has been show to be no better than placebo in the control of agitation in AD.[86] A Cochrane review concluded that there was insufficient evidence to recommend the use of trazadone for the control of agitation in dementia.[107] A meta-analysis concluded that antidepressant agents have not been found to be effective in the management of symptoms other than depression in people with dementia.[103]

Depression

See Chapter 3. Nonpharmacological interventions that may be beneficial to depressed patients with dementia include increasing social activities, reminiscing about previous pleasurable life events and adapting formerly enjoyed activities to fit in with their current functional levels.[69]

Reduced oral intake

A reduction in oral intake may be produced by a concurrent depressive episode or be the result of either the loss of desire to eat or the loss of cerebral co-ordination of the swallowing mechanism. These latter causes usually herald the terminal phase of dementia. Therefore it is important to try to exclude or treat a depressive illness (*see* Chapter 3). An antidepressant that may also cause stimulation of appetite, such as mirtazepine, could be tried.

Nasogastric and percutaneous endoscopic gastrostomy (PEG) tubes are used to bypass abnormal swallowing mechanisms to prevent malnutrition (*see* p 121). Nasogastric tubes are usually only a temporary measure (days to weeks), with PEG tubes being more appropriate for long-term use. They have also been utilised in patients with end-stage dementia with reduced oral intakes.

The insertion is often justified by the notion that suffering will be alleviated, life will be prolonged or on grounds that not providing nutrition is morally wrong.[108] Evidence from available studies does not support tube feeding as beneficial in terms of quality of life, prolonging survival or nutritional status.[109,110] An improved survival following PEG insertion has only been demonstrated in patients with cerebrovascular disease or oropharyngeal cancer.[111] If the patient is physically able but choosing not to eat, and a reversible condition such as depression has been excluded, then it is questionable how forcibly feeding them would improve their quality of life. At the most extreme, patients may actually be restrained to prevent them from pulling an irritating tube out.[108]

There is an argument that denying nutrition in the setting of palliative care is causing patients suffering. This is, obviously, hard to assess in advanced dementia but evidence from patients with other terminal conditions suggests that comfort can be achieved despite minimal oral intake (*see* p 288).

Another common reason for PEG insertion is to prevent aspiration pneumonia.[112] However, PEG insertion has not been found to prevent aspiration pneumonia and may even make it more likely to occur.[113] This latter scenario could be due to a reduced lower oesophageal sphincter efficacy following gastrostomy insertion.[110] One study found that 57% of PEG-fed patients with dementia had had an episode of aspiration pneumonia in the preceding six months.[114]

Patients with dementia who have PEG tubes inserted have poorer survivals than age-matched controls without PEG tubes.[115,116] Feeding tube placement has not been associated with a survival advantage in patients with dementia compared to demented people without feeding tubes.[117,118] The mortality following PEG insertion is higher in patients with dementia than those without. The 30-day mortality rate for procedures within elderly hospitalised demented people is around 54% and the one-year mortality 90%[119] (compared to 24–28% and 63%, respectively (*see* p 121)). There are also complication rates associated with tube feeding, including blockage of the tube and infection at the insertion site. Another harm that should be considered is the removal of the pleasurable sensation of the taste of food.

In summary, there is no convincing evidence that feeding tubes result in any beneficial effects in advanced dementia and there is good reason to think that they cause harm. Techniques that may improve oral intake and feeding safety include ensuring an upright position when feeding, small and frequent meals, and increased supervision during feed times.[110]

Ethical and legal issues

The following text refers to law within the UK at the time of writing. This may be subject to change over time and will also vary in different countries (although general principles are likely to be very similar). The components are also relevant to conditions other than dementia (e.g. delirium). Box 1.3 provides links to some information relating to countries outside the UK.

Box 1.3   Ethical guidance in countries outside the UK

Although principles remain similar, variance occurs in ethical issues between countries and sometimes between states. The information below is intended to act as a starting point for those seeking more information.

Australia
The website of the Office of the Public Advocate of South Australia contains some useful information on capacity, power of attorney and guardianship legislation (www.opa.sa.gov.au/ACFbooklet.pdf). The Australian Medical Association's code of ethics (2004) can be found on its website (www. ama.com.au/web.nsf/doc/WEEN-5WW598).

Canada
The website of the Canadian Medical Association contains an article with some information relating to ethical issues in the elderly (www.cma.ca/multimedia/CMA/Content_Images/Insite_cma/WhatWePublish/LeadershipSeries/English/pg23EC.pdf).

USA
The American Medical Association website (www.ama-assn.org/ama/pub/category/8457.html) contains an article 'Withholding or Withdrawing Life-Sustaining Medical Treatment'. The University of Washington School of Medicine website contains information around end of life decisions including the assessment of mental capacity (depts.washington.edu/bioethx/topics/term life.html#comp quest).

Box 1.4 offers some clarification about legislation regarding mental health in the UK.

Box 1.4   Mental health law

Legislation regarding mental health (e.g. the Mental Health Bill) is for the detainment ('sectioning') and treatment of psychiatric illness in people with mental health disorders (e.g. depression, schizophrenia ...) and not organic conditions (e.g. delirium, dementia ...). For this reason it is rarely relevant to general geriatric practice.

Mental capacity

There comes a point when cognitive function becomes so impaired that individuals are no longer able to make reasonable decisions regarding their own care – this is termed 'lacking mental capacity'. Medical practitioners are commonly asked to make decisions as to whether this has occurred. This is often very difficult as we are asked to make a decision in a black and white manner about a process that represents shades of grey. Standard cognitive assessments, such as the MMSE, do not evaluate a person's mental capacity to make decisions about their welfare. A patient who makes what appear to be irrational decisions due to personal idiosyncrasy does not necessarily lack mental capacity.

Capacity assessments should be judged for each matter to be evaluated, that is, they are decision-specific. For example, if a patient is judged not to have the capacity to handle their finances, it does not automatically follow that they are incapable of choosing where they wish to live. The assessments should also be made when the patient is functioning at their best. This may be particularly relevant to people who have fluctuating conditions (e.g. DLB (*see* p 76)). When a patient is judged to lack capacity to make a particular decision for him or herself, then a decision is made 'in their best interests'. This decision is usually made by agreement between different members of a multi-disciplinary team. What constitutes 'best interests' is not exclusively based on medical evidence, and factors such as the person's previously expressed opinions regarding their healthcare and their religious beliefs should also be considered.[120] In some instances this may include the information contained in a living will. It is advised that the option chosen should be the least restrictive for the patient.[121]

Relatives or carers cannot make such decisions for an individual who lacks capacity (except in the case of a 'Lasting Power of Attorney' order (*see* below)). However, their opinions as to what the person would have chosen for themself, if they were able, are clearly very relevant and important in deciding what represents 'best interests' for that individual. This would include information from a living will (*see* below). Ideally, medical staff and family members should be in agreement with regard to the appropriateness of any decision. When conflict occurs a second opinion may be sought, and occasionally a court judgment is required.

Assessing mental capacity

In situations where what the patient wishes to do and what would be in the patient's best interests are the same, then assessing capacity is irrelevant. Capacity assessments can be performed by any doctor but are usually best done by the doctor who knows the patient best. In difficult cases the opinion of someone with more expertise in making these decisions, such as a psychiatrist, may also be sought. In order to have mental capacity, a patient should comply with the following three points:

- understand the information that they are being told
- believe that the information is true
- be able to retain the information long enough to 'weigh it in the balance'.

They must also have the ability to communicate their decision to others (this may be in spoken words, written language or some other means, e.g. for those with dysphasia). All of these things must occur in the absence of coercion from others.

In practical terms, when a specific decision is to be made then the patient's knowledge of this subject should be explored. For example, if this is a decision to return to their home then the patient should be asked to describe their home. If they provide grossly inaccurate information (such as living with their parents) then they are unlikely to be able to base a decision on sound data. Next, the benefits and risks of each option should be discussed. Following this, the patient should be asked to repeat the information given so as to assess their ability to retain it. Information from other members of the medical team (e.g. nursing staff, physiotherapists and occupational therapists) may also be useful. As a general principle, when there is substantial doubt, it is best to assume that the patient does have mental capacity.

Living wills/advance directives

Living wills or advance directives are oral or written instructions made by a person, at a time when they are well, in regard to their preferences for future care. These are only relevant if appropriate to the current clinical situation. If a patient has made a decision to refuse a particular treatment, then this is legally binding. If the decision is in favour of receiving a specific treatment, then this should be taken into consideration by the medical team but it is not legally binding that they must receive it.[119]

Power of Attorney

- *Enduring Power of Attorney* is a legally binding appointment of another person to take responsibility for financial matters of an individual at some point in the future when they no longer have the mental capacity to do this for themselves. It does not apply to non-financial matters. It cannot be set up for individuals who have already lost the capacity to make such a decision. In this instance they have to apply for 'Court of Protection' – a more difficult and costly procedure. For this reason it is advisable for all people to appoint someone with an Enduring Power of Attorney responsibility early in the course of a dementia illness.
- *Lasting Power of Attorney* is similar to Enduring Power of Attorney in most aspects, except that it allows the appointed person to also make decisions regarding social and health care. This is already possible in Scotland and may soon also be incorporated into the law within the rest of the UK (at the time of writing it is speculated to come into force in April 2007).[122]

Guardianship

Guardianship refers to the legal allocation of another person to make decisions in an individual's best interests for the foreseeable future. This person may be a relative or a publicly appointed person. This procedure is usually unnecessary, but in some cases a guardian's input can help to enforce the 'best interests' upon the patient. For example, a person judged to lack capacity who repeatedly tries to leave a care home that has been chosen to be the best living environment for them can be returned against their will if the guardian is in agreement.

Palliative care

Dementia is a progressive disorder, and ultimately the palliation of symptoms will be the most appropriate intervention (*see* Chapter 18). Currently, palliative care services and medications are underutilised within this patient group.[123]

Further reading

Mendez M, Cummings JL. *Dementia: a clinical approach*, 3rd Ed. Boston, MA: Butterworth Heinemann, 2003.

Andersen G. *Caring for People with Alzheimer's Disease: a training manual for direct care providers.* Baltimore, MD: Health Professional Press, 1995.

References

1 Skoog I, Nilsson L, Palmertz B *et al.* A population-based study of dementia in 85-year-olds. *NEJM*, 1993; **328**: 153–158.
2 Lobo A, Launer LJ, Fratiglioni L *et al.* Prevalence of dementia and major subtypes in Europe: a collaborative study of population-based cohorts. *Neurology*, 2000; **54** (Suppl 5): S4–9.
3 Rocca WA, Bonaiuto S, Lippi A *et al.* Prevalence of clinically diagnosed Alzheimer's disease and other dementing disorders: a door-to-door survey in Appignano, Macerata Province, Italy. *Neurology*, 1990; **40**: 626–631.

4   Ferri CP, Prince M, Brayne C *et al.* Global prevalence of dementia: a Delphi consensus study. *Lancet*, 2005; **366**: 2112–2117.

5   Graham JE, Rockwood K, Beattie BL *et al.* Prevalence and severity of cognitive impairment with and without dementia in an elderly population. *Lancet*, 1997; **349**(9068): 1793–1796.

6   Budson AE and Price BH. Memory dysfunction. *NEJM*, 2005; **352**(7): 692–699.

7   Ancelin ML, Artero S, Portet F *et al.* Non-degenerative mild cognitive impairment in elderly people and the use of anticholinergic drugs: longitudinal cohort study. *BMJ*, 2006; **332**: 455–458.

8   Wolf-Klein GP, Silverstone FA, Levy AP *et al.* Screening for Alzheimer's disease by clock drawing. *JAGS*, 1989; **37**: 730–734.

9   Mathuranath PS, Nestor PJ, Berrios GE *et al.* A brief cognitive test battery to differentiate Alzheimer's disease and frontotemporal dementia. *Neurology*, 2000; **55**: 1613–1620.

10 Tweedy J, Reding M, Garcia C *et al.* Significance of cortical disinhibition signs. *Neurology*, 1982; **32**: 169–173.

11 Owen G and Mulley GP. The palmomental reflex: a useful clinical sign? *J Neurol Neurosurg Psy*, 2002; **73**: 113–115.

12 Huff FJ, Boller F, Lucchelli F *et al.* The neurologic examination in patients with probable Alzheimer's disease. *Arch Neurol*, 1987; **44**: 929–932.

13 Burns A, Jacoby R and Levy R. Neurological signs in Alzheimer's disease. *Age Ageing*, 1991; **20**: 45–51.

14 Warren JD, Schott JM, Fox NC *et al.* Brain biopsy in dementia. *Brain*, 2005; **128**: 2016–2025.

15 Flood JM, Weinstock HS, Guroy ME *et al.* Neurosyphilis during the AIDS epidemic, San Francisco, 1985–1992. *J Inf Dis*, 1998; **177**: 931–940.

16 Kraybill ML, Larson EB, Tsuang W *et al.* Cognitive differences in dementia patients with autopsy-verified AD, Lewy body pathology or both. *Neurology*, 2005; **64**: 2069–2073.

17 Nyenhuis DL and Gorelick PB. Vascular dementia: a contemporary review of epidemiology, diagnosis, prevention and treatment. *JAGS*, 1998; **46**: 1437–1448.

18 Mega MS, Cummings JL, Fiorello T *et al.* The spectrum of behavioral changes in Alzheimer's disease. *Neurology*, 1996; **46**: 130–135.

19 Assal F and Cummings JL. Neuropsychiatric symptoms in the dementias. *Curr Op Neurol*, 2002; **15**(4): 445–450.

20 Prusiner SB. Shattuck Lecture – neurodegenerative diseases and prions. *NEJM*, 2001; **344**(20): 1516–1526.

21 Cummings JL. Alzheimer's disease. *NEJM*, 2004; **351**: 56–67.

22 Henon H, Durieu I, Guerouaou D *et al.* Poststroke dementia: incidence and relationship to prestroke cognitive decline. *Neurology*, 2001; **57**: 1216–1222.

23 Barba R, Martinez-Espinosa S, Rodriguez-Garcia E *et al.* Poststroke dementia: clinical features and risk factors. *Stroke*, 2000; **31**: 1494–1501.

24 Desmond DW, Moroney JT, Paik MC *et al.* Frequency and clinical determinants of dementia after ischaemic stroke. *Neurology*, 2000; **54**: 1124–1131.

25 Zekry D, Hauw J and Gold G. Mixed dementia: epidemiology, diagnosis and treatment. *JAGS*, 2002; **50**: 1431–1438.

26 Snowdon DA, Greiner LH, Mortimer JA *et al.* Brain infarction and the clinical expression of Alzheimer disease. The Nun Study. *JAMA*, 1997; **277**(10): 813–817.

27 Stevens M, Van Duijn CM, Kamphorst W *et al.* Familial aggregation in frontotemporal dementia. *Neurology*, 1998; **50**: 1541–1545.

28 Chow TW, Miller BL, Hayashi VN *et al.* Inheritance of frontotemporal dementia. *Arch Neurol*, 1999; **56**: 817–822.

29 The Lund and Manchester Groups. Clinical and neuropathological criteria for fronto-temporal dementia. *J Neurol Neurosurg Psy*, 1994; **57**: 416–418.

30 Thomas VC and Rockwood KJ. Alcohol abuse, cognitive impairment, and mortality among older people. *JAGS*, 2001; **49**(4): 415–420.

31 Dugbartey A. Neurocognitive aspects of hypothyroidism. *Arch Int Med*, 1998; **158**: 1413–1418.

32 Toh B, van Driel IR and Gleeson PA. Pernicious anaemia. *NEJM*, 1997; **337**(20): 1441–1448.

33 Carmel R. Prevalence of undiagnosed pernicious anaemia in the elderly. *Arch Int Med*, 1996; **156**: 1097–1100.

34 Glatzel M, Stoeck K, Seeger H et al. Human prion diseases: molecular and clinical aspects. Arch Neurol, 2005; **62**: 545–552.

35 De Silva R, Findlay C, Awad I et al. Creutzfeldt–Jakob disease in the elderly. Postgrad Med J, 1997; **73**: 557–559.

36 Johnson RT and Gibbs CJ. Creutzfeldt–Jakob disease and related transmissible spongiform encephalopathies. NEJM, 1998; **339**(27): 1994–2004.

37 Tschampa HJ, Neumann M, Zerr I et al. Patients with Alzheimer's disease and dementia with Lewy bodies mistaken for Creutzfeldt–Jakob disease. J Neurol Neurosurg Psy, 2001; **71**: 33–39.

38 Zerr I, Pocchiari M, Collins S et al. Analysis of EEG and CSF 14–3–3 proteins as aids to the diagnosis of Creutzfeldt–Jakob disease. Neurology, 2000; **55**: 811–815.

39 Lemstra AW, van Meegen MT, Vreyling JP et al. 14–3–3 testing in diagnosing Creutzfeldt–Jakob disease: a prospective study of 112 patients. Neurology, 2000; **55**: 514–516.

40 Schroter A, Zerr I, Henkel K et al. Magnetic resonance imaging in the clinical diagnosis of Creutzfeldt–Jakob disease. Arch Neurol, 2000; **57**: 1751–1757.

41 Shiga Y, Miyazawa K, Sato S et al. Diffusion-weighted MRI abnormalities as an early diagnostic marker for Creutzfeldt–Jakob disease. Neurology, 2004; **63**: 443–449.

42 Poser S, Mollenhauer B, Kraub A et al. How to improve the clinical diagnosis of Creutzfeldt–Jakob disease. Brain, 1999; **122**: 2345–2351.

43 Massman PJ, Sims J, Cooke N et al. Prevalence and correlates of neuropsychological deficits in amyotrophic lateral sclerosis. J Neurol Neurosurg Psy, 1996; **61**: 450–455.

44 Ruitenberg A, van Swieten JC, Witteman JCM et al. Alcohol consumption and risk of dementia: the Rotterdam study. Lancet, 2002; **359**: 281–286.

45 Mukamal KJ, Kuller LH, Fitzpatrick AL et al. Prospective study of alcohol consumption and risk of dementia in older adults. JAMA, 2003; **289**(11): 1405–1413.

46 Ganguli M, Vander Bilt J, Saxton JA et al. Alcohol consumption and cognitive function in late life: a longitudinal community study. Neurology, 2005; **65**: 1210–1217.

47 Truelsen T, Thudium D and Gronbaek M. Amount and type of alcohol and risk of dementia: the Copenhagen City Heart Study. Neurology, 2002; **59**: 131–139.

48 Stampfer MJ, Kang JH, Chen J et al. Effects of moderate alcohol consumption on cognitive function in women. NEJM, 2005; **352**(3): 245–253.

49 Hein HO, Suadicani P and Gyntelberg F. Alcohol consumption, serum low density lipoprotein cholesterol concentration, and risk of ischaemic heart disease: six year follow up in the Copenhagen male study. BMJ, 1996; **312**: 736–741.

50 Whitmer RA, Gunderson EP, Barrett-Connor E et al. Obesity in middle age and future risk of dementia: a 27 year longitudinal population based study. BMJ, 2005; **330**: 1360–1362.

51 Gustafson D, Lissner L, Bengtsson C et al. A 24-year follow-up of body mass index and cerebral atrophy. Neurology, 2004; **63**: 1876–1881.

52 Whitmer RA, Sidney S, Selby J et al. Midlife cardiovascular risk factors and risk of dementia in late life. Neurology, 2005; **64**: 277–281.

53 Hofman A, Ott A, Breteler MMB et al. Atherosclerosis, apolipoprotein E, and prevalence of dementia and Alzheimer's disease in the Rotterdam study. Lancet, 1997; **349**: 151–154.

54 Forette F, Seux M, Staessen JA et al. Prevention of dementia in randomised double-blind placebo-controlled Systolic Hypertension in Europe (Syst-Eur) trial. Lancet, 1998; **352**: 1347–1351.

55 Launer LJ, Masaki K, Petrovitch H et al. The association between midlife blood pressure levels and late-life cognitive function: the Honolulu-Asia Aging Study. JAMA, 1995; **274**(23): 1846–1851.

56 Petersen RC, Thomas RG, Grundman M et al. Vitamin E and donepezil for the treatment of mild cognitive impairment. NEJM, 2005; **352**: 2379–2388.

57 Miller ER, Pastor-Barriuso R, Dalal D et al. Meta-analysis: high-dosage vitamin E supplementation may increase all-cause mortality. Ann Int Med, 2005; **142**(1): 37–46.

58 Shumaker SA, Legault C, Kuller L et al. Conjugated equine estrogens and incidence of probable dementia and mild cognitive impairment in postmenopausal women: Women's Health Initiative Memory Study. JAMA, 2004; **291**(24): 2947–2958.

59 Larson EB, Wang L, Bowen JD et al. Exercise is associated with reduced risk for incident dementia among persons 65 years of age and older. Ann Int Med, 2006; **144**(2): 73–81.

60 Doody RS, Stevens JC, Beck C et al. Practice parameter: management of dementia (an evidence-based review). Neurology, 2001; **56**: 1154–1166.

61 Mittleman MS, Ferris SH, Shalman E *et al.* A family intervention to delay nursing home placement of patients with Alzheimer disease: a randomized controlled trial. *JAMA*, 1996; **276**(21): 1725–1731.

62 Fitten LJ, Perryman KM, Wilkinson CJ *et al.* Alzheimer and vascular dementias and driving. *JAMA*, 1995; **273**(17): 1360–1365.

63 Small GW, Rabins PV, Barry PP *et al.* Diagnosis and treatment of Alzheimer disease and related disorders. *JAMA*, 1997; **278**: 1363–1371.

64 AD2000 Collaborative Group. Long-term donepezil treatment in 565 patients with Alzheimer's disease (AD2000): randomised double-blind trial. *Lancet*, 2004; **363**: 2105–2115.

65 Morton V and Torgerson DJ. Effect of regression to the mean on decision making in health care. *BMJ*, 2003; **326**: 1083–1084.

66 Kaduszkiewicz H, Zimmermann T, Beck-Bornholdt H *et al.* Cholinesterase inhibitors for patients with Alzheimer's disease: systematic review of randomised clinical trials. *BMJ*, 2005; **331**: 321–323.

67 Areosa Sastre A, Sherriff F and McShane R. Memantine for dementia. Cochrane Database Syst Rev 2005, Volume (3).

68 Ballard C and O'Brien J. Treating behavioural and psychological signs in Alzheimer's disease. *BMJ*, 1999; **319**: 138–139.

69 Teri L, Logsdon RG and McCurry SM. Nonpharmacologic treatment of behavioral disturbance in dementia. *Med Clin N Am*, 2002; **86**: 641–656.

70 Rovner BW, Steele CD, Shmuely Y *et al.* A randomized trial of dementia care in nursing homes. *JAGS*, 1996; **44**(1): 7–13.

71 Ballard CG, O'Brien JT, Reichelt K *et al.* Aromatherapy as a safe and effective treatment for the management of agitation in severe dementia: the results of a double-blind, placebo-controlled trial with Melissa. *J Clin Psych*, 2002; **63**(7): 553–558.

72 Sutherland D, Woodward Y, Byrne J *et al.* The use of light therapy to lower agitation in people with dementia. *Nurs Times*, 2004; **100**(45): 32–34.

73 Neil W, Curran S and Wattis J. Antipsychotic prescribing in older people. *Age Ageing* 2003; **32**: 475–483.

74 McShane R, Keene J, Gedling K *et al.* Do neuroleptic drugs hasten cognitive decline in dementia? Prospective study with necropsy follow up. *BMJ*, 1997; **314**: 266–270.

75 Ballard C, Margallo-Lana M, Juszczak E *et al.* Quetiapine and rivastigmine and cognitive decline in Alzheimer's disease: randomised double blind placebo controlled trial. *BMJ*, 2005; **330**: 874–877.

76 Devanand DP, Sackeim HA, Brown RP *et al.* A pilot study of haloperidol treatment of psychosis and behavioural disturbance in Alzheimer's disease. *Arch Neurol*, 1989; **46**: 854–857.

77 Wirshing DA, Spellberg BJ, Erhart SM *et al.* Novel antipsychotics and new onset diabetes. *Biol Psychiatry*, 1998; **44**: 778–783.

78 Wirshing DA. Adverse effects of atypical antipsychotics. *J Clin Psychiatry*, 2001; **62**(Suppl. 21): 7–10.

79 Wooltorton E. Risperidone (Risperdal): increased rate of cerebrovascular events in dementia trials. *CMAJ*, 2002; **167**(11): 1269–1270.

80 Wooltorton E. Olanzapine (Zyprexa): increased incidence of cerebrovascular events in dementia trials. *CMAJ*, 2004; **170**(9): 1395.

81 Gill SS, Rochon PA, Herrmann N *et al.* Atypical antipsychotic drugs and risk of ischaemic stroke: population based retrospective cohort study. *BMJ*, 2005; **330**: 445.

82 Schneider LS, Dagerman KS and Insel P. Risk of death with atypical antipsychotic drug treatment for dementia: meta-analysis of randomized placebo-controlled trials. *JAMA*, 2005; **294**(15): 1934–1943.

83 Wang PS, Schneeweiss S, Avorn J *et al.* Risk of death in elderly users of conventional vs. atypical antipsychotic medications. *NEJM*, 2005; **353**(22): 2335–2341.

84 De Deyn PP, Rabheru K, Rasmussen A *et al.* A randomized trial of risperidone, placebo, and haloperidol for behavioral symptoms of dementia. *Neurology*, 1999; **53**: 946–955.

85 Schneider LS, Pollock VE and Lyness SA. A metaanalysis of controlled trials of neuroleptic treatment in dementia. *JAGS*, 1990; **38**(5): 553–563.

86 Teri L, Logsdon RG, Peskind E *et al.* Treatment of agitation in AD: a randomised placebo-controlled clinical trial. *Neurology,* 2000; **55**: 1271–1278.

87 Devanand DP, Marder K, Michaels KS *et al.* A randomized, placebo-controlled dose-comparison trial of haloperidol for psychosis and disruptive behaviors in Alzheimer's disease. *Am J Psych,* 1998; **155**(11): 1512–1520.

88 Brodaty H, Ames D, Snowdon J *et al.* A randomized placebo-controlled trial of risperidone for the treatment of aggression, agitation and psychosis of dementia. *J Clin Psychiatry,* 2003; **64**(2): 134–143.

89 Katz IR, Jeste DV, Mintzer JE *et al.* Comparison of risperidone and placebo for psychosis and behavioural disturbances associated with dementia: a randomized, double-blind trial. *J Clin Psychiatry,* 1999; **60**(2): 107–115.

90 Schneider LS, Tariot PN, Dagerman KS *et al.* Effectiveness of atypical antipsychotic drugs in patients with Alzheimer's disease. *NEJM,* 2006; **355**(15): 1525–1538.

91 Street JS, Clark WS, Gannon KS *et al.* Olanzapine treatment of psychotic and behavioral symptoms in patients with Alzheimer's disease in nursing care facilities. *Arch Gen Psychiatry,* 2000; **57**: 968–976.

92 Lonergan E, Luxenberg J and Colford J. Haloperidol for agitation in dementia. Cochrane Database Syst Rev 2002, Issue 2. Art. No.: CD002852. DOI: 10.1002/14651858.CD002852.

93 Ray WA, Taylor JA, Meador KG *et al.* Reducing antipsychotic drug use in nursing homes. *Arch Int Med,* 1993; **153**: 713–721.

94 Fossey J, Ballard C, Juszczak E *et al.* Effect of enhanced psychosocial care on antipsychotic use in nursing home residents with severe dementia: cluster randomised trial. *BMJ,* 2006; **332**: 756–761.

95 Gurwitz JH, Field TS, Avorn J *et al.* Incidence and preventability of adverse drug events in nursing homes. *Am J Med,* 2000; **109**: 87–94.

96 Bronskill SE, Anderson GM, Sykora K *et al.* Neuroleptic drug therapy in older adults newly admitted to nursing homes: incidence, dose, and specialist contact. *JAGS,* 2004; **52**: 749–755.

97 McGrath AM and Jackson GA. Survey of neuroleptic prescribing in residents of nursing homes in Glasgow. *BMJ,* 1996; **312**: 611–612.

98 Lee PE, Gill SS, Freedman M *et al.* Atypical antipsychotic drugs in the treatment of behavioural and psychological symptoms of dementia: systematic review. *BMJ,* 2004; **329**: 75–78.

99 American Geriatric Society and American Association for Geriatric Psychiatry. Consensus statement on improving the quality of mental health care in U.S. nursing homes: management of depression and behavioral symptoms associated with dementia. *JAGS,* 2003; **51**: 1287–1298.

100 Holmes C, Wilkinson D, Dean C *et al.* The efficacy of donepezil in the treatment of neuropsychiatric symptoms in Alzheimer disease. *Neurology,* 2004; **63**: 214–219.

101 McKeith I, Del Ser T, Spano P *et al.* Efficacy of rivastigmine in dementia with Lewy bodies: a randomised, double-blind, placebo-controlled international study. *Lancet,* 2000; **356**: 2031–2036.

102 Onofrj M and Thomas A. Severe worsening of parkinsonism in Lewy body dementia due to donepezil. *Neurology,* 2003; **61**: 1452.

103 Sink KM, Holden KF and Yaffe K. Pharmacological treatment of neuropsychiatric symptoms of dementia: a review of the evidence. *JAMA,* 2005; **293**(5): 596–608.

104 Tariot PN, Erb R, Podgorski CA *et al.* Efficacy and tolerability of carbamazepine for agitation and aggression in dementia. *Am J Psychiatry,* 1998; **155**(1): 54–61.

105 Lonergan ET and Luxenberg J. Valproate preparations for agitation in dementia. Cochrane Database Syst Rev 2005, Volume (3).

106 Christensen DB and Benfield WR. Alprazolam as an alternative to low-dose haloperidol in older, cognitively impaired nursing facility patients. *JAGS,* 1998; **46**(5): 620–625.

107 Martinon-Torres G, Fioravanti M and Grimley Evans J. Trazodone for agitation in dementia. Cochrane Database Syst Rev 2005, Volume (3).

108 Gillick MR. Rethinking the role of tube feeding in patients with advanced dementia. *NEJM,* 2000; **342**(3): 206–210.

109 Dharmarajan TS, Unnikrishnan D and Pitchumoni CS. Percutaneous endoscopic gastrostomy and outcome in dementia. *Am J Gastroent,* 2001; **96**(9): 2256–2263.

110   Finucane TE, Christmas C and Travis K. Tube feeding in patients with advanced dementia: a review of the evidence. *JAMA*, 1999; **282**(14): 1365–1370.

111   Sanders DS, Anderson AJ and Bardhan KD. Percutaneous endoscopic gastrostomy: an effective strategy for gastrostomy feeding in patients with dementia. *Clin Med*, 2004; **4**(3): 235–241.

112   Mitchell SL, Berkowitz RE, Lawson FME *et al.* A cross-national survey of tube-feeding decisions in cognitively impaired older persons. *JAGS*, 2000; **48**: 391–397.

113   Finucane TE and Bynum JPW. Use of tube feeding to prevent aspiration pneumonia. *Lancet*, 1996; **348**: 1421–1424.

114   Peck A, Cohen CE and Mulvihill MN. Long-term enteral feeding of aged demented nursing home patients. *JAGS*, 1990; **38**(11): 1195–1198.

115   Nair S, Hertan H and Pitchumoni CS. Hypoalbuminemia is a poor predictor of survival after percutaneous endoscopic gastrostomy in elderly patients with dementia. *Am J Gastroent*, 2000; **95**(1): 133–136.

116   Abuksis G, Mor M, Segal N *et al.* Percutaneous endoscopic gastrostomy: high mortality rates in hospitalised patients. *Am J Gastroent*, 2000; **95**(1): 128–132.

117   Meier DE, Ahronheim JC, Morris J *et al.* High short-term mortality in hospitalized patients with advanced dementia. *Arch Int Med*, 2001; **161**: 594–599.

118   Mitchell SL, Kiely DK and Lipsitz LA. The risk factors and impact on survival of feeding tube placement in nursing home residents with severe cognitive impairment. *Ann Int Med*, 1997; **157**: 327–332.

119   Sanders DS, Carter MJ, D'Silva J *et al.* Survival analysis in percutaneous endoscopic gastrostomy feeding: a worse outcome in patients with dementia. *Am J Gastroent*, 2000; **95**(6): 1472–1475.

120   Department of Health. *Seeking Consent: working with older people.* London: DoH, 2001. (Available at: www.doh.gov.uk/consent)

121   Hotopf M. The assessment of mental capacity. *Clinical Med*, 2005; **5**(6): 580–584.

122   The Mental Capacity Act 2005. (Available at: www.opsi.gov.uk/acts/acts2005/20050009. htm)

123   Sampson EL, Gould V, Lee D *et al.* Differences in care received by patients with and without dementia who died during acute hospital admission: a retrospective case note study. *Age Ageing*, 2006; **35**(2): 187–189.

Chapter 2

Delirium

Clinical features

Delirium is an acute confusional state. Its key features are listed below:

- acute onset
- fluctuating course
- cognitive impairments: short-term memory, orientation, attention and consciousness.

It is characterised by an onset that is usually a matter of hours to days. There is also a fluctuation in severity that is typically worse in the evening or night time ('sun downing'). Cognitive function shows a reduction in memory and impairments in orientation, attention, planning skills and consciousness. In this context consciousness refers to awareness of one's surroundings rather than a Glasgow Coma Scale (GCS) score. Misinterpretation of events or objects is common. This may be associated with full-blown hallucinations – usually visual and involving animals such as spiders. There may also be delusions, often of persecution. Disturbances in mood may be associated. Alterations in psychomotor activity commonly occur, which may result either in an agitated or a hypo-alert state.[1] Patients in this hypo-alert variant are more likely to be missed and neglected than are those who have behavioural problems due to an agitated state. Accordingly, they are noted to have less favourable clinical outcomes and so extra vigilance is required.

Differential diagnoses commonly include dementia and psychiatric disorders (mainly psychotic depression and schizophrenia). Patients with a hypo-alert delirium have a high chance of being misdiagnosed as having depression.[2] (*See* Table 1.1 for a comparison of the core features of delirium, dementia and depression.)

The cognitive impairment is traditionally thought of as fully reversible (but *see* p 46). The duration is variable from just one day to several months. Typical episodes last around eight to 12 days but are often prolonged in the elderly.[1,3] In some patients delirium may cause lasting cognitive impairment but this is hard to evaluate because of the possibility of preceding, undetected dementia. Delirium results in worse outcomes and longer lengths of stay. The worse outcomes include complications, such as falls and pressure sores, and a higher rate of institutionalisation. There is also an increased mortality rate.[4]

Epidemiology

Delirium is more common with advancing age. The mean age of acute medical patients with delirium is 75–82 years.[5–7] Estimates of prevalence among acutely hospitalised elderly patients vary widely due to differing diagnostic criteria used, but appear to be between 10% and 40%.[3,8–10] It is even more common among elderly people admitted with hip fractures (between 30% and 60%).[10] Lower figures are probably noted in clinical practice due to high rates of underdiagnosis.[4,5] Patients may be mislabelled as 'poor historians' without any thought as to the underlying cause.[11] A significant number of cases develop during a hospital stay. One study found that 15% of patients over the age of 65 years on medical or surgical wards developed delirium during their admission. Another found that 15–18% of those over the age of 70 developed delirium within nine days of admission.[12]

Risk factors

Multiple risk factors for the development of delirium have been identified. Some of the more common ones are listed below.

- *Advanced age.*
- *Pre-existing dementia.*
- *Co-morbidity*: one study found a mean of 6.3 medical diagnoses per person.[7]
- *Post-operative period*: in a cohort of patients (mean age 68 years) without a baseline deficit who underwent major surgery, 26% had cognitive dysfunction at one week after surgery, falling to 10% after three months.[13] Associated risk factors were older age, longer duration of anaesthesia and the occurrence of post-operative complications. It is also more likely if benzodiazepines are used in this period.[14]
- *Terminal illness.*
- *Sensory impairment*: visual and hearing deficits are significantly more prevalent in those with delirium.[6]
- *Polypharmacy*: one study found a mean of 6.9 medications per person.[7]

Causes

The cause of an episode of delirium in the elderly is usually multifactorial,[4] and the more frail the individual at baseline, the less noxious the insults that are required to induce it.[12] Often an acute illness is superimposed on potentially causative medication in a person with a low threshold, for example due to background cognitive impairment. Drug (e.g. benzodiazepine) and alcohol withdrawal are also aetiologically important. Almost any illness can potentially precipitate delirium. A list of common causative factors is given in Table 2.1. Hospitalisation itself is associated with the induction of delirium. Precipitating factors have been found to include commencing multiple medications, and bladder catheterisation.[12] Rarer causes that are easily missed include non-convulsive seizures and subdural haematomas.[11] Despite extensive investigation, the cause of delirium will remain undiagnosed in around 5–10% of patients.[3,7]

Pathophysiology

'Acute brain failure' is a term that has been used to describe delirium. There appears to be a relative reduction in acetylcholine (ACh) and an increase in dopamine

Table 2.1 Common causes of delirium in the elderly

Causative factor	Comments
Drugs: there are multiple potential agents; some of the more common offenders are listed here	*Anticholinergics* (e.g. tricyclic antidepressants (TCAs), oxybutynin and tolterodine); other agents or their metabolites have also been found to have some anticholinergic activity (e.g. prednisolone, theophylline and digoxin[15]); such drugs may increase the chance of toxity when taken with other drugs with anticholinergic properties *Sedatives*: especially benzodiazepines – a meta-analysis found that cognitive adverse events were 4.8 (95% CI 1.5–15.5) times more likely with sedative hypnotics than placebo[16] *Opioid analgesics* *Anti-Parkinsonian drugs*: including levodopa, dopamine agonists, selegiline and amantadine
Alcohol and drug withdrawal	Benzodiazepines should not be discontinued abruptly in the elderly as this may induce delirium[17]
Medical illnesses	Especially infection (found to be the cause of delirium in 34% of cases in one study[6]) and stroke
Metabolic disturbances	For example, dehydration, hypercalcaemia, hypoglycaemia and hypoxia
Environmental factors	Including the sudden change that occurs when patients are admitted to hospital

activity. This idea is supported by the facts that anticholinergic and dopaminergic medications frequently cause delirium, whereas antidopaminergic agents (e.g. haloperidol) are sometimes used to reduce the clinical features. There may also be disturbances in other transmitter types, such as serotinergic. It is thought to be mediated by an acute stress response with resultant increased cortisol levels, sympathetic activation and elevated cytokines. Many brain regions are impaired by this disorder, but prefrontal, non-dominant parietal and anterior thalamic processes appear to be particularly affected.

Assessment

Obtaining an accurate history from the patient and performing a thorough examination are often not possible due to the confusion and agitation. A background history obtained from a friend or carer is highly valuable and should be specifically sought. This may confirm the acute nature of symptom onset and give an impression of background cognition and functional status. An assessment of cognition may be made with a screening tool such as the Mini Mental State Examination (MMSE) or Abbreviated Mental Test (AMT) (*see* Appendix A). Even more brief screening tools, for example the Confusion Assessment Method (CAM) (*see* Appendix A) composed of approximately four questions, have also been developed in order to improve the recognition of this condition by a wider range of healthcare workers. Attention deficits may be demonstrated by simple bedside tests such as listing the months of the year backwards (*see* p 8).[11] Taking accurate medication and alcohol histories is also important.

Investigations

The basic tests that should be performed in all patients with suspected delirium are listed below.

- *Blood tests*: full blood count, electrolytes, urea, creatinine, calcium, glucose, liver function tests, C-reactive protein or erythrocyte sedimentation rate, thyroid function and blood cultures.
- *Urinalysis and culture.*
- *Oxygen saturation* ± arterial blood gas analysis.
- *Chest X-ray.*

Other tests may be indicated according to the clinical situation. They include vitamin B_{12} and folate estimation, serum drug levels (e.g. digoxin), CT/MRI scanning, lumbar puncture and electroencephalogram (EEG) recording. EEGs often show generalised slowing, but the absence of an abnormality does not exclude delirium.[1] These tests may be especially helpful in diagnosing suspected non-convulsive status epilepticus.

Management

Patients in an agitated state of delirium may be resistant to hospital admission and medical treatment. It is important to establish whether they have the mental capacity to reliably make decisions about these issues (*see* p 32). If the patient is judged to not have mental capacity at that time then treatment may be undertaken against his or her wishes under common law; that is, administering a treatment that a reasonable person would wish to receive. The use of 'sectioning' under the Mental Health Act is rarely applicable as delirium is not usually classified as a mental disorder. It is important to remember that as cognition characteristically fluctuates in delirium, so may a patient's mental capacity. Therefore, multiple assessments may need to be made during the course of an illness.

Guidelines have been developed to try and improve physicians' management of this problem (e.g. those of the British Geriatrics Society and Royal College of Physicians[18]), but they do not appear to have a dramatic effect alone.[5] There are few controlled trials in the management of delirium. Accordingly the best clinical practice is not well defined. Surveys have demonstrated much variation in the practices of physicians.[8] Trials of multifactorial interventions have suggested a benefit.[9,10] These usually include components of improvement in the recognition of delirium, staff education, medication review and management on specialised units.

A study that assessed a total of 374 patients over the age of 75 years (mean age 81) before and then four and nine months after the inception of such a multifactorial intervention found that the in-hospital prevalence of delirium fell from 41% to 19% nine months later.[9] There was an associated reduction in the prescribing of benzodiazepines, opiates and antihistamines, and an increase in neuroleptic and antidepressant use.

Another study randomised 400 patients aged 70 years or above (mean age 80 years) to either an intervention or a control ward.[10] Components of the intervention were educational sessions for doctors and nurses, and reorganisation of the care and staffing of the ward (to include better continuity of care and interaction with patients). Both wards had a prevalence of delirium of around 31% in the 24 hours following admission. A smaller proportion of those people on the intervention ward remained delirious after seven days (30% vs 60%; $p = 0.001$). Both length of stay and mortality rates were lower in those with delirium on the intervention ward (11 vs 21 days; $p < 0.001$, and 3% vs 15%; $p = 0.03$, respectively). However, the assessors were not blinded to the allocation and there were significant differences in patient composition between the wards. For example, there were more patients who had been admitted due to stroke on the control ward.

The management of delirium can be divided into four basic components:

- identify and reverse any underlying causes
- environmental and supportive factors
- symptom control
- clinical review and follow-up.

Identify and reverse any underlying causes

The initial assessment is aimed at identifying underlying causes. Where possible these deficits should be corrected. For those in whom alcoholism is suspected, thiamine supplementation is appropriate.[11] This should initially be given intravenously (two pairs of Pabrinex vials given three times daily for at least 48 hours).[19]

Environmental and supportive factors

Continuity of staff should be promoted whenever possible. Generally, a quiet and calm environment is best. This may be most reliably achieved in a side room. Low wattage night lighting can help to reduce confusion and misinterpretation of sounds and noises overnight. Orientation aids, such as clearly visible clocks and calendars, may help. Potentially dangerous objects should be removed. Sensory deficits should be corrected. This may simply be ensuring the patient has their glasses or hearing aid fitted. Familiar people such as family members help to calm an agitated patient. Multiple ward moves are counterproductive and should be avoided. However, these steps are often difficult to achieve at the time of acute hospitalisation due to the transitory nature of admission units.[5] Education of patients and their relatives about the condition is important.

Some physicians have suggested the development of specialised delirium units to improve management. It may not be feasible to set up such units in most hospitals, many of which already struggle to develop and maintain the requirement for discrete stroke units (*see* p 120). The components of good delirium care can usually be incorporated into standard acute geriatric wards.[20]

Bed rails (or cot sides) have been used to try and reduce the risk of falls. Evidence for their efficacy is lacking and they may be associated with increased harm (*see* p 190). Despite this, they are used in around a third of delirious patients.[5] In those who are very agitated and at high risk of falls, a mattress placed directly on the floor is probably the safest option. Hospital beds that can be lowered to ground level may become available in the near future.

Symptom control

For mild to moderate delirium a non-pharmacological approach is preferable. Drugs should be used with caution. Paradoxically, they may worsen confusion and make the situation harder to manage. They also have other adverse effects, including an increased risk of falls (*see* p 185). Additionally, there are no randomised controlled trials comparing medications to placebo in the treatment of delirium, and evidence of any benefit is mainly anecdotal.[21] In those in whom it is deemed necessary, it is preferable to give medication regularly rather than as required as this is more likely to prevent the development of problem behaviours. A response to oral medication may take three to four hours. It is important to remember the fluctuating nature of symptoms and that they tend to be worse overnight. A patient may be asleep during the ward round but then cause pandemonium for the staff on the night shift. It is also important to try and restore normal sleep patterns by non-pharmacological measures.

In those with associated hepatic impairment, some medications will not be metabolised effectively and will tend to accumulate within the patient. The anti-psychotic agent haloperidol, and the benzodiazepine lorazepam do not require much hepatic clearance and are therefore relatively safe to use in this situation.[1]

Oral medication

There are very few trial data on the pharmacological treatment of delirium. Thus the best management strategy is unclear. The one trial that compared the use of antipsychotic agents to benzodiazepines (in 30 AIDS patients with a mean age of 39 years) found evidence of efficacy with haloperidol or chlorpromazine but no benefit from lorazepam.[22]

- *Antipsychotics*: haloperidol is the usual first choice. It has a high potency, few anticholinergic effects and no active metabolites.[1] Generally, cardiac safety with this medication is good but there is a possibility of QT prolongation and torsade de pointes.[1] In older people low starting doses (0.25–0.5 mg once or twice a day) are necessary.[8] Atypical antipsychotics have been used in delirium and do appear to have a similar efficacy to typical agents.[23] They are more expensive but cause fewer extrapyramidal side effects, but with their short-term use in delirium this may not be relevant. The many potential side effects of these agents are discussed on p 26.
- *Benzodiazepines*: these agents are useful when the delirium is due to either alcohol or benzodiazepine withdrawal, or when there are associated seizures.[4] In other situations they are likely to be ineffective.[8,22] Shorter-acting agents without active metabolites, such as lorazepam, tend to be favoured.[1] Occasionally anti-psychotic medications are inappropriate (e.g. patients with dementia with Lewy bodies (DLB)) (*see* p 76) and so benzodiazepines are then used in preference.

Parenteral medication

In emergency situations it is occasionally necessary to rapidly sedate a patient. This is associated with significant risks and should be considered a last resort when harm is otherwise likely to be caused to the patient or others. Options in this situation include intravenous (IV) or intramuscular (IM) haloperidol or IV lorazepam. The IM route has the benefit that a cannula is not required; however, it will have a slower onset of action (around 30 minutes). As with most medications in the elderly, lower doses are usually required than those for younger people. It is best to start small and gradually increase if necessary. Starting doses of 0.5 to 1 mg for both haloperidol and lorazepam are usually appropriate.[11] Any adverse effects are generally those seen with oral preparations. Lorazepam has a rapid onset of action and is more likely to cause respiratory depression than haloperidol. In this situation the antagonist flumazenil may be necessary.

Review and follow-up

Communication with the patient and the relatives is an important component of management. A significant number of patients will still have cognitive deficits at the time of discharge (*see* below). The patient's medication requirements should be reviewed before discharge. Alternative medications to replace those that precipitated a delirium episode may be appropriate. If medications were commenced to control symptoms, their discontinuation should now be considered. Multi-disciplinary team assessment is useful for most patients. Referral to psychiatry-of-old-age services should be considered for those who have residual cognitive deficits.

Outcome

The symptoms of delirium commonly take a long time to fully resolve in the elderly, and in some cases they do not resolve at all.[11] The actual number of patients who have some lasting impairment is hard to calculate because of the common association with background dementia. Typically, more than half of elderly delirious patients will have ongoing impairment at the time of discharge. In one study of such people (mean age 82 years), admission MMSE scores averaged 12 and rose to 17 at discharge.[3] A meta-analysis of studies found that one month after admission 47% of elderly patients were in institutions and only 55% had improved mentally.[24]

During episodes of delirium the risk of medical complications, such as pressure ulcers (*see* p 266), is increased.[1] Following an episode there is a higher chance of admission to institutional care.[6] Delirium is also associated with increased mortality: rates of 10–30% have been seen in the setting of acute medical patients with delirium.[5,6,24]

Prevention

Ideally it would be possible to identify those patients at risk and take steps to prevent the occurrence of delirium. One trial stratified 852 patients over the age of 70 (mean age 80 years) into intervention and usual care groups.[25] The trial targeted interventions to try to improve or correct for six proposed risk factors: cognitive impairment; sleep disorders; immobility; dehydration; visual impairments; and hearing impairments. This resulted in a lower incidence of delirium in the intervention arm (10% vs 15%).

Another study randomised patients over the age of 65 (mean age 79 years) with a fractured hip, who had been admitted to an orthopaedic ward to receive either geriatrician consultation or usual care.[26] The geriatrician input involved making recommendations to enhance the patients' care based on a structured protocol. Interventions included actions to restore normal physiological values (e.g. oxygen saturation), appropriate medication use and care environment, and steps to im-prove the early detection of complications. The incidence of delirium was reduced to 32% in the intervention group compared to 50% among the control subjects (RR 0.64, 95% CI 0.37–0.98). Thus pro-active specialist input to non-medical units may reduce the rate of development of delirium.

References

1   American Psychiatric Association. Practice guideline for the treatment of patients with delirium. *Am J Psychiatry*, 1999; **156**(5 Suppl): 1–20.
2   Farrell KR and Ganzini L. Misdiagnosing delirium as depression in medically ill elderly patients. *Arch Intern Med*, 1995; **155**: 2459–2464.
3   Rockwood K. The occurrence and duration of symptoms in elderly patients with delirium. *J Gerontol*, 1993; **48**(4): M162–M166.
4   Meagher DJ. Delirium: optimising management. *BMJ*, 2001; **322**: 144–149.
5   Young LJ and George J. Do guidelines improve the process and outcomes of care in delirium? *Age Ageing*, 2003; **32**: 525–528.
6   George J, Bleasdale S and Singleton SJ. Causes and prognosis of delirium in elderly patients admitted to a district general hospital. *Age Ageing*, 1997; **26**: 423–427.
7   Rudberg MA, Pompei P, Foreman MD *et al.* The natural history of delirium in older hospitalized patients: a syndrome of heterogeneity. *Age Ageing*, 1997; **26**: 169–174.
8   Carnes M, Howell T, Rosenberg M *et al.* Physicians vary in approaches to the clinical management of delirium. *JAGS*, 2003; **51**: 234–239.
9   Naughton BJ, Saltzman S, Ramadan F *et al.* A multifactorial intervention to reduce the prevalence of delirium and shorten hospital length of stay. *JAGS*, 2005; **53**: 18–23.
10   Lundstrom M, Edlund A, Karlsson S *et al.* A multifactorial intervention program reduces the duration of delirium, length of hospitalization, and mortality in delirious patients. *JAGS*, 2005; **53**: 622–628.
11   Nayeem K and O'Keeffe ST. Delirium. *Clin Med*, 2003; **3**: 412–415.
12   Inouye SK and Charpentier PA. Precipitating factors for delirium in hospitalized elderly patients: predictive model and interrelations with baseline vulnerability. *JAMA*, 1996; **275**(11): 852–857.
13   Moller JT, Cluitmans P, Rasmussen LS *et al.* Long-term postoperative cognitive dysfunction in the elderly: ISPOCD1 study. *Lancet*, 1998; **351**: 857–861.
14   Marcantonio ER, Juarez G, Goldman L *et al.* The relationship of postoperative delirium with psychoactive medications. *JAMA*, 1994; **272**: 1518–1522.
15   Tune L, Carr S, Hoag E *et al.* Anticholinergic effects of drugs commonly prescribed for the elderly: potential means for assessing risk of delirium. *Am J Psychiatry*, 1992; **149**: 1393–1394.
16   Glass J, Lanctot KL, Herrmann N *et al.* Sedative hypnotics in older people with insomnia: meta-analysis of risks and benefits. *BMJ*, 2005; **331**: 1169–1173.
17   Foy A, Drinkwater V, March S *et al.* Confusion after admission to hospital in elderly patients using benzodiazepines. *BMJ*, 1986; **293**: 1072.
18   Potter J and George J. Guidelines for the prevention, diagnosis and management of delirium in older people in hospital. The British Geriatrics Society and the Royal College of Physicians,

2005. (Available at: www.bgs.org.uk/Publications/Publication%20Downoads/Delirium-2006.doc)

19 Thomson AD, Cook CCH, Touquet R *et al*. The Royal College of Physicians report on alcohol: guidelines for managing Wernicke's encephalopathy in the accident and emergency department. *Alcohol and Alcoholism*, 2002; **37**(6): 513–521.

20 Rozzini R, Sabatini T, Trabucchi M *et al*. Do we need delirium units? *JAGS*, 2005; **53**(5): 914–915.

21 Ryan CS. Placebo controlled trials of pharmacological treatments are needed. *BMJ*, 2001; **322**: 1602.

22 Breitbart W, Marotta R, Platt MM *et al*. A double-blind trial of haloperidol, chlorpromazine, and lorazepam in the treatment of delirium in hospitalized AIDS patients. *Am J Psychiatry*, 1996; **153**: 231–237.

23 Tune L. The role of antipsychotics in treating delirium. *Curr Psych Reports*, 2002; **4**: 209–212.

24 Cole MG and Primeau FJ. Prognosis of delirium in elderly hospital patients. *Can Med Assoc J*, 1993; **149**(1): 41–46.

25 Inouye SK, Bogardus ST, Charpentier PA *et al*. A multicomponent intervention to prevent delirium in hospitalized older patients. *NEJM*, 1999; **340**(9): 669–676.

26 Marcantonio ER, Flacker JM, Wright RJ *et al*. Reducing delirium after hip fracture: a randomized trial. *JAGS*, 2001; **49**(5): 516–522.

Chapter 3

Depression

Epidemiology

The World Health Organization (WHO) has reported that each year 5.8% of men and 9.5% of women will suffer a depressive episode.[1] Major depression has been estimated to have a prevalence of between 2% and 4% in those over the age of 65 years.[2,3] The figure rises to 15% of those in long-term care and 40% of those in acute hospital beds.[4] It is more common in people with chronic illnesses, especially neurodegenerative disorders. It has been estimated to occur in up to 50% of those with Parkinson's disease,[5] and 20–40% of those with Alzheimer's disease.[6,7] Post-stroke depression has been found to have a prevalence of about 30% in the first two years following an event.[8] 'Vascular depression' is a term for a mood disorder that accompanies generalised cerebrovascular disease. It is associated with subcortical hyperintensities and the theory is that such lesions disrupt the neural circuits that influence mood.

There is a genetic component in some depressive and bipolar disorders; however, this is more common in younger presentations. A prior history of psychiatric illness may be elicited. Major adverse life events, such as loss of spouse or onset of serious illness, are common precipitants. Untreated depression has been associated with increased risk of medical conditions such as heart attack and stroke.[4] Despite this, physicians generally appear to be undertreating depression.[9]

Subtypes of depression

Major depression

According to the DSM criteria,[10] major depression is defined as depressed mood or marked loss of interest experienced most of the time for more than two weeks' duration, plus four or more of the symptoms listed below.

- *Vegetative*: weight or appetite loss, insomnia/hypersomnia, loss of energy, psychomotor agitation/retardation, ↓ concentration.
- *Cognitive*: worthlessness/guilt, suicidal ideation, loss of interest.

Psychotic depression

Psychotic depression refers to the association of depression with delusions, paranoia and auditory hallucinations, or both. This seems to occur more commonly in older people.[4] Such people are at an increased risk of self-harm. They should be managed by specialists and may require a combination of antidepressant and antipsychotic medications, or electroconvulsive therapy (ECT).

Bipolar disorder

Bipolar disorder is defined as depression plus one or more episodes of mania. It is less likely to present in older individuals. A manic episode is a period of abnormally elevated mood plus three or more of:[10]

- delusions of grandeur
- ↓ sleep
- pressured speech
- flight of ideas
- distractibility
- ↑ activity
- excessive involvement in pleasurable activities.

Suicide

Suicide is more common in males, in those with a history of previous mental illness, and in association with alcohol abuse. It is also more likely in those with inadequate emotional support.

Assessment

The problem with the assessment of older adults with concomitant disease is that many of the vegetative symptoms are non-specific for depression. For example, slowing down is also a feature of Parkinson's disease, and fatigue may be caused by anaemia. The gold standard of diagnosis is the psychiatric interview. A number of screening tools suitable for use by the non-specialist with limited time have been developed. These include the Hospital Anxiety and Depression Scale (HAD) and the Geriatric Depression Scale (GDS). They are discussed further in Appendix A. The use of a single question ('Are you depressed?') has also been found to have a reasonable efficacy in detecting depression in a cohort of terminally ill patients.[11]

Simple blood tests should be performed to exclude possible physical causes of depressive symptoms. These include the conditions listed below.

- Hypothyroidism.
- ↓ Vitamin B_{12}.
- ↑ Calcium.

Depression and dementia

Depressive 'pseudo-dementia'

Depression may mimic dementia and therefore be a cause of a reversible cognitive impairment.[6] (See Table 1.1 for a comparison of the features of depression and dementia.) However, the conditions are associated and often occur together within individuals. Also, there is an increased risk of developing a dementia in the years following a depressive presentation with memory impairment. One study found that depressed people with a reversible cognitive deficit (an initial Mini Mental State Examination (MMSE) score of 19 rising to 26 after treatment for depression) had a 4.7 times higher risk of subsequent irreversible dementia in the following three years than similar-aged (mean 74 years) control subjects with depression alone (43% vs 12% developed dementia).[12] This raises the possibility that depression may be an aetiological factor in the development of some dementias.[6]

Compared to a genuine dementia, there are thought to be more 'I don't know' rather than incorrect answers during cognitive testing, but this feature may not be common in the elderly.[12] Patients usually retain awareness of their memory loss. Speech and response times tend to be slowed. There may be associated neuro-vegetative changes (e.g. altered sleep and eating patterns). Pseudo-dementia is more common in people with a prior history of depression.

Depression occurring in people with dementia

Depression occurs more commonly in people with dementia. This is probably due to the interruption of mood-related neural circuits. Alzheimer's disease often affects norepinephrinergic and serotinergic pathways of the locus ceruleus and dorsal raphe nuclei.

Screening for depression in patients with dementia is more challenging than in cognitively normal populations. It is made harder by both the difficulty of reliable history from those with memory impairment and the overlap of physical symptoms such as apathy. There may be an increased tendency for delusions and agitation in depressed patients with dementias,[6] making it an important, treatable factor in such people. Patients with only mild dementia may be assessed with standard screening tests (e.g. the GDS). It has been estimated that these remain valid down to an MMSE score of 15.[6] Those with moderate or severe dementia are better assessed with the Cornell Scale for depression in dementia (a 19-item clinician administered test that incorporates information from carers).[13] The prevalence of depression appears to reduce with more advanced disease but this may reflect the greater difficulty of diagnosis in this group.

It is generally accepted among clinicians that medications with more anti-cholinergic activity (e.g. tricyclic antidepressants (TCAs)) be avoided in favour of alternative agents (e.g. selective serotonin reuptake inhibitors (SSRIs)) in these patients.[14] Specialist psychiatry input is advised when there is associated suicidal ideation, psychotic features or a failure to respond after six weeks of treatment.

Treatment

The therapeutic options of psychotherapy, pharmacotherapy and ECT are discussed below. There is some evidence that, at least in primary care, an integrated approach involving a depression care manager, a general practitioner (GP) and a psychiatrist can lead to improvements in patients' symptoms and quality of life.[15] A system such as this may incorporate patient education, psychotherapy, antidepressant drugs and relapse prevention strategies.

Psychotherapy

Psychotherapy alone may be considered as a first-line management strategy in mild, but not severe, depression. It may be used in combination with other modalities for more serious mood disorders. It is thought to be most useful when background personality disorders, psychosocial factors or interpersonal stressors are prominent.[16] Cognitive therapy tries to identify and correct negative thought patterns. Behavioural therapy aims to promote the positive reinforcement of pleasurable activities and the negative reinforcement of harmful behaviours. It may have a role in reducing suicide rates among those who have made previous suicide attempts.[17] Meta-analyses suggest that they may have a similar efficacy to pharmacological agents.[18] However, a recent trial that compared the use of psychotherapy, paroxetine, or both, for the maintenance of remission in older adults (mean age 77 years) found a far lower rate with paroxetine (37%) compared to psychotherapy alone (68%).[19] Also, there was no significant benefit from adding psychotherapy to paroxetine. These treatment modalities have the advantage of avoiding the risk of side effects and drug interactions but their use may be dictated by local access to such services.

Pharmacotherapy

The majority of antidepressant agents act by potentiating the effects of serotonin and/or norepinephrine within the brain. There is insufficient evidence to reliably compare all of the available antidepressant medications with one another. From meta-analyses, there appears to be little difference in either efficacy or number of adverse events between any of the SSRIs, TCAs and atypical agents.[19,20] However, a review of studies performed in primary care patients has suggested that SSRIs are better tolerated than TCAs.[21] The decision on which agent to choose may be based on side-effect profiles (*see* Table 3.1). Those with more anticholinergic properties (e.g. TCAs) are usually best avoided in the elderly.[22]

Table 3.1   Key properties of commonly used antidepressant agents

Drug class (examples)	Comments
TCAs (amitriptyline, doxepin, nortriptyline)	Block the reuptake of norepinephrine and serotonin; antidepressants with the most anticholinergic effects (*see* Table 3.2); may cause cardiac arrythmias (sinus tachycardias due to pro-adrenergic and anticholinergic effects, also ventricular tachycardia secondary to QT prolongation); may be lethal in overdose; sedating
SSRIs (citalopram, paroxetine, sertraline, fluoxetine)	Serotinergic mechanism of action (block reuptake); may cause gastrointestinal side effects (e.g. nausea and diarrhoea), sexual dysfunction and gastrointestinal bleeding; less cardiac toxicity
Atypical agents trazadone	Serotinergic mechanism of action; sedating; may cause priapism; generally similar to TCAs but with less anticholinergic effects
mirtazepine	Appetite-stimulating property: may have a role in people with reduced dietary intake
venlafaxine	Similar to SSRIs; best avoided in people with heart disease, electrolyte disturbance or hypertension
MAOIs (phenelzine)	Rarely used in the current treatment of depression; one of the reasons for this is the need for a low tyramine diet to avoid provoking the serotonin syndrome (*see* Box 3.1); another reason is the high potential for drug interactions; they may be lethal in overdose

TCA = tricyclic antidepressant; SSRI = selective serotonin reuptake inhibitor; MAOI = monoamine oxidase inhibitor.

A period of six to eight weeks on treatment is usually required to achieve substantial improvement.[16] Six months after the resolution of symptoms the drugs may be gradually withdrawn. If treatment is deemed to have been unsuccessful after a period of at least four weeks on a reasonable dose of the drug, an alternative class of agent may be considered. When switching between agents it is preferable to have a period of around two days off all antidepressant medications. This time period should be increased when switching to or from monoamine oxidase inhibitors (MAOIs) or fluoxetine due to the prolonged half-lives of these drugs or their metabolites. If there is still no improvement, specialist input is necessary to consider alternative strategies such as combinations of antidepressant agents or ECT.

A trial of 4041 younger adult patients with depression found that a remission rate of approximately 30% was seen after treatment with citalopram at a mean dose of 42 mg and mean duration of 47 days.[23] Two further trials were performed on patients from the initial cohort who failed to respond to or were intolerant of citalopram after up to 12 weeks of treatment. The first recruited 727 patients (mean age 42 years) who agreed to participate in a randomised change in therapeutic agent to either bupropion-MR, venlafaxine-XR, or an alternative SSRI (sertraline).[24] Bupropion is thought to act by blocking the neuronal reuptake of dopamine and norepinephrine. It has a tendency to lower seizure thresholds and so should be avoided in patients at risk. It is also used in smoking cessation (*see* p 113). The study found that around 25% of patients had a remission of their depressive symptoms irrespective of which agent was used.

The second study enrolled patients willing to add a second agent to citalopram.[25] Here 565 patients (mean age 41 years) were randomised to citalopram plus either bupropion-MR or buspirone (a selective serotonin receptor agonist). Similar remission rates of around 30% were seen in both groups. Withdrawal rates due to intolerance were a little lower with bupropion (13% vs 21%). However, a placebo group was not used in either of the secondary studies and so true effect sizes cannot be calculated. Taken together these studies suggest that about 50% of younger patients with severe, recurrent depression will not achieve remission with pharmacotherapy.

Other drugs

St John's Wort (hypericum extract WS 5570) is a herbal remedy that has been proposed to have antidepressant properties. It appears to be as effective as SSRIs in the management of moderate to severe depression.[26] It may have interactions with other medications. Mood stabilisers are additional agents used in the management of bipolar disorder. They include lithium and some anticonvulsant drugs (e.g. sodium valproate). Antipsychotic agents are occasionally used in the management of depression with psychotic features (which is usually best done by a specialist on an inpatient basis).

Side effects

All antidepressants appear to be associated with an increased risk of falls (*see* p 185). The elimination of TCAs is slowed in older people, leading to lower doses causing higher serum levels than those seen in younger people.[22] SSRIs have been associated with an increased risk of gastrointestinal haemorrhage and so caution should be taken when combining with other such agents, such as non-steroidal anti-inflammatory drugs (NSAIDs). The SSRIs, MAOIs and venlafaxine more commonly cause insomnia or agitation.[27] The TCAs, mirtazepine and trazadone are more likely to cause sedation.[16] Of the newer agents, venlafaxine appears to be associated with a higher rate of nausea (30%). Paroxetine, sertraline and mirtazepine appear to have a higher rate of sexual-type side effects. Mirtazepine is associated with the greatest amount of weight gain (an average of 2 kg over an eight-week period).[20] This effect is probably mediated by a histamine receptor-blocking action. The TCAs appear to have the most anticholinergic effects (*see* Table 3.2). Of the SSRIs, paroxetine is thought to be more anticholinergic.

Table 3.2   Anticholinergic side effects

Central nervous system	Sedation
	Cognitive impairment (*see* p 148)
	Delirium (*see* p 42)
Gastrointestinal	↓ Saliva production (which increases the risk of dental decay)
	Constipation
Ophthalmic	Mydriasis (which may precipitate glaucoma)
	Impaired accommodation (which may cause blurred vision)
Cardiovascular	Arrhythmias (especially if underlying cardiac disease)
	Tachycardia
	Orthostatic hypotension
Urinary	Retention (which may lead to overflow incontinence)

Other side effects seen with antidepressants include hyponatraemia (probably secondary to syndrome of inappropriate secretion of antidiuretic hormone (SIADH)), which appears to be more common with SSRIs, and the serotonin syndrome[28] – *see* Box 3.1.

Electroconvulsive therapy

Electroconvulsive therapy involves the passing of an electric current through the cerebrum of anaesthetised patients. It has been found to be an effective treatment for depression in the short term, probably more effective than drug therapy, but data on the elderly are limited.[29] ECT treatment, given by specialists, is suitable for either refractory depression or when severe symptoms need to be addressed rapidly. Examples of indications include high suicide risk, self-starving, catatonia and psychotic delusions.[16]

   ECT usually involves two or three treatments per week with a total of six to 12 treatments. Response rates of between 30% and 55% have been reported in case series.[30,31] In those who do respond there is a high relapse rate, overall affecting around two-thirds of the patients treated this way.[30] The number relapsing can be reduced by maintenance pharmacological treatment. A study that compared such maintenance treatment with placebo found relapse rates of 39% in those receiving a combination of a TCA and lithium, 60% in those on a TCA alone and 84% in those on placebo medication over a 24-week period.[31]

The major side effects following treatment are memory impairment and confusion. These usually improve over a period of days to weeks. Cognitive adverse effects are more common with higher electrical doses, bilateral application and more frequent sessions.[29] The risk of these may be reduced by less frequent or unilateral treatments in those with baseline cognitive impairment, which places them at a higher chance of problems.[6]

Box 3.1   The serotonin syndrome

The serotonin syndrome occasionally occurs following the ingestion of pro-serotinergic agents. It has a rapid onset. Clinical features range from mild cases of tremor and diarrhoea to severe cases of potentially fatal neuromuscular rigidity, hyperthermia and delirium.[28] Metabolic changes that may occur include rhabdomyolysis, acidosis and disseminated intravascular coagulation (DIC).

The range of clinical manifestations of serotinergic syndrome:

MILD	MODERATE	SEVERE
Tremor	Pyrexia (38–40°C)	Pyrexia (>40°C)
Tachycardia	Hypertension	Hypertension/hypotension
Mydriasis	Hyper-reflexia	Rigidity
Diarrhoea	Clonus	Delirium
	Increased bowel sounds	
	Agitation	

Causative agents include all antidepressants, but especially SSRIs and MAOIs, and some other agents with pro-serotinergic activity, such as tramadol, sumatriptan, ondansetron and 'ecstasy' (MDMA). It may be more likely to occur with combinations of serotinergic drugs or in the presence of agents that block the hepatic degradation of serotinergic agents, for example erythromycin or valproate. Tryptophan is the precursor of serotonin (5-HT) and the ingestion of large quantities can also provoke the syndrome.

The diagnosis is made by the combination of a history of recent serotinergic drug ingestion in tandem with characteristic clinical features. The differential diagnosis includes neuroleptic malignant syndrome (*see* p 81), malignant hyperthermia (hypertonicity, hyperthermia and acidosis following inhalational anaesthetic agent administration) and anticholinergic toxicity (mydriasis, delirium, dry erythematous skin, urinary retention and reduced bowel sounds).

Treatment involves removing the causative agents, intravenous fluids and benzodiazepines. Severe cases may need sedation and ventilation. The 5-HT$_{2A}$ antagonist cyproheptadine has been utilised but no randomised controlled trial evidence of efficacy is available, and an alternative is the atypical anti-psychotic olanzapine.[28] Hypertension and tachycardia may be controlled with intravenous beta-blockers.

Anxiety

Anxiety is commonly seen in association with depression. There are a variety of clinical presentations, for example generalised anxiety disorder, obsessive-compulsive disorder, and post-traumatic stress disorder. It may be accompanied by physical symptoms such as shortness of breath, palpitations, dizziness, tingling and chest pain.

Assessment should be aimed at trying to exclude physical causes. The more common of these are listed in Table 3.3.

Table 3.3 Physical causes of anxiety disorders

Drugs
    antidepressants
    lithium toxicity
    digoxin toxicity
    anticholinergics
    steroids
    theophylline
    calcium channel blockers
    benzodiazepine withdrawal
    alcohol withdrawal

Hypoglycaemia

Thyroid disorders

Management

SSRI antidepressants have been found to be effective in reducing anxiety. An analysis of studies of the SSRI-like agent venlafaxine found a 66% response rate in those aged over 60 years compared to 41% of those in the placebo group.[32] Benzodiazepines have also been used and may have a quicker onset of action; however, their multiple associated side effects makes them unsuitable for most elderly people (*see* pp 185 and 275). Behavioural therapies may be appropriate in some patients, depending on local availability.

References

1 World Health Organization. (Available at: www.who.int/mediacentre/factsheets/fs265/en)
2 Copeland JR, Dewey ME, Wood N *et al*. The range of mental illness among the elderly in the community: prevalence in Liverpool using the GMS-AGECAT package. *Br J Psychiatry*, 1987; **150**: 815–823.
3 Livingston G, Hawkins A, Graham N *et al*. The Gospel Oak Study: prevalence rates of dementia, depression and activity limitation among elderly residents in inner London. *Psychol Med*, 1990; **20**: 137–146.
4 Raj A. Depression in the elderly: tailoring medical therapy to their special needs. *Postgrad Med*, 2004; **115**(6): 26–42.
5 Dooneief G, Mirabello E, Bell K *et al*. An estimate of the incidence of depression in idiopathic Parkinson's disease. *Arch Neurol*, 1992; **49**: 305–307.
6 Katz IR. Diagnosis and treatment of depression in patients with Alzheimer's disease and other dementias. *J Clin Psychiatry*, 1998; **59**(Suppl. 9): 38–44.

7   Lazarus LW, Newton N, Cohler B *et al.* Frequency and presentation of depressive symptoms in patients with primary degenerative dementia. *Am J Psychiatry,* 1987; **144**(1): 41–45.

8   Robinson RG, Bolduc PL and Price TR. Two-year longitudinal study of poststroke mood disorders: diagnosis and outcome at one and two years. *Stroke,* 1987; **18**: 837–843.

9   Hirschfeld RMA, Keller MB, Panico S *et al.* The National Depressive and Manic-Depressive Association consensus statement on the undertreatment of depression. *JAMA,* 1997; **277**: 333–340.

10 American Psychiatric Association. *Diagnostic and Statistical Manual of Mental Disorders,* 4th Ed. Washington, DC: American Psychiatric Association, 1994.

11 Chochinov HM, Wilson KG, Enns M *et al.* "Are you depressed?" Screening for depression in the terminally ill. *Am J Psychiatry,* 1997; **154**(5): 674–676.

12 Alexopoulos GS, Meyers BS, Young RC *et al.* The course of geriatric depression with "reversible dementia": a controlled study. *Am J Psychiatry,* 1993; **150**(11): 1693–1699.

13 Alexopoulos GS, Abrams RC, Young RC *et al.* Cornell scale for depression in dementia. *Biological Psychiatry,* 1988; **23**(3): 271–284.

14 American Geriatric Society and American Association for Geriatric Psychiatry. Consensus statement on improving the quality of mental health care in U.S. nursing homes: management of depression and behavioral symptoms associated with dementia. *JAGS,* 2003; **51**: 1287–1298.

15 Hankeler EM, Katon W, Tang L *et al.* Long term outcomes from the IMPACT randomised trial for depressed elderly patients in primary care. *BMJ,* 2006; **332**: 259–262.

16 Mann JJ. The medical management of depression. *NEJM,* 2005; **353**: 1819–1834.

17 Brown GK, Ten Have T, Henriques GR *et al.* Cognitive therapy for the prevention of suicide attempts: a randomized controlled trial. *JAMA,* 2005; **294**(5): 563–570.

18 Bartels SJ, Dums AR, Oxman TE *et al.* Evidence-based practices in geriatric mental health care: an overview of systematic reviews and meta-analyses. *Psychiatr Clin N Am,* 2003; **26**: 971–990.

19 Reynolds CF, Dew MA, Pollock BG *et al.* Maintenance treatment of major depression in old age. *NEJM,* 2006; **354**(11): 1130–1138.

20 Hausen RA, Gartlehner G, Lohr KN *et al.* Efficacy and safety of second-generation antidepressants in the treatment of major depressive disorder. *Ann Int Med,* 2005; **143**: 415–426.

21 MacGillivray S, Arroll B, Hatcher S *et al.* Efficacy and tolerability of selective serotonin reuptake inhibitors compared with tricyclic antidepressants in depression treated in primary care: systematic review and meta-analysis. *BMJ,* 2003; **326**: 1014–1017.

22 Chutka DS, Takahashi PY and Hoel RW. Inappropriate medications for elderly patients. *Mayo Clin Proc,* 2004; **79**: 122–139.

23 Trivedi MH, Rush AJ, Wisniewski SR *et al.* Evaluation of outcomes with citalopram for depression using measurement-based care in STAR*D: implications for clinical practice. *Am J Psychiatry,* 2006; **163**: 28–40.

24 Rush AJ, Trivedi MH, Wisniewski SR *et al.* Bupropion-SR, sertraline, or venlafaxine-XR after failure of SSRIs for depression. *NEJM,* 2006; **354**(12): 1231–1242.

25 Trivedi MH, Fava M, Wisniewski SR *et al.* Medication augmentation after failure of SSRIs for depression. *NEJM,* 2006; **354**(12): 1243–1252.

26 Szegedi A, Kohnen R, Dienel A *et al.* Acute treatment of moderate to severe depression with hypericum extract WS 5570 (St John's Wort): randomised controlled double-blind non-inferiority trial versus paroxetine. *BMJ,* 2005; **330**: 503–506.

27 Anonymous. Do SSRIs cause gastrointestinal bleeding? *Drug and Therapeutics Bulletin,* 2004; **42**(3): 17–18.

28 Boyer EW and Shannon M. The serotonin syndrome. *NEJM,* 2005; **352**(11): 1112–1120.

29 The UK ECT Review Group. Efficacy and safety of electroconvulsive therapy in depressive disorders: a systematic review and meta-analysis. *Lancet,* 2003; **361**: 799–808.

30 Prudic J, Olfson M, Marcus SC *et al.* Effectiveness of electroconvulsive therapy in community settings. *Biol Psychiatry,* 2004; **55**: 301–312.

31 Sackeim HA, Haskett RF, Mulsant BH *et al.* Continuation pharmacotherapy in the prevention of relapse following electroconvulsive therapy. *JAMA,* 2001; **285**(10): 1299–1307.

32 Katz IR, Reynolds CF, Alexopoulos GS *et al.* Venlafaxine ER as a treatment for generalized anxiety disorder in older adults: polled analysis of five randomized placebo-controlled clinical trials. *JAGS,* 2002; **50**: 18–25.

Chapter 4

Movement disorders

This chapter does not include all movement disorders but instead specifically covers those conditions that more commonly present in the elderly. There is some overlap of clinical features with other diagnoses. For example, patients with advanced Alzheimer's disease often develop some extrapyramidal signs (*see* p 14).

Movement disorders are predominantly caused by lesions affecting the basal ganglia. The main components of this system are shown in Figure 4.1. Complex interconnections, both excitatory and inhibitory, exist between the various ganglia. A review of these is beyond the scope of this book and is of questionable relevance to clinical practice. Their overall effect is modulation of the motor cortex output via connections from the venterolateral thalamus.

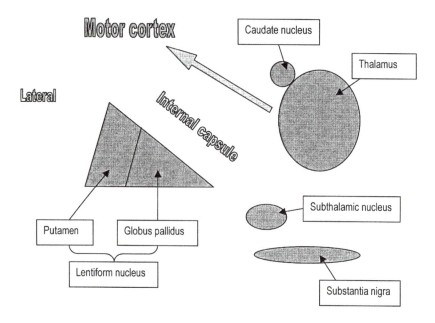

Figure 4.1 Basic anatomy of the basal ganglia (coronal view of the right-sided structures from an anterior aspect).

Assessment

History

The assessment of patients with suspected movement disorders clearly requires a careful history plus a neurological and gait examination. A thorough medication history may reveal potentially causative agents. Previous stroke and vascular risk factors may suggest a vascular aetiology. Some conditions have a genetic basis and a family history should be sought. Movement disorders are commonly associated with depression and cognitive impairment and so screening for these problems is appropriate. Enquiry should be made about related complications, including constipation and urinary incontinence. These may be part of an autonomic disturbance, which could also include postural hypotension and male impotence. Disturbed sleep patterns, including REM sleep disorder, may be associated with movement disorders. Hallucinations can be caused by some movement disorders or they may occur as secondary to prescribed medications. The timing of the occurrence of gait problems and falls within the illness can give clues to the diagnosis. Other symptoms and signs may be looked for according to the suspected condition, as discussed later.

Examination

In patients with Parkinson's disease (PD) the classic Parkinsonian tremor may not be present at rest. Distracting the patient can sometimes induce it. This can be achieved by asking the patient to rest their hands on their knees, palms facing upwards, and then recite the months of the year backwards. It may also become more apparent whilst the patient is walking during the gait assessment.

Bradykinesia (slow movement) is a key clinical feature of Parkinsonism. Its detection is somewhat subjective. There are various techniques that have been proposed to test it. One of these is shown in Figure 4.2. In the feet it can be demonstrated by asking the patient to repeatedly tap the foot on the floor as fast as they can.

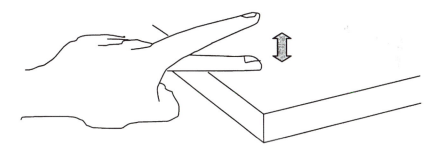

Figure 4.2 Testing for bradykinesia. The patient is asked to tap the index and middle fingers, in turn, onto a desk surface or the back of the other hand, as fast as they can.

Increased tone can be made more obvious by asking the patient to perform voluntary movements with the contralateral limb at the same time. This is termed 'reinforcement'. Increased tone in Parkinsonism is usually described as 'lead pipe' (present throughout the range of movement) or cog-wheeling (a tremor superimposed on underlying increased tone). The glabellar tap is one of the frontal release signs (*see* p 10). It is not specific for any diagnosis and has limited value in the assessment of such patients.

A gait examination should be performed. The classic Parkinsonian 'festinating' gait is described in Figure 4.3. More subtle changes may be loss of arm swing or unsteadiness/difficulty turning around. A small-stepping gait ('marche à petits pas') without other characteristic abnormalities is suggestive of a vascular cause. A method for testing for postural instability is shown in Figure 4.4.

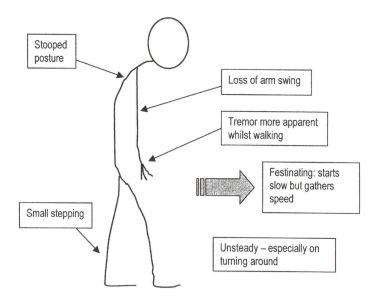

Stooped posture

Loss of arm swing

Tremor more apparent whilst walking

Festinating: starts slow but gathers speed

Small stepping

Unsteady – especially on turning around

Figure 4.3   The classic Parkinsonian gait.

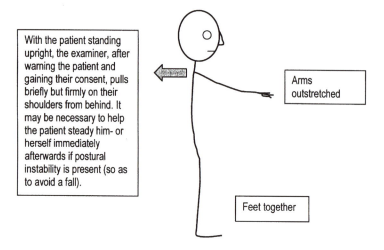

With the patient standing upright, the examiner, after warning the patient and gaining their consent, pulls briefly but firmly on their shoulders from behind. It may be necessary to help the patient steady him- or herself immediately afterwards if postural instability is present (so as to avoid a fall).

Arms outstretched

Feet together

Figure 4.4   Testing for postural instability.

Eye signs may occur with movement disorders. Supranuclear palsy is a particular feature of progressive supranuclear palsy (PSP) (*see* p 77). More subtle, and less specific, signs include abnormal saccades and square wave jerks. The assessment of saccades is shown in Figure 4.5. Square wave jerks are movements of the eyes (saccadic intrusions) whilst the patient is trying to maintain a fixed gaze on an object. They are deemed abnormal when they occur at a rate of more than 10 per minute. They are more commonly seen in people with PSP or multiple system atrophy (MSA) than those with PD.[1]

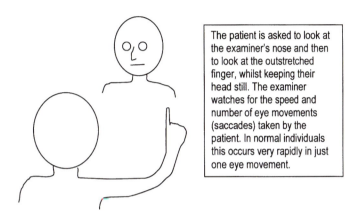

The patient is asked to look at the examiner's nose and then to look at the outstretched finger, whilst keeping their head still. The examiner watches for the speed and number of eye movements (saccades) taken by the patient. In normal individuals this occurs very rapidly in just one eye movement.

Figure 4.5   Assessment of visual saccades.

Investigations

Blood tests can occasionally exclude other causes of tremor (e.g. hyperthyroidism or hypoglycaemia). Computerised tomography (CT) and magnetic resonance imaging (MRI) scans may be suggestive of a vascular aetiology or hydrocephalus. They are not usually helpful in the diagnosis of other movement disorders. Regional cerebral atrophy is associated with some conditions but these changes are rare in early disease. Positron emission tomography (PET) scans may show reduced uptake of (18F) fluorodopa in the substantia nigra in subjects with Parkinson's disease. This technique, like most diagnostic tests, has a sensitivity and specificity well below 100%, and it is expensive and not readily obtained. For these reasons, its clinical utility has not been established. Longer-term follow-up and the response to a trial of levodopa therapy is a common method of distinguishing Parkinsonian syndromes.

Parkinson's disease

- Prevalence: 100–190 per 100 000 people.
- Survival: approximately 13 years.[2]
- Mean age of onset: 62 years.[2,3]

Key clinical features: bradykinesia, resting tremor, rigidity and postural instability.

The prevalence of PD rises with increasing age (*see* Figure 4.6[4]). It is the second most common neurodegenerative disorder after Alzheimer's disease. Parkinsonism refers to the presence of clinical features of PD, which may be due to other causes (e.g. drug-induced or vascular); these are discussed later in this chapter. The overall population prevalence is in the region of 100–190 cases per 100 000 in the Western world. It is probably marginally more common in men than women.

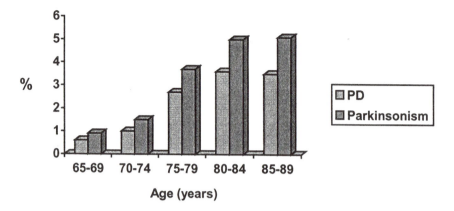

Figure 4.6 The rising prevalence of Parkinsonism with age.

A non-specific prodromal illness such as depression or anxiety may precede the motor symptoms.[5] Initial onset is almost always unilateral and affects the arms first. The typical progression is next to affect the ipsilateral leg after around one year and then the contralateral arm two to three years later.[6]

The characteristic pill-rolling resting tremor is a common early sign but 25% of PD patients will never develop a tremor.[5] The tremor may be suppressed in some situations and can be induced by distraction or whilst the patient is walking. Hallucinations occur in 10–40% of patients treated for PD,[7] mainly secondary to dopaminergic medications but other factors such as depression and cognitive or visual impairments increase the risk.[8] They are typically visual but may be auditory. Speech is affected with a tendency to develop a quiet, monotonous voice. Hand-writing may become small and irregular. Early falls (occurring within the first two to three years from diagnosis) are very uncommon in PD and suggest an alternative diagnosis, for example PSP or MSA (*see later*).

The clinical accuracy of diagnosing PD is less than perfect. Experts in PD implementing standard diagnostic criteria and with a prolonged follow-up period can expect to have around a 90% accuracy.[3]

Several disease rating scales have been developed to try and assess severity of PD. These are used primarily in research trials and are of limited clinical value. They include the Hoehn and Yahr, and Unified Parkinson's Disease Rating Scale (UPDRS) (*see* Appendix A).

Pathogenesis

Pathological changes of PD include neuronal loss in the substantia nigra and Lewy body deposition. Inherited forms of PD have been identified but they account for less than 10% of all cases;[9] they are more frequently associated with younger-onset PD. However, they do provide some insight into the pathogenic mechanisms of PD. Implicated genes are multiple but include those that encode parkin and alpha-synuclein. Parkin is involved in assisting the action of the ubiquitin-proteasome system that degrades protein. Alpha-synuclein is a major component of Lewy bodies. It is postulated that the accumulation of abnormal proteins is key to the development of PD (and many other neurodegenerative disorders). These proteins may affect mitochondrial function with resultant oxidative stress damage rather than be directly toxic to neurons.[9]

So far, no particular environmental agent has been strongly implicated in the development of typical PD. Extrinsic agents such as MPTP (a street drug contaminant) and following viral encephalitis (post-encephalitic Parkinsonism) can, rarely, result in conditions mimicking PD. Smoking and caffeine intake seem to confer a small protective advantage in epidemiological studies but the mechanism of these possible effects is unclear.[10–12] Rural living has also been associated with PD in some epidemiological studies.

Dementia associated with PD

Dementia occurs more commonly in people with PD than age-matched control subjects. It has been estimated that around 75% of people with PD will develop some degree of dementia.[13] However, a significant dementia appears to develop in around 30%.[14] Using a definition of a Mini Mental State Examination (MMSE) score <25, cognitive impairment was found to have a prevalence of 23% in a PD population (mean age 75 years).[15] People with early hallucinations or an akinetic-rigid or symmetrical pattern at onset appear to be most at risk.[13] These latter features are often seen in dementia with Lewy bodies (DLB) and suggest a common mechanism. The major distinction between PD dementia (PDD) rather than DLB is the timing of onset of symptoms. In the latter condition, motor and cognitive features must occur within one year of each other to meet current diagnostic criteria (*see* p 76). The pattern of cognitive deficit is very similar to that seen in DLB.[16] Both PDD and DLB are associated with Lewy bodies in the cerebral cortex. They appear to be differing presentations of the same process. Given the older age of most patients with PD and the prevalence of AD (*see* p 14) in this age group, it is reasonable to assume that a number of people diagnosed with PDD will have AD-type cerebral pathology. An autopsy study has found AD pathology in 33% of PD patients.[17] Conditions such as PSP (*see* p 77) may also be misdiagnosed as PDD.

Treatment of Parkinson's disease

Motor symptoms

Symptomatic treatments for PD motor features do not affect disease progression and so there is usually no rush to initiate them. The right time to commence therapy is arbitrary. It usually happens when symptoms begin to significantly affect the patient's life. This may occur earlier in the disease process if the dominant hand is the first involved. Ultimately, this decision will vary according to individual patients' preferences. A number of agents have been proposed as neuroprotective but, to date, the evidence is unconvincing.[18] Early-stage disease is relatively easy to treat. As the condition progresses the response to pharmacologic agents diminishes and additional complications such as wearing-off phenomena and dyskinesias present. This aspect of PD management is very challenging. A range of agents is available for use in PD. Much uncertainty still exists regarding the optimal ones to use.[14] Many of the drug trials involved only small patient numbers and inadequate follow-up.[19] An additional dilemma for the geriatrician is the absence of data regarding the use of such agents in older people with comorbidities. A suggested scheme for choice of therapy as disease progresses is shown in Figure 4.7.

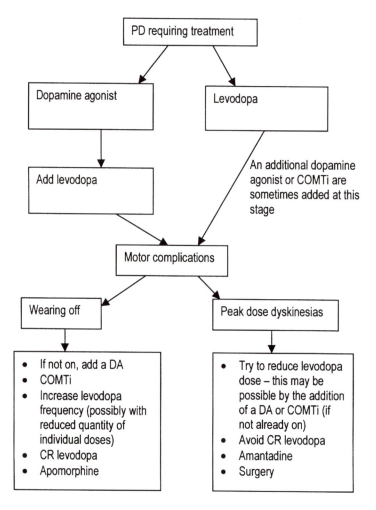

Figure 4.7 A Parkinson's disease treatment flow diagram. DA = dopamine agonist; COMTi = catecholamine-o-methyl transferase (COMT) inhibitor; CR = controlled-release.

Levodopa

Levodopa remains the most effective anti-Parkinsonian treatment available. Almost all patients will have a marked response to this agent, so much so that this has become a supportive diagnostic feature of PD. Exactly what constitutes a reasonable trial of levodopa before declaring a failed response is unclear. Most physicians would advocate several weeks of therapy on at least 300 mg a day. No improvement after this time suggests an alternative diagnosis but occasionally patients require higher doses of levodopa, up to 1500mg per day.[14]

Pharmacology

The rationale for the use of levodopa is that it is converted to dopamine within the surviving neurons of the basal ganglia to help compensate for the causative loss of dopaminergic cells (giving dopamine would be ineffective as it cannot cross the blood–brain barrier). It is always given with a decarboxylase inhibitor (carbidopa or benzeraside) to prevent excessive peripheral conversion of levodopa to dopamine, which would reduce cerebral availability and produce excessive side effects (mainly nausea, vomiting and orthostatic hypotension) (*see* Figure 4.8).

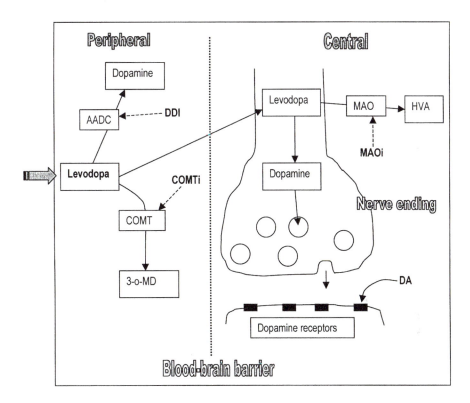

Figure 4.8   Sites of action of dopaminergic therapies. DDI = dopa decarboxylase inhibitor; AADC = aromatic amino acid decarboxylase; COMT = catecholamine-o-methyl transferase; COMTi = COMT inhibitor; MAO = monoamine oxidase; MAOi = MAO inhibitor; HVA = homovanillic acid; 3-o-MD = 3-o-methyldopa; DA = dopamine agonist; broken arrows = inhibitory effects.

Levodopa is absorbed in the small intestine and reaches peak plasma concentrations after about 30 minutes. This onset is slower if gastric emptying is delayed, for example by food or anticholinergic drugs, or as a result of accompanying autonomic neuropathy. This may account for some variation in dose response in later-stage disease. Its absorption from the gut and movement across the blood–brain barrier are dependent on an amino acid transporter system. This system can become saturated after eating a meal containing protein, which can reduce drug availability in the central nervous tissues. Therefore, levodopa should be taken with small meals low in protein content.

Doses are titrated up slowly to avoid precipitating side effects, namely nausea, vomiting and orthostatic hypotension. The dosage times of levodopa should also take into account the duration of action of the drug and the times of activity during the day. In early disease levodopa can be expected to work for four or more hours but this time will reduce with disease progression (*see below*). The first dose should be taken immediately on waking and subsequent doses at four-hourly intervals, for example 7 am, 11 am and 3 pm. The last dose should not be taken too late in the day as motor improvements are, generally, not beneficial whilst asleep.

Usually levodopa is more effective at reducing bradykinesia and rigidity than tremor. It continues to be an effective treatment for PD for several decades in many individuals.[20] However, complications do develop – as discussed below. Non-oral formulations of levodopa, including intravenous and intraduodenal, have also been proposed.[21] Such formulations are associated with various practical difficulties and have, so far, rarely been used in clinical practice.

Controlled-release preparations

Specialised formulations of levodopa have been developed that give a slow, sustained release of the drug over a 12-hour period, but the onset of action is delayed. It is particularly useful for nocturnal problems – such as reduced mobility that limits getting out of bed to use the toilet. Other benefits may include reducing motor fluctuations. It is usually used in combination with rapid-acting preparations to prevent a delay in onset, especially first thing in the morning. Because of poorer absorption, around a 30% higher total dose equivalent is needed for controlled-release (CR) preparations compared to standard-release formulations.[14] They may be associated with more psychiatric adverse effects and prolonged dyskinesias compared to standard levodopa in advanced disease.[14]

Dispersible preparations

Dispersible levodopa has the advantage of a faster onset of action (20–30 minutes vs 30–60 minutes with standard formulations).[20] This may be useful to rapidly control Parkinsonism at key times, such as when first waking in the morning.

Side effects

- *Non-motor complications*: combining levodopa with a peripheral decarboxylase inhibitor mainly prevents nausea caused by the peripheral conversion of levodopa to dopamine. When it does occur, it can be minimised by slow dose titration. Alternatively, the dopamine receptor antagonist domperidone can be used to block peripheral dopamine-induced adverse effects as it has a very poor penetration of the blood–brain barrier. It is usually possible to reduce this medication after a few weeks on levodopa therapy. Other complications include hallucinations, orthostatic hypotension (*see* p 201), delirium and hypersexuality.
- *Motor complications*: dose response variations to levodopa occur late in the disease. They affect around half of patients after five years of levodopa treatment and nearly all after 10 years.[22,23] They seem to be at least partly related to levodopa

use rather than PD alone as animal model studies suggest that they can be induced in normal individuals following levodopa administration.[24] However, they do not tend to occur in other diseases treated with levodopa (e.g. some dystonias).[23] They have also been developed in a small number of patients receiving dopamine agonists alone, with no prior levodopa exposure.[25,26] They include motor fluctuations (wearing off and on–off phenomena) and dyskinesias. Their mechanisms are not well understood. Patients are described as being in the 'on' state when their Parkinsonism is controlled by medication and in the 'off' state when this is not the case. In general, the therapeutic window becomes narrower and the pharmacodynamics of levodopa within the brain tissue change as time progresses, *see* Figure 4.9.

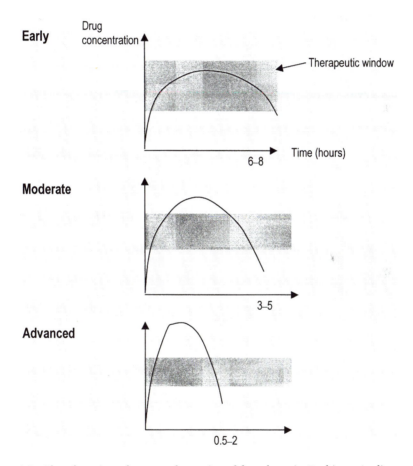

Figure 4.9 The changing pharmacodynamics of levodopa in Parkinson's disease after prolonged exposure.

One theory to explain this phenomenon is that therapeutic levodopa acts through being converted to dopamine within surviving nigrostriatal neurons and is stored pre-synaptically. It is then released as required. As the disease progresses there are fewer available neurons to store dopamine, leading to shorter treatment effects of levodopa doses.[23] Eventually there is almost no dopamine storage capacity and cerebral dopamine availability is directly related to peripheral levodopa concentrations. This leads to the need for very regular drug dosing or continuous infusions.

An alternative theory is that there are changes in the post-synaptic response to dopamine stimulation as the disease progresses. This concept is supported by an observed shortening of duration of action of a bolus infusion of apomorphine (a post-synaptic acting dopamine agonist) in advanced disease.[27] This may be partially mediated by changes in N-methyl-D-aspartate (NMDA) pathways – as supported by the apparent beneficial action of amantadine (an NMDA receptor blocker; *see* p 73). The reality is probably a combination of both pre- and post-synaptic mechanisms.

There has been concern that the increased dopamine metabolism induced by giving exogenous levodopa may lead to oxidative stress within the remaining nigrostriatal neurons and thereby worsen the condition. However, available evidence does not strongly support this idea.[18] Some of the motor complications may be worsened by pulsatile stimulation of the neuronal pathways. There is evidence that they can be improved by continuous dopamine stimulation.[28] Therefore, there may be some logic in using CR preparations of levodopa in this population. However, a trial comparing the use of CR to standard-release levodopa did not find a difference in the development of motor complications after five years.[29] Alternative strategies include the use of more frequent doses of standard-release levodopa or the addition of a catecholamine-o-methyl transferase (COMT) inhibitor (*see* p 69). Lower doses of levodopa may reduce the tendency to develop dyskinesias. A maximum daily levodopa dose of 600 mg is probably appropriate.[20] Despite these side effects levodopa remains an important and effective treatment for PD. Most patients would choose to accept some dyskinesia than be stuck in the 'off' state.

- *'Wearing off'* is a term for the re-emergence of Parkinsonian features as plasma levodopa levels fall. It occurs more frequently as the disease progresses and is caused by a shortening of the effective time of each dose of levodopa. It is usually defined as being present once levodopa doses are effective for less than four hours.[14]
- *'Freezing'* describes the sudden onset of the inability to initiate gait, which gives the appearance of being frozen in time. It may be provoked by actions such as turning round or by environmental factors such as doorways. The provision of visual cues such as a striped pattern on floors can sometimes reduce this phenomenon.[30] Occasionally, movements such as stamping the feet or walking sideways can allow normal walking to resume. It is usually poorly responsive to pharmacologic manipulation.
- *'On–off'* is an expression for the pattern whereby patients suddenly change from the 'on' state to the 'off' state unrelated to medication doses or plasma levodopa concentrations. It is usually poorly responsive to pharmacologic manipulation.

Dyskinesia

There are several subtypes of dyskinesia associated with PD. The most common is a chorea (rapid, irregular movements) associated with peak dose drug levels, but diphasic and 'off' phase types have also been described.[31] These may present as dystonia (sustained contractions), stereotypy (repetitive movements) or myoclonus (muscular jerks). More than one of these may occur at the same time. The diphasic type causes dyskinesia when drug levels are either rising or falling – thereby occurring twice with each levodopa dose. 'Off' dystonia usually presents as early morning or nocturnal cramps that most commonly affect the distal legs, which may be painful. Most patients would rather accept a degree of dyskinesia than suffer immobility related to underdosing. They are more likely to develop in younger rather than older patients.[31]

Peak dose dyskinesias may be improved by smaller, more frequent levodopa doses. Diphasic ones may be improved by using dopamine agonists in preference to levodopa. Off dystonias may be reduced by using long-acting agents overnight (e.g. CR levodopa or dopamine agonists).

COMT inhibitors

COMT inhibitors (COMTi) act by blocking one of the degradation pathways of levodopa (to 3-o-methyldopa) (see Figure 4.8). Tolcapone has both central and peripheral actions but due to cases of hepatoxicity it has been withdrawn from widespread use.[32] Entacapone does not cross the blood–brain barrier. It has a half-life of just one hour and is taken with each dose of levodopa. It increases the half-life of levodopa without increasing the maximum concentration and so, in theory, it should not worsen dyskinesias. The benefit is in the order of an additional 30 minutes 'on' time with each levodopa dose.[33] It appears to be helpful in patients who are experiencing motor fluctuations.[34] A 15–30% reduction in levodopa dose is recommended at the initiation of entacapone therapy.[14] It has not been associated with hepatic toxicity. Patients should be warned that an orange discolouration of their urine could occur. It occasionally causes diarrhoea. Preparations containing levodopa, a decarboxylase inhibitor and entacapone are available.

Dopamine agonists

Dopamine agonists act directly on post-synaptic dopamine receptors (see Figure 4.8), of which there are at least five subtypes (D_1–D_5). The agonists can be subdivided into two groups; those that are derived from ergot (e.g. bromocriptine, cabergoline and pergolide) and those that are not (e.g. ropinirole and pramipexole). Generally, there seems little to choose between the various dopamine agonists in terms of efficacy at any stage of the disease.[18,35–38]

Side effects

Pulmonary, pericardial, heart valve, and retroperitoneal fibrosis are infrequent side effects associated with the ergot-derived agents, occurring, on average, two years after commencement.[39–41] For these reasons it has been suggested that all patients should undergo baseline investigations when starting these medications (e.g. ESR, U&E, CXR and lung function tests) and they should be carefully monitored.[42] Problematic side effects with all dopamine agonists include somnolence, hallucinations and leg oedema. Somnolence is a feature of advanced PD irrespective of treatment but does appear to be made worse by dopamine agonists.[43] Rarely, sudden episodes of sleep have resulted in motor vehicle accidents.[44] This should be considered when initiating treatment in patients who still drive. The leg oedema is characteristically poorly responsive to diuretic therapy but is rapidly reversed by stopping the offending medication.[45]

Dopamine appears to have a central role in the normal brain reward system. This mechanism can, rarely, be affected by dopaminergic therapies. Recently there have been reports of an association between dopamine agonists and gambling addiction.[46] Problems seem to present within three months of maintaining a target dose and resolve on drug withdrawal. There may also be associated compulsive eating, alcoholism and hypersexuality. The most commonly implicated agent is pramipexole but others include pergolide and ropinirole. Pramipexole is the most potent agonist of D_3 receptors, which may explain its stronger association with gambling behaviour. Hedonistic homeostatic dysregulation is a form of behavioural disorder that is associated with substance addiction, which can rarely occur with dopaminergic agents in PD patients.[47] Young-onset males are most likely to develop it. Patients tend to increase their own medications and resist attempts to reduce doses. Severe dyskinesias are associated. There are varying degrees of severity of this condition. A form of mania, hypersexuality, changes in food intake, social isolation and drug hoarding can develop. The commencement of apomorphine may trigger this, and some patients develop a rapid onset of a 'high' with this agent. Management is difficult as withdrawal of these drugs may lead to unacceptable motor effects. Although rare these are potentially serious adverse events that should be monitored for and which patients and their carers should be warned about.

Dopamine agonists in early PD

Dopamine agonists are often advocated for the initial treatment of PD due to concerns that levodopa use may be associated with increased neuronal toxicity. Additionally, they may reduce dopamine turnover and subsequent oxidative stress due to their direct post-synaptic action. However, these issues remain a matter of ongoing debate.[48,49] They are less effective than levodopa but may delay its introduction for several years. This is particularly important in patients with a younger age of onset, who are at a higher risk of motor complications due to the long duration of their illness.

A study randomised 268 patients (mean age 63 years) with early PD to receive either ropinirole or levodopa over a five-year period.[25] Both groups of patients were allowed additional open label levodopa doses as required. After five years, 20% of the ropinirole group had developed dyskinesia compared to 45% of the levodopa group. Similar degrees of benefit were not seen for motor fluctuations. However, UPDRS scores were better in the levodopa arm. Around half of the patients in both groups withdrew prematurely (mainly due to adverse events). Side effects occurring more commonly with ropinirole compared to levodopa included somnolence (27% vs 19%), hallucinations (17% vs 6%) and leg oedema (14% vs 6%).

A similar study compared pramipexole to levodopa:[26] 301 patients were randomised (mean age 61 years) and followed up for a two-year period. After this time 28% of the pramipexole group had developed either motor fluctuations or dyskinesias compared to 51% of the levodopa group. This benefit was offset by better UPDRS and quality of life scores in the levodopa group. Side effects more commonly seen with pramipexole also included somnolence (32% vs 17%), hallucinations (9% vs 3%) and leg oedema (15% vs 4%). Results for studies involving cabergoline and pergolide appear to show similar trends.[50]

Studies of 10-year duration have failed to show a mortality benefit of initial dopamine agonist therapy compared to initial levodopa use.[51,52] Also, the evidence that dyskinesias are less severe with agonists after 10 years of treatment is less convincing. One study found that the numbers with moderate to severe dyskinesias were similar in both groups after this length of time despite early results in favour of the agonist arm.[52] Again the patients treated with levodopa had lower levels of disability. So, the use of these agents may not significantly reduce motor complication rates after prolonged treatment.[20]

The dilemma is whether the reduced risk of motor complications seen with dopamine agonists early in the disease justifies their use despite poorer efficacy and associated side effects. The trials, so far, have recruited cohorts of young patients who are more likely to develop motor complications than older people. The occurrence of side effects, particularly psychiatric ones, could be different in the elderly. Many physicians are currently advising the use of dopamine agonists as initial therapy in biologically younger patients and levodopa in the older, more frail.[14,50] This distinction is fairly arbitrary and the best practice may only be determined by the results of future clinical trials.

Dopamine agonists in advanced PD

Dopamine agonists have also been tried as supplementary therapy to levodopa in advanced PD. A study randomised 360 patients (mean age 63 years) with sub-optimally controlled advanced PD plus motor fluctuations to receive either pramipexole or placebo over a 32-week period.[53] There were significant improvements in UPDRS scores with pramipexole compared to placebo for motor scores (25% vs 12%) and reduction in 'off' time (31% vs 7%). Resting tremor, rigidity and bradykinesia were improved. Side effects seen more commonly with pramipexole included dyskinesia (61%), hallucinations (19%) and confusion (11%). Similar results have been found with studies of both pergolide and ropinirole.[54,55]

The addition of these agents to levodopa often allows a reduction in levodopa dose of around 30%.[54,55] This levodopa-sparing effect may lower the incidence of future motor fluctuations.

Apomorphine

Apomorphine is a dopamine agonist that needs to be taken by a parenteral route. It appears to activate mainly D_1 and D_2 receptors. When given subcutaneously it has an onset of action after 5–15 minutes.[56] The initial concomitant use of domperidone limits (but may not remove) the associated nausea, vomiting and postural hypotension. It is indicated for use in patients with advanced PD plus motor fluctuations.

It is usually given as either a continuous subcutaneous infusion, via a portable infusion pump, or as intermittent subcutaneous injections that are self-administered. To select patients who are likely to benefit an 'apomorphine test' is given. This involves increasing bolus doses of apomorphine at 90-minute intervals, with careful monitoring, until either an anti-Parkinsonian effect or unacceptable side effects occur.[56] The threshold dose that leads to benefit is recorded and is used to calculate a reasonable starting dose for individual patients. It may be possible to slowly reduce, and occasionally withdraw, levodopa therapy once a continuous infusion has been established.[57]

With continuous infusions, patients appear to benefit in terms of reduction in the percentage of day spent in the 'off' state (from around 50% to around 25%)[56] and in the incidence of dyskinesias.[57] Minor local reactions, including nodules, may occur at injection sites. Psychiatric side effects, including psychosis and hallucinations, and sedation may limit the use of apomorphine in many older people.

A trial of intermittent apomorphine injections compared to placebo injections has demonstrated a benefit in UPDRS scores with this treatment when administered in the 'off' state (a 24- vs 0-point reduction – *see* Appendix A).[58] Side effects occurring more commonly in the treatment group included yawning, dyskinesias, somnolence, nausea/vomiting, postural dizziness, rhinorrhoea (runny nose), hallucinations/confusion, and leg oedema. The benefit lasts for around one hour with each dose.

Monoamine oxidase inhibitors

The monoamine oxidase inhibitor (MAOI) selegiline (also known as deprenyl) has been used both as a putative neuroprotective agent and as a treatment for PD. The enzyme monoamine oxidase type B is involved in the degradation of dopamine (as compared to type A that degrades serotonin and norepinephrine, and is targeted in the treatment of depression – *see* p 52). The theory is that blocking this enzyme will increase the available dopamine within the brain (*see* Figure 4.8). Selegiline has a specific action on the type B enzyme and so has a low risk of 'cheese reaction' or serotonin syndrome (*see* Box 3.1). However, there have been rare cases of serotonin syndrome with combinations of selegiline and antidepressant drugs, necessitating caution with this combination.[59] Given the high incidence of depression in PD, this is potentially very important.

It has been speculated that inhibition of this enzyme could prevent the formation of harmful free radicals from dopamine metabolism. Thus it could have a neuroprotective effect and this has been suggested by several trials.[60] However, there is controversy as to whether this apparent effect could be explained by a mild symptomatic benefit allowing a delay in the need for levodopa.

A meta-analysis of 17 randomised trials (involving 3525 patients) of selegiline use in early PD found evidence to support a small beneficial effect on disability, the need for levodopa and motor fluctuations.[61] Side effects did not appear to be a significant problem. The DATATOP study did not demonstrate a survival benefit in 800 patients receiving either selegiline or placebo after 13 years of follow-up.[62] Unfortunately, there are no data comparing selegiline with dopamine agonists, the main alternative levodopa-sparing therapy in early PD.

The drug has amphetamine metabolites that may cause insomnia. Data from the Parkinson's Disease Research Group study suggests that selegiline may be associated with an increased incidence of falls and dementia.[63] It seems logical to avoid this medication in patients with cognitive impairment, significant orthostatic hypotension or a history of falls.

A fast-absorbed sublingual preparation of this medication is available which may help patients with swallowing difficulties. There is some trial evidence of a symptomatic benefit when it is used in combination with levodopa therapy in patients with motor fluctuations.[64] A newer MAOI called rasagiline is also available. A trial has found a similar reduction in daily off time with this agent in people with advanced PD to that seen with entacapone.[65]

Amantadine

Amantadine was initially introduced as an anti-viral agent but was subsequently found to have anti-Parkinsonian properties. It has an NMDA receptor-blocking action, which leads to an anti-glutaminergic effect. In patients with PD this is thought to help by inhibiting excitatory pathways within the basal ganglia. It may also have dopaminergic and cholinergic effects. It has been found to lead to a modest improvement in Parkinsonism. Studies recruiting small numbers of patients (14–24) over short durations (six weeks) and using crossover designs have suggested a beneficial role in the control of dyskinesias and motor fluctuations when used in combination with levodopa in advanced PD.[66,67] This benefit is maintained to at least one year.[68] A six-week trial of amantadine may be tried in those patients with disabling dyskinesias.[20] It may also have some neuroprotective properties. Observational data have suggested an association between amantadine use and improved survival in PD.[69] This notion needs to be confirmed in a controlled trial setting. Side effects include confusion, hallucinations and leg oedema. Cognitive side effects often limit the use of this drug in the elderly.

Anticholinergic drugs

Anticholinergic agents (e.g. benzhexol, procyclidine and orphenadrine) are associated with cognitive impairment, particularly in the elderly (*see* p 148), and are now very rarely used for the management of PD. There is evidence that they are associated with increased rates of Alzheimer-type pathology formation (amyloid plaques and neurofibrillary tangles).[70] These agents may have a place in the control of tremor-predominant PD in younger people.[20]

Surgical techniques

Surgical interventions for PD are usually performed with stereotactic techniques under local anaesthesia in order to assess motor response during the procedure. Due to the associated complications, they are usually reserved for those with advanced disease that causes significant disability that can no longer be controlled with medical therapy alone. This normally equates to patients with severe motor fluctuations and dyskinesias. Successful positioning requires intra-operative feedback from the patient and so significant cognitive impairment is a contraindication. Evaluation of these techniques in randomised controlled studies is difficult due to ethical considerations with placebo surgery. To date they have almost exclusively been performed in people under the age of 75 years. They are probably only suitable for a small number of highly selected, younger PD patients.

Deep brain stimulation

Deep brain stimulation (DBS) is a technique that involves the implantation of a device much like a cardiac pacemaker but with the electrode sited in the basal ganglia. This device then uses low-current, high-frequency electrical stimulation to inhibit local neuronal functioning. The effects are reversed if the device is switched off. The most common target sites are the subthalamic nucleus (STN) and globus pallidus interna (GPi). Both sites are associated with improvements in dyskinesias and both on and off period symptoms. A crossover study of 143 patients (mean age 58 years) who had received DBS devices compared motor symptoms with the devices turned on and off.[71] It was found that stimulation of the subthalamic nucleus or pars interna of the globus pallidus was associated with median improvements of 49% and 37% in motor scores, respectively. Fifty-eight adverse events occurred in 143 patients (undergoing 277 procedures). These included haemorrhage, seizures and infection. Four patients (2.8%) had lasting neurological deficits.

After insertion it may be possible to reduce drug doses. A study found that 50% of patients were able to come off levodopa altogether and in these patients dyskinesias were markedly reduced.[72] The motor benefits appear be maintained, at least in part, to beyond five years from implantation.[73] Thalamic stimulation has been used to treat tremor associated with both PD and essential tremor with some success.[74] When the effects of DBS have been compared between patients over the age of 70 years and younger patients, the benefits are less clear.[75] Both groups had reduced dyskinesias but the older patients had a tendency toward worsening of axial signs (including gait impairment, which led to increased rates of falls).

Stereotactic surgery

Surgery for PD is usually performed using radiofrequency ablation. Thalamotomy has had some success in the treatment of tremor in the past but has now been outmoded by DBS, which has had similar success rates with fewer complications.[76] Pallidotomy, usually unilateral, appears to reduce the occurrence of dyskinesias (mainly contralateral). This benefit is maintained up to at least four years.[77] Side effects are not inconsiderable. Around 14% will have an adverse event with 5% of these being rated as severe (e.g. persisting neurological deficit) and the mortality rate is around 0.4%.[78] Bilateral pallidotomy is associated with cognitive, behavioural and motor complications.[79]

Growth factors

Glial cell-derived neurotrophic factor (GDNF) is a naturally occurring growth factor that has poor penetration of the blood–brain barrier. It has been delivered directly to the brains of patients with PD via a continuous infusion through a catheter placed into the putamen in two small, non-controlled studies ($n = 5$ and $n = 10$).[80,81] There were apparent improvements in motor scores on the UPDRS in the order of around 30%. These improvements seem to be maintained to at least two years.[82] Clearly, these trials were uncontrolled and recruited extremely small numbers and so further data are still required.

Neuronal transplantation

Human embryonic dopamine neuron transplants have been tried in the treatment of advanced PD. When they have been compared to sham surgery the results have not demonstrated clinically significant benefit and they have been associated with worsening of dyskinesia.[83,84] There is also concern that the transplanted tissues may contain non-neuronal cells that could grow out of control and cause complications.[85] The transplantation of porcine tissues has also been tried.[86] Such a method could result in the transmission of zoonoses. Currently these techniques are for research only and are not used in standard clinical practice.

Non-motor symptoms

Depression is a frequent component of PD, perhaps affecting as many as 50% of patients.[87] The clinical features of Parkinsonism (e.g. psychomotor retardation) can mimic depression and its diagnosis in these patients is not always easy. Sedating antidepressants, such as tricyclic antidepressants (TCAs), taken at night may aid sleep pattern restoration. Their anticholinergic properties may reduce salivation (and so improve drooling) but may also worsen cognition, orthostatic hypotension (OH) and falls. Selective serotonin reuptake inhibitors (SSRIs) have occasionally been associated with worsening of tremor.[88] All these agents could potentially interact with selegiline and so caution is needed with such a combination. The management of depression is discussed further in Chapter 3.

Cognitive impairment and psychotic features are not easily treated. It is important to limit contributory drugs. It is suggested that sedating medications, then anticholinergics or amantadine, then selegiline, and then dopamine agonists are withdrawn in that order.[14] Lastly, it may be necessary to reduce levodopa doses. Hallucinations, if distressing to the patient, may be similarly reduced by the above medication changes. If this fails it is occasionally necessary to try a low dose of an antipsychotic agent in combination with levodopa. Of the available agents, quetiapine appears to have a lower incidence of worsened Parkinsonism than either risperidone or olanzapine.[89,90] This class of agent has many side effects (*see* p 26) and should be used with caution.

Cholinesterase inhibitors have been tried in the treatment of PDD. A group of 541 patients with PDD (mean age 73 years, mean MMSE score 19/30) received either rivastigmine or placebo over a 24-week period.[91] There was a small but statistically significant difference in ADAS-cog scores (*see* Appendix A) of 2.8 (out of 70) in favour of the rivastigmine group. However, the clinical significance of this degree of change is questionable and differential drop-out rates may have accounted for some of the difference. Also, there were significantly more side effects observed in the treatment arm. Those occurring more commonly with rivastigmine compared to placebo included nausea (29% vs 11%), vomiting (17% vs 2%) and tremor (10% vs 4%). The cost–benefit ratio does not appear to justify the use of cholinesterase inhibitors in PDD.

Falls are more common in patients with PD due to the combination of a gait and balance disorder, postural instability and OH due to both autonomic neuropathy and medication-induced. They have been found to occur in 68% of a cohort of patients with PD over a one-year period.[92] A history of previous falls, the presence of cognitive impairment and loss of arm swing are associated with a higher risk. Adequate motor control is clearly important. The management of OH is discussed on p 203. Physiotherapy may help patients learn safer methods of mobilisation in difficult situations such as turning around. Gait and balance training is likely to be appropriate. Other causes of falls should also be considered (*see* Chapter 9).

Sleep disturbance is common in PD.[93] Excessive daytime sleepiness is a feature of the disease and is made worse by dopaminergic treatments, especially dopamine agonists. Nocturia, restless legs syndrome or the inability to turn over in bed may disturb night-time sleep. These latter two factors may improve with long-acting dopaminergic agents taken before bed. Depression may also be causative. Steps to improve nocturnal sleep may reduce daytime sleepiness.

Drooling (sialorrhoea) is caused by a reduction in swallowing frequency and efficacy, not by an increase in saliva production. It has been successfully improved by botulinium toxin injections to the salivary glands.[94] Constipation is a common manifestation in PD due to both autonomic neuropathy and levodopa. Its management is discussed in Chapter 7. Urinary frequency and incontinence may occur in advanced disease (*see* Chapter 6). Erectile dysfunction may be managed with sildenafil but this treatment can precipitate OH.[95]

Specialties allied to medicine

PD nurse specialists are often employed in a variety of components of patient care, including education, counselling and monitoring of treatments. Their use has been found to improve patients' sense of well-being with no additional overall cost, but does not appear to affect patient outcomes.[96] Speech therapy may have a role in improving the quality of patients' speech.[97,98] The management of swallowing disorders is discussed on p 261. Physiotherapy has been found to improve motor and activities of daily living (ADL) UPDRS scores but this effect was not maintained once therapy was discontinued.[99] It may well have a role in improving mobility and reducing falls, as mentioned previously.

Dementia with Lewy bodies

- Percentage of all dementia: 10–15.[100]
- Mean age of onset: 66 years.[101]
- Male:female ratio = 2:1.
- Core clinical features are: Parkinsonism, fluctuating cognitive impairment and visual hallucinations.

Other suggestive features are early falls, episodes of reduced consciousness, neuroleptic sensitivity, REM sleep disorder and other hallucinations or delusions.[102] The cognitive impairment and Parkinsonism may not occur simultaneously at the onset; however, they should occur within 12 months of each other to meet standard diagnostic criteria.[102] Some autopsy-confirmed cases have been identified that did not develop Parkinsonism during the course of their illness.[100] The episodes of reduced consciousness are probably autonomically mediated due to Lewy body pathology within the autonomic centres of the brainstem. Three or more of daytime drowsiness, daytime sleeping > 2 hours, staring into space for long periods and episodes of disorganised speech occur in 63% of people with DLB compared to 12% of people with AD and only 0.5% of normal elderly people.[103]

The features of the cognitive impairment are generally those of other subcortical dementias (*see* p 12) but typically it is fluctuating in severity (*see* Figure 1.2). In the early stages, patients may function at a near-normal level between fluctuations. The duration of these may vary from hours to weeks. Problems with frontal-executive functions, attention and visuospatial tests are characteristic. A study comparing clinical features with autopsy pathology in a cohort of people with cognitive impairment found that, in comparison to AD, DLB patients tend to perform worse in tests of executive function and attention but better in tests of memory and verbal skills.[104] However, they also found that a large percentage of patients have mixed cerebral pathology with a combination of the plaques and tangles of AD plus Lewy bodies in the substantia nigra or amygdala. This group of patients with mixed pathology tended to do similarly to the AD group in neuropsychological testing but had a worse prognosis, with an average annual decline in MMSE score of 5.0 points compared to 3.5 and 3.4 for the AD and Lewy body pathology only groups, respectively.

Neuroleptic sensitivity occurs in around 60–80% of patients with DLB compared to <10% of those with AD, and about half of these reactions appear to be severe.[105] They usually present as a sudden onset of confusion, sedation and rigidity. A number will develop neuroleptic malignant syndrome (*see* p 81) and some reactions are fatal. Visual hallucinations usually take the form of animals or people. Neuroleptic agents can reduce them, but given the risk of sensitivity, this should only be undertaken if they are distressing to the patient. Available observational evidence suggests that quetiapine may be the safest agent in this patient group.[89] The lowest effective dose should be used for the shortest possible length of time.

Pathologic findings include Lewy bodies. These are spherical, eosinophilic, intracytoplasmic inclusion bodies. They may be found throughout the brain but appear more commonly in the basal ganglia and limbic system. There are some pathological similarities to AD (*see* p 15): beta amyloid plaques are commonly associated, but neurofibrillary tangles are infrequent.[102]

Treatment

Treatment of the cognitive and behavioural aspects of this condition is similar to that of other dementias and is discussed on p 22. The treatment of the movement disorder aspects is similar to those of PD as discussed earlier. Dopaminergic agents may worsen hallucinations and cognitive impairment, making it difficult to find the right therapeutic balance.

Progressive supranuclear palsy

- Prevalence: 5–6/100 000.[106,107]
- Mean survival: six years.[108,109]
- Mean age of onset: 63 years.[108]
- Male:female ratio = 2:1.
- Key clinical features: supranuclear gaze palsy, axial rigidity, pseudobulbar palsy, subcortical dementia, early gait abnormality, postural instability and falls.

PSP (formerly known as Steele–Richardson–Olszewski syndrome) is more common in men than women. Pathological features include atrophy of the upper brainstem with tau protein deposition and neurofibrillary tangles. The cause is unknown, however, some cases are inherited in an autosomal dominant manner and may be linked to mutations affecting the tau protein gene.[110] Diagnostic criteria have been published.[111]

The most common presenting complaint is of gait unsteadiness or falls.[109] When falls occur within the first year of diagnosis in patients with Parkinsonism, PSP is highly likely.[112] Classically the gaze palsy affects up and down gaze, which can present as problems negotiating flights of stairs. The earliest ophthalmic feature is usually impairment of saccadic movements, commonly seen as slowing of vertical saccades.[5] A method for demonstrating this is shown in Figure 4.5. Other ophthalmic features that may be present include lid retraction, blepharospasm (abnormal eyelid contractions), reduced convergence and internuclear ophthalmoplegia.

The axial rigidity causes an extended posture with neck hyperextension commonly present. The pseudobulbar palsy manifests as dysarthria and dysphagia. Generalised hyper-reflexia, a positive jaw jerk and frontal release signs (see p 10) may be present on examination. Cognitive signs are those of a subcortical dementia. There may also be palalia (repetition of words) and emotional lability. There appears to be an increased incidence of hypertension in patients with PSP, possibly due to involvement of the brainstem adrenergic nuclei.[113] Urinary incontinence commonly develops. The onset of the condition is usually symmetric in distribution. It is often misdiagnosed before the development of characteristic signs such as gaze palsy. A non-specific prodromal illness may precede motor and cognitive impairment.

MRI scanning may demonstrate atrophy of the upper brainstem, temporal and frontal lobes. These changes are unlikely to occur in early disease and so are rarely helpful in the diagnosis. Falls occurring within the first year of presentation, absence of a tremor-predominant pattern and poor levodopa response all suggest PSP rather than PD.[101]

Treatment

Generally patients do not respond to levodopa. Around 20% will have a small benefit that is usually only short-lived.[5] Cholinesterase inhibitors have not produced significant cognitive benefits in PSP and also appear to impair mobility and functional status.[114] Botulinium toxin may help with rigidity.[115] Physiotherapy and fall-prevention strategies (see p 187) may be beneficial. Swallowing assessment and intervention may reduce the risk of aspiration pneumonia.

Multiple system atrophy

- Prevalence: 4/100 000.[106]
- Survival: nine years.[116]
- Mean age of onset: 53 years.[116]
- Male:female ratio = 2:1.
- Key clinical features: Parkinsonism, one or more of pyramidal tract signs, cerebellar signs, autonomic dysfunction.

Multiple system atrophy (MSA) is a heterogeneous condition with a variety of clinical manifestations. It was initially classified as three separate conditions – striatonigral degeneration, olivopontocerebellar atrophy and Shy–Drager syndrome – depending on whether Parkinsonian, cerebellar or autonomic features predominated, respectively. More recently these have been considered as parts of the spectrum of this condition and much overlap, both clinically and pathologically, is observed.

The onset of motor symptoms is usually symmetrical. Autonomic dysfunction is seen in 97% of cases with male impotence, OH and urinary incontinence being the most commonly seen features.[116] Parkinsonism is present in around 90% of cases, pyramidal tract signs in 60% and cerebellar signs in 50%.[116] The Parkinsonism is more commonly of an akinetic rigid type, but two-thirds of patients will have a tremor though not usually the classic pill-rolling variety. Dysarthria (95%), stridor (30%) and myoclonus (30%) may also be present.[116] Some patients develop obstructive sleep apnoea. There is an association between MSA and peripheral neuropathy. Cognition is usually not affected but a mild subcortical type dementia may develop. There is a high rate of misdiagnosis even amongst specialists. Early autonomic, cerebellar and gait disorders in the absence of marked cognitive impairment are suggestive of MSA.[117]

MRI scanning may demonstrate cerebellar and brainstem atrophy. The putamen may show relative signal hypointensity and atrophy with signal hyperintensity at its lateral margin. These changes are specific for MSA but are not very sensitive and may not be apparent until late in the disease.[118] Functional imaging studies may show reduced metabolism in the cerebellum and putamen. The role of these investigations in the diagnosis of MSA is not fully established.

Treatment

Around 30% of patients will have a significant response to levodopa therapy[116] so a trial of therapy is usually warranted. However, any response is usually only short-lived and the majority are poorly responsive. The management of orthostatic hypotension and urinary incontinence are discussed in Chapters 10 and 6, respectively. Erectile dysfunction may be managed with sildenafil but this treatment can precipitate or aggravate orthostatic hypotension.[95]

Corticobasal degeneration

- Prevalence: <1/100 000.
- Survival: eight years.[119]
- Mean age of onset: 63 years.[119]
- Key clinical features: asymmetric Parkinsonism, dystonia and myoclonus, ideomotor apraxia, subcortical dementia, alien limb phenomena.

Corticobasal degeneration (CBD) is a neurodegenerative condition of unknown aetiology. It shares pathological similarities with both PSP and frontotemporal dementia (FTD).[120] It is also associated with abnormal tau protein processing.

The most common presenting signs are unilateral limb clumsiness or rigidity, bradykinesia, ideomotor apraxia, postural imbalance and arm dystonia. The ideomotor apraxia can be demonstrated by asking the patient to mime activities such as combing their hair or cutting a piece of paper with a pair of scissors. The myoclonus usually can be induced ('stimulus-sensitive'). Around 50% will develop an 'alien limb'. This may present as spontaneous limb elevation, uncontrollable reaching for objects or intermanual conflict when performing tasks. This is not specific for CBD and may occur in other neurodegenerative disorders. Cortical sensory signs such as astereognosis (the inability to recognise objects by touch – e.g. keys placed in the hand), agraphaesthesia (the inability to distinguish numbers or letters 'drawn' on the palm) and reduced two-point discrimination may occur. Approximately one-third of patients will have early cognitive impairment.[121] There may also be clinical features similar to PSP, such as pseudobulbar palsy and ophthalmic signs. Clinical variants of this condition also exist. It can initially present as a focal cortical degenerative syndrome, for example primary progressive aphasia, or similarly to FTD.

Diagnostic accuracy is low (less than 50%) in comparison to autopsy pathology.[119] This is probably due to the clinical heterogeneity of CBD and the large degree of overlap both clinically and pathologically between all of the neuro-degenerative disorders.[121] MRI scanning may demonstrate focal cortical atrophy or atrophy of the corpus callosum in later disease.[5]

Treatment

Around 25% of those with Parkinsonism will have a small response to levodopa. This medication should not be continued in the absence of a continued benefit due to potential adverse effects. Benzodiazepines may help reduce myoclonus in about 25%. Botulinium toxin may be useful for dystonia.

Drug-induced movement disorders

Drug-induced movement disorders include Parkinsonism, acute dystonia, neuro-leptic malignant syndrome and tardive dyskinesia. Antipsychotic medications most commonly cause them. The indications for these medications, given their multiple harmful effects, should be carefully reviewed (*see* p 26). The mainstay of diagnosis and treatment is to identify potentially causative agents and attempt to withdraw them where possible.

Parkinsonism

Drug-induced Parkinsonism accounts for around 9% of all Parkinsonism.[122] It usually presents as a rapid onset of symmetrical bradykinesia.[5] A Parkinsonian tremor can occur but is uncommon. It is usually reversible over weeks to months on discontinuation of the offending agent. Typical antipsychotic medications are more likely to induce Parkinsonism than atypical ones (*see* p 26). A long list of other potentially causative agents has been produced. Most of these are very rare. Anti-dopaminergic anti-emetics (e.g. metoclopramide), monoamine depletors (e.g. res-erpine) and some calcium channel blockers (e.g. cinnarizine) are occasionally implicated.

The use of levodopa in combination with the offending neuroleptic agent to treat drug-induced Parkinsonism is ineffective and illogical. Anticholinergic agents have been used previously to control such symptoms but they are associated with cognitive impairment in the elderly and should be avoided (*see* Table 2.1 and p 148).

Tardive dyskinesia

Tardive dyskinesia (TD) is a term for choreioathetoid movements that develop after a period of months to years on neuroleptic agents. The likelihood of its development appears to be related to cumulative exposure. It is often precipitated or worsened by drug dose reductions or withdrawal. It is frequently permanent but may slowly improve once the causative agent has been discontinued. The most common manifestation is orofacial dyskinesia but athetosis or dystonia is possible.

The relative risk of the development of TD with typical or atypical agents is controversial. One study compared matched groups of 61 patients (mean age 66 years) on haloperidol or risperidone for the development of tardive dyskinesia over a nine-month period.[123] A higher rate was seen with haloperidol compared to risperidone (RR 4.1, 95% CI 2.5–5.7). However, the study included patients with a mixture of diagnoses and variable previous neuroleptic exposure. It cannot be excluded that some of the dyskinesias were induced by changes in medication or dose adjustments.

An open-label study of 330 patients with dementia (mean age 83 years) on various doses of risperidone (mean dose 0.96 mg/day) found an annual incidence of TD of 2.6%.[124] This figure is lower than the previous estimates of around 25% per year for those on typical agents. However, a retrospective review of 21 835 older adults with dementia (mean age 83 years) who had been started on neuroleptic medication found that there were 5.24 cases of drug-induced movement disorders other than Parkinsonism per 100 person-years with typical agents compared to 5.19 cases with atypical agents.[125] This difference was not statistically significant (RR 0.99, 95% CI 0.86–1.15).

Neuroleptic malignant syndrome

Key clinical features:

- muscle rigidity
- hyperthermia (>37.5°C)
- autonomic instability, for example tachycardia, hypertension or a labile blood pressure
- altered level of consciousness
- ↑ creatine kinase (CK).

Neuroleptic malignant syndrome (NMS) should be suspected in patients with a combination of the above clinical features whilst on a potentially causative medication. It has been seen most frequently with typical antipsychotic medications, especially haloperidol.[126,127] But it has also been described in patients taking atypical antipsychotic agents,[128–130] and occasionally in patients taking metoclopramide.[126] Rarely, it is seen in patients with PD who have been rapidly withdrawn from their medication.[131] It may, very infrequently, be induced by antidepressants and pro-cholinergic medications (e.g. cholinesterase inhibitors).[132] Polypharmacy may be an important factor in many patients. It also appears to be more likely to occur in those who become dehydrated whilst on causative drugs.[133]

NMS is an idiosyncratic reaction (irrespective of drug dose or duration of therapy), which usually occurs within the first four weeks of commencement of the causative drug but occasionally only after several months of therapy. Estimates of incidence amongst those on antipsychotic medications vary between 0.1% and 2%,[133] probably reflecting differing populations studied. It is seen much more commonly in younger schizophrenic patients than older patients with dementia.[127] It is mostly likely caused by a relative deficit in dopamine within the brain but shares similarities with the serotonin syndrome (*see* Box 3.1) and so this neurotransmitter may also be involved. An important differential diagnosis is the neuroleptic sensitivity seen in DLB (*see* p 77).

Investigations

Serum levels of CK and a full blood count (FBC) should be performed. An elevated CK is a common, but non-specific, finding. It may also be seen simply with sepsis. An elevated white cell count (WCC) is supportive, but, obviously, not specific for a diagnosis of NMS. Urinary myoglobin will usually be elevated. Tests to exclude alternative diagnoses may be considered.

DSM-IV diagnostic criteria

A Rigidity and hyperthermia on neuroleptic medication.
B Two or more of: diaphoresis, dysphagia, tremor, incontinence, confusion/coma, mutism, tachycardia, increased/labile blood pressure (BP), increased WCC, increased CK.
C Not caused by other drug/condition.
D Not better accounted for by a mental disorder.

Complications

There are many potential complications of this condition and significant ones have been reported in around 30% of cases.[126] Some of the more common are listed below:

- myoglobinuric renal failure (rhabdomyolysis)
- respiratory failure ($\pm$ aspiration)
- thromboembolism
- dehydration.

Treatment

The first step is to stop the antipsychotic (or other suspected causative) medication, ensure adequate hydration and control pyrexia. As may be expected in such a rare and sporadic condition, large-scale randomised controlled trials of treatment modalities have not been performed.

The pro-dopaminergic medications bromocriptine and dantrolene have been proposed to reduce hyperthermia and rigidity in these patients, but this approach is controversial. Their use is usually unnecessary when the disorder is detected early and the offending agent is discontinued. There is also some evidence that bromocriptine or dantrolene may actually worsen or prolong the duration of episodes.[133] Mechanical ventilation is sometimes required for those with respiratory failure.

Outcome

The length of episodes varies widely, but they typically last around 7–10 days, and it has a mortality rate of around 20%.[133,134] Recommencement of causative medications, if necessary, should be delayed until at least two weeks after the event.[135] After this time, a low dose of a low-potency drug (e.g. an atypical rather than a typical antipsychotic agent) should be used and the patient should be carefully monitored for signs of recurrence.

Vascular Parkinsonism

Parkinsonism induced by vascular lesions is an important cause in the elderly, and accounts for around 8% of all Parkinsonism.[122] It more commonly affects the legs than the arms ('lower-body Parkinsonism') and rarely causes the characteristic 'pill-rolling' tremor of PD. The onset is usually rapid or step-wise, and clinical features are bilateral and symmetrical, with rigidity, a small-stepping gait ('marche à petits pas') and a mask-like face.[136] The history usually reveals vascular risk factors (especially hypertension and diabetes) or prior strokes. Non-Parkinsonian neurological signs may also be present (e.g. pyramidal tract). Any of dysarthria, dysphagia, emotional lability, incontinence and cognitive impairment may be early features. Table 4.1 compares some of the distinguishing features of vascular Parkinsonism and PD.

Table 4.1   Vascular Parkinsonism vs Parkinson's disease

	Vascular Parkinsonism	*Parkinson's disease*
Onset	Bilateral and symmetrical	Unilateral
Progression	Rapid or step-wise	Slow and insidious
'Pill-rolling' tremor	Rare	Frequent
Gait	Upright stance, broad-based and small-stepping	Stooped and festinating
Other features	History of strokes or vascular risk factors; pyramidal tract signs; early emotional lability; incontinence or cognitive impairment	Good response to levodopa therapy

Multiple lacunar strokes or basal ganglia infarction are thought to be causative. CT imaging may show vascular changes. The role of functional imaging is controversial. The response to levodopa is poor or non-existent (this feature often helps support a diagnosis). Other PD therapeutic strategies are not indicated. Treatment includes addressing vascular risk factors, and commencing antiplatelet agents and statins where indicated (*see* p 109).

Normal pressure hydrocephalus

Normal pressure hydrocephalus (NPH) is a rare but potentially reversible cause of cognitive impairment (<1% of cases of dementia). It may be idiopathic or occur secondarily to intracerebral pathology, for example meningitis, subarachnoid haemorrhage or tumour. It is a clinical syndrome with a characteristic triad of features:

- gait disturbance
- cognitive impairment
- urinary incontinence.

The presenting feature is usually a gait disorder. Classically this is of a 'foot stuck to the floor' nature. Alternatively the gait may be simply unsteady and broad-based with small steps and low floor clearance. The legs and bladder are affected more than the upper limbs due to the positioning of their fibres within the motor cortex. As they lie inferomedially, they are more stretched by the ventricular enlargement. The urinary incontinence is urge in nature (*see* p 141). Cognitive deficits are usually of a subcortical type (*see* p 12).

Examination may show upper motor neuron signs in the legs. The upper limbs may show reduced co-ordination and a fine action tremor. Classic Parkinsonism may be present. Papilloedema is absent.

CT scanning reveals enlarged ventricles usually with sulcal effacement. This latter feature helps to distinguish NHP from the ventricular enlargement seen with brain atrophy but this is not absolute (*see* Figure 4.10). Lumbar puncture opening pressure is not elevated. It is believed that the damage is caused by initial raised intracranial fluid pressure, which then normalises once the ventricles have become dilated.

The removal of 40–50 ml of cerebrospinal fluid (CSF) followed by repeat assessment of walking speed or cognition has been used to identify those patients likely to respond to a shunting procedure. It is a fair predictor of those who will have cognitive improvement.[137] A better test appears to be external lumbar drainage (ELD). Here a drain is placed into the spinal canal and 10 ml of CSF is drained each hour through a valve over a three-day period. An improvement in walking or cognition following this test has a 92% sensitivity to detect those who will improve with a shunting procedure.[138] Such an improvement appears to occur in patients of all ages.

Treatment

Ventriculoperitoneal (VP) shunting is the usual treatment for this condition; however, there is no randomised controlled trial evidence demonstrating that shunting is effective.[139] Patients with idiopathic NPH do less well than those with an underlying disorder after shunting. Approximately 30% of patients with the idiopathic variant will improve following shunting at the expense of a 38% complication rate, with a 6% incidence of serious complications (permanent neurological deficit and death).[140] Patients with a known underlying cause have around a 70% response rate to shunting.[141] Predictors of shunt response include early gait disturbance, the presence of all three of the classic features and a recent onset of symptoms. Dementia is the least likely feature to improve post-shunting.[138]

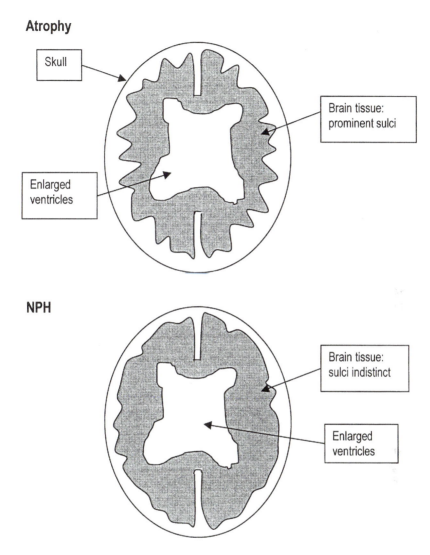

Figure 4.10 A comparison of the CT appearance of cerebral atrophy and that of normal pressure hydrocephalus.

Essential tremor

Essential tremor (ET) is a very common movement disorder, affecting around 5% of people over the age of 65 years.[142] Characteristically it causes a tremor when maintaining a fixed body position (postural) or on movement (action). It does not usually cause a resting tremor and never causes the classic pill-rolling tremor of PD. Nor does it characteristically cause a tremor that worsens on approaching a target (intention), which is seen with cerebellar disorders. It may be confused with an exaggerated physiological tremor, which is seen with metabolic disorders (e.g. thyrotoxicosis and alcohol withdrawal) or medication-induced (e.g. sodium valproate, beta-agonists, lithium and antidepressants). Previously, the prefix 'benign' was attached to ET. This was misleading as some patients may become severely disabled due to this disorder.

Approximately 50% of patients have affected family members, and it is thought to be autosomal dominantly inherited.[142] The causative gene (or genes) has not been identified and the pathogenesis of ET is unknown. It causes a bilateral tremor in the hands of almost all patients. In smaller numbers the head (34%), legs (20%), and voice (12%) are affected.[142] There are no symptoms or neurological signs other than tremor. Patients usually give a history of having been tremulous for many years. They may improve following drinking alcohol.

Treatment

Not all patients with ET will require treatment and many will be asymptomatic. Some patients will self-medicate with alcohol, and alcoholism is a potential, but uncommon, association. When intervention is required, no treatment strategy has proven beneficial to all patients. Response rates are variable. The more commonly used techniques are discussed below.

Medications

- *Beta-blockers*: beta-blockers have been shown to reduce the severity of tremor in 40–50% of patients.[143] This is probably mediated by a peripheral mechanism. Less lipophilic drugs that do not cross the blood–brain barrier (e.g. atenolol and metoprolol) appear to be as effective as ones that do (e.g. propranolol). They are contraindicated in some patients (e.g. those with reversible airways disease).
- *Primidone*: the mechanism of action of primidone is unclear. It may have a direct effect or it may be predominantly due to its barbiturate metabolites. It has been evaluated in several small randomised controlled trials mainly recruiting patients in their 50s and 60s. The mean tremor-reduction efficacy is in the region of 40–50%.[143] The main side effects are sedation, dizziness and unsteadiness. It is likely to increase the risk of falls within the elderly. Similar to barbiturates, it is probably best avoided in older, frailer patients.
- *Anticonvulsants*: gabapentin has a GABA-mediated mechanism of action. Results of small trials have suggested a probable mild benefit.[144] Topiramate is an anticonvulsant medication believed to have a broad spectrum of actions. It was found to have a mild benefit in ET in a small crossover-designed trial.[145]
- *Botulinium toxin*: injections of botulinium toxin into the wrist flexors and extensors have been used in patients with ET of disabling severity.[146] This was associated with reductions in the tremor severity but induced some hand weakness and very little functional improvement.

Surgery

DBS of the thalamic nuclei has been used to successfully reduce tremor and improve functional disability in non-randomised studies using small numbers of patients.[147,148] The high associated complication rate is unlikely to make this a common treatment modality for this condition.

Further reading

Jankovic J and Tolosa E. *Parkinson's Disease and Movement Disorders*. 4th edition. Philadelphia, PA: Lippincott Williams & Wilkins, 2002.

Playfer JR and Hindle JV. *Parkinson's Disease in the Older Patient*. London: Arnold, 2001.

References

1   Rascol O, Sabatini U, Simonetta-Moreau M *et al.* Square wave jerks in Parkinsonian syndrome. *J Neurol Neurosurg Psy,* 1991; **54**: 599–602.

2   Hughes AJ, Daniel SE, Blankson S *et al.* A clinicopathologic study of 100 cases of Parkinson's disease. *Arch Neurol,* 1993; **50**: 140–148.

3   Hughes AJ, Daniel SE and Lees AJ. Improved accuracy of clinical diagnosis of Lewy body Parkinson's disease. *Neurology,* 2001; **57**: 1497–1499.

4   De Rijk MC, Tzourio C, Breteler MMB *et al.* Prevalence of parkinsonism and Parkinson's disease in Europe: the EUROPARKINSON collaborative study. *J Neurol Neurosurg Psy,* 1997; **62**: 10–15.

5   Chadwick WC and Aminoff MJ. Clinical differentiation of parkinsonian syndromes: prognostic and therapeutic relevance. *Am J Med,* 2004; **117**: 412–419.

6   Poewe WH and Wenning GK. The natural history of Parkinson's disease. *Ann Neurol,* 1998; 44(Suppl. 1): S1–9.

7   Barnes J and David AS. Visual hallucinations in Parkinson's disease: a review and phenomenological survey. *J Neurol Neurosurg Psy,* 2001; **70**: 727–733.

8   Holroyd S, Currie L and Wooten GF. Prospective study of hallucinations and delusions in Parkinson's disease. *J Neurol Neurosurg Psy,* 2001; **70**: 734–738.

9   Eriksen JL, Wszolek Z and Petrucelli L. Molecular pathogenesis of Parkinson disease. *Arch Neurol,* 2005; **62**: 353–357.

10 Gorell JM, Rybicki BA, Johnson CC *et al.* Smoking and Parkinson's disease: a dose-response relationship. *Neurology,* 1999; **52**: 115–119.

11 Beneditti MD, Bower JH and Maraganore DM. Smoking, alcohol, and coffee consumption preceding Parkinson's disease: a case-control study. *Neurology,* 2000; **55**: 1350–1358.

12 Ross GW, Abbott RD, Petrovitch H *et al.* Association of coffee and caffeine intake with the risk of Parkinson disease. *JAMA,* 2000; **283**: 2674–2679.

13 Aarsland D, Andersen K, Larsen JP *et al.* Prevalence and characteristics of dementia in Parkinson disease: an 8-year prospective study. *Arch Neurol,* 2003; **60**: 387–392.

14 Olanow CW, Watts RL and Koller WC. An algorithm (decision tree) for the management of Parkinson's disease (2001): treatment guidelines. *Neurology,* 2001; **56** (Suppl. 5): S1–S88.

15 Athey RJ, Porter RW and Walker RW. Cognitive assessment of a representative community population with Parkinson's disease (PD) using the Cambridge Cognitive Assessment-Revised (CAMCOG-R). *Age Ageing,* 2005; **34**: 268–273.

16 Press DZ. Parkinson's disease dementia – a first step? *NEJM,* 2004; **351**(24): 2547–2549.

17 Boller F, Mizutani T, Roessmann U *et al.* Parkinson disease, dementia, and Alzheimer disease: clinicopathological correlations. *Ann Neurol,* 1980; **7**: 329–335.

18 Horn S and Stern MB. The comparative effects of medical therapies for Parkinson's disease. *Neurology,* 2004; **63** (Suppl. 2): S7–12.

19 Wheatley K, Stowe RL, Clarke CE *et al.* Evaluating drug treatments for Parkinson's disease: how good are the trials? *BMJ,* 2002; **324**: 1508–1511.

20 Lees AJ. Drugs for Parkinson's disease: oldies but goodies. *J Neurol Neurosurg Psy,* 2002; **73**: 607–610.

21 Mouradian MM. Should levodopa be infused into the duodenum? *Neurology,* 2005; **64**: 182–183.

22 Riley D and Lang AE. The spectrum of levodopa-related fluctuations in Parkinson's disease. *Neurology,* 1993; **43**: 1459–1463.

23 Thanvi BR and Lo TCN. Long term motor complications of levodopa: clinical features, mechanisms, and management strategies. *Postgrad Med J,* 2004; **80**: 452–458.

24 Togasaki DM, Tan L, Protell P *et al.* Levodopa induces dyskinesias in normal squirrel monkeys. *Ann Neurol,* 2001; **50**: 254–257.

25 Rascol O, Brooks DJ, Korczyn AD *et al.* A five-year study of the incidence of dyskinesia in patients with early Parkinson's disease who were treated with ropinirole or levodopa. *NEJM,* 2000; **342**: 1484–1491.

26 Parkinson Study Group. Pramipexole vs levodopa as initial treatment for Parkinson disease: a randomized controlled trial. *JAMA,* 2000; **284**(15): 1931–1938.

27 Bravi D, Mouradian MM, Roberts JW *et al.* Wearing-off fluctuations in Parkinson's disease: contribution of postsynaptic mechanisms. *Ann Neurol,* 1994; **36**(1): 27–31.

28 Mouradian MM, Heuser IJE, Baronti F *et al.* Modification of central dopaminergic mechanisms by continuous levodopa therapy for advanced Parkinson's disease. *Ann Neurol,* 1990; **27**: 18–23.

29 Koller WC, Hutton JT, Tolosa E *et al.* Immediate-release and controlled-release carbidopa/levodopa in PD: a 5-year randomized multicenter study. *Neurology,* 1999; **53**: 1012–1019.

30 Jiang Y and Norman KE. Effects of visual and auditory cues on gait initiation in people with Parkinson's disease. *Clin Rehabil,* 2006; **20**: 36–45.

31 Fahn S. The spectrum of levodopa-induced dyskinesias. *Ann Neurol,* 2000; **47**(Suppl. 1): S2–11.

32 Assal F, Spahr L, Hadengue A *et al.* Tolcapone and fulminant hepatitis. *Lancet,* 1998; **352**: 958.

33 Merello M, Lees AJ, Webster R *et al.* Effect of entacapone, a peripherally acting catechol-O-methyltransferase inhibitor, on the motor response to acute treatment with levodopa in patients with Parkinson's disease. *J Neurol Neurosurg Psy,* 1994; **57**: 186–189.

34 Parkinson Study Group. Entacapone improves motor fluctuations in levodopa-treated Parkinson's disease patients. *Ann Neurol,* 1997; **42**: 747–755.

35 Inzelberg R, Nisipeanu P, Rabey JM *et al.* Double-blind comparison of cabergoline and bromocriptine in Parkinson's disease patients with motor fluctuations. *Neurology,* 1996; **47**: 785–788.

36 Guttman M and the International Pramipexole-Bromocriptine Study Group. Double-blind comparison of Pramipexole and bromocriptine treatment with placebo in advanced Parkinson's disease. *Neurology,* 1997; **49**: 1060–1065.

37 Korczyn AD, Brunt ER, Larsen JP *et al.* A 3-year randomized trial of ropinirole and bromocriptine in early Parkinson's disease. *Neurology,* 1999; **53**: 364–370.

38 Bonuccelli U. Comparing dopamine agonists in Parkinson's disease. *Curr Op Neurol,* 2003; **16** (Suppl. 1): S13–19.

39 Shaunak S, Wilkins A, Pilling JB *et al.* Pericardial, retroperitoneal, and pleural fibrosis induced by pergolide. *J Neurol Neurosurg Psy,* 1999; **66**: 79–81.

40 Van Camp G, Flamez A, Cosyns B *et al.* Treatment of Parkinson's disease with pergolide and relation to restrictive valvular heart disease. *Lancet,* 2004; **363**: 1179–1183.

41 Pinero A, Marcos-Alberca P and Fortes J. Cabergoline-related severe restrictive mitral regurgitation. *NEJM,* 2005; **353**(18): 1976–1977.

42 Committee on Safety of Medicines. Fibrotic reactions with pergolide and other ergot-derived dopamine receptor agonists. *Curr Problems Pharmacovigilance,* 2002; **28**: 3.

43 Ondo WG, Dat Vuong K, Khan H *et al.* Daytime sleepiness and other sleep disorders in Parkinson's disease. *Neurology,* 2001; **57**: 1392–1396.

44 Frucht S, Rogers JD, Greene PE *et al.* Falling asleep at the wheel: motor vehicle mishaps in persons taking pramipexole and ropinirole. *Neurology,* 1999; **52**: 1908–1910.

45 Tan E and Ondo W. Clinical characteristics of pramipexole-induced peripheral edema. *Arch Neurol,* 2000; **57**: 729–732.

46 Dodd ML, Klos KJ, Bower JH *et al.* Pathological gambling caused by drugs used to treat Parkinson disease. *Arch Neurol,* 2005; **62**: 1377–1381.

47 Giovannoni G, O'Sullivan JD, Turner K *et al.* Hedonistic homeostatic dysregulation in patients with Parkinson's disease on dopamine replacement therapies. *J Neurol Neurosurg Psy,* 2000; **68**: 423–428.

48 Weiner WJ. The initial treatment of Parkinson's disease should begin with levodopa. *Movement Disorders,* 1999; **14**(5): 716–724.

49 Montastruc JL, Rascol O and Senard J. Treatment of Parkinson's disease should begin with a dopamine agonist. *Movement Disorders,* 1999; **14**(5): 725–730.

50   Clarke C and Guttman M. Dopamine agonist monotherapy in Parkinson's disease. *Lancet,* 2002; **360**: 1767–1769.

51   Hely MA, Morris JGL, Traficante R *et al.* The Sydney multicentre study of Parkinson's disease: progression and mortality at 10 years. *J Neurol Neurosurg Psy,* 1999; **67**: 300–307.

52   Lees AJ, Katzenschlager R, Head J *et al.* Ten-year follow-up of three different initial treatments in de-novo PD: a randomized trial. *Neurology,* 2001; **57**: 1687–1694.

53   Lieberman A, Ranhosky A and Korts D. Clinical evaluation of pramipexole in advanced Parkinson's disease: results of a double-blind, placebo-controlled, parallel-group study. *Neurology,* 1997; **49**: 162–168.

54   Lieberman A, Olanow CW, Sethi K *et al.* A multicenter trial of ropinirole as adjunct treatment for Parkinson's disease. *Neurology,* 1998; **51**: 1057–1062.

55   Onalow CW, Fahn S, Muenter M *et al.* A multicenter double-blind placebo-controlled trial of pergolide as an adjunct to Sinemet in Parkinson's disease. *Movement Disorders,* 1994; **9**(1): 40–47.

56   Pietz K, Hagell P and Odin P. Subcutaneous apomorphine in late stage Parkinson's disease: a long term follow up. *J Neurol Neurosurg Psy,* 1998; **65**: 709–716.

57   Colzi A, Turner K and Lees AJ. Continuous subcutaneous waking day apomorphine in the long term treatment of levodopa induced interdose dyskinesias in Parkinson's disease. *J Neurol Neurosurg Psy,* 1998; **64**: 573–576.

58   Dewey RB, Hutton JT, LeWitt PA *et al.* A randomized, double-blind, placebo-controlled trial of subcutaneously injected apomorphine for parkinsonian off-state events. *Arch Neurol,* 2001; **58**: 1385–1392.

59   Richard IH, Kurlan R, Tanner C *et al.* Serotonin syndrome and the combined use of deprenyl and an antidepressant in Parkinson's disease. *Neurology,* 1997; **48**: 1070–1077.

60   Palhagen S, Heinonen EH, Hagglund J *et al.* Selegiline delays the onset of disability in de novo parkinsonian patients. *Neurology,* 1998; **51**: 520–525.

61   Ives NJ, Stowe RL, Marro J *et al.* Monoamine oxidase type B inhibitors in early Parkinson's disease: meta-analysis of 17 randomised trials involving 3525 patients. *BMJ,* 2004; **329**: 593–596.

62   Marras C, McDermott MP, Rochon PA *et al.* Survival in Parkinson disease: thirteen-year follow-up of the DATATOP cohort. *Neurology,* 2005; **64**: 87–93.

63   Ben-Shlomo Y, Churchyard A, Head J *et al.* Investigation by Parkinson's Disease Research Group of United Kingdom into excess mortality seen with combined levodopa and selegiline treatment in patients with early, mild Parkinson's disease: further results of randomised trial and confidential enquiry. *BMJ,* 1998; **316**: 1191–1196.

64   Waters CH, Sethi KD, Hauser RA *et al.* Zydis selegiline reduces off time in Parkinson's disease patients with motor fluctuations: a 3-month randomized, placebo-controlled study. *Movement Disorders,* 2004; **19**(4): 426–432.

65   Rascol O, Brooks DJ, Melamed E *et al.* Rasagiline as an adjunct to levodopa in patients with Parkinson's disease and motor fluctuations (LARGO, lasting effect in adjunct therapy with rasagiline given once daily, study): a randomised, double-blind, parallel-group trial. *Lancet,* 2005; **365**: 947–954.

66   Verhagen Metman L, Del Dotto P, van den Munckhof P *et al.* Amantadine as treatment for dyskinesias and motor fluctuations in Parkinson's disease. *Neurology,* 1998; **50**: 1323–1326.

67   Snow BJ, Macdonald L, Mcauley D *et al.* The effect of amantadine on levodopa-induced dyskinesias in Parkinson's disease: a double-blind, placebo-controlled study. *Clin Neuropharm,* 2000; **23**(2): 82–85.

68   Verhagen Metman L, Del Dotto P, LePool K *et al.* Amantadine for levodopa-induced dyskinesias: a 1-year follow-up study. *Arch Neurol,* 1999; **56**: 1383–1386.

69   Uitii RJ, Rajput AH, Ahlskog JE *et al.* Amantadine treatment is an independent predictor of survival in Parkinson's disease. *Neurology,* 1996; **46**: 1551–1556.

70   Perry EK, Kilford L, Lees AJ *et al.* Increased Alzheimer pathology in Parkinson's disease related to antimuscarinic drugs. *Ann Neurol,* 2003; **54**: 235–238.

71   The Deep-Brain, Stimulation for Parkinson's Disease Study Group. Deep-brain stimulation of the subthalamic nucleus or the pars interna of the globus pallidus in Parkinson's disease. *NEJM,* 2001; **345**(13): 956–963.

72   Vingerhoets FJG, Villemure JG, Temperli R *et al.* Subthalamic DBS replaces levodopa in Parkinson's disease: two-year follow-up. *Neurology,* 2002; **58**: 396–401.

73 Krack P, Batir A, Van Blercom N *et al.* Five-year follow-up of bilateral stimulation of the subthalamic nucleus in advanced Parkinson's disease. *NEJM,* 2003; **349**(20): 1925–1934.

74 Koller W, Pahwa R, Busenbark K *et al.* High-frequency unilateral thalamic stimulation in the treatment of essential tremor and parkinsonian tremor. *Ann Neurol,* 1997; **42**: 292–299.

75 Russmann H, Ghika J, Villemure JG *et al.* Subthalamic nucleus deep brain stimulation in Parkinson's disease patients over age 70 years. *Neurology,* 2004; **63**: 1952–1954.

76 Schuurman PR, Bosch DA, Bossuyt PMM *et al.* A comparison of continuous thalamic stimulation and thalamotomy for suppression of severe tremor. *NEJM,* 2000; **342**: 461–468.

77 Fine J, Duff J, Chen R *et al.* Long-term follow-up of unilateral pallidotomy in advanced Parkinson's disease. *NEJM,* 2000; **342**: 1708–1714.

78 Alkhani A and Lozano AM. Pallidotomy for Parkinson disease: a review of contemporary literature. *J Neurosurg,* 2001; **94**: 43–49.

79 Ghika J, Ghika-Schmid F, Frankhauser F *et al.* Bilateral contemporaneous posteroventral pallidotomy for the treatment of Parkinson's disease: neuropsychological and neurological side effects: report of four cases and review of the literature. *J Neurosurg,* 1999; **91**: 313–321.

80 Gill SS, Patel NK, Hotton GR *et al.* Direct brain infusion of glial cell line-derived neurotrophic factor in Parkinson disease. *Nature Med,* 2003; **9**(5): 589–595.

81 Slevin JT, Gerhardt GA, Smith CD *et al.* Improvement of bilateral motor functions in patients with Parkinson disease through the unilateral intraputaminal infusion of glial cell line-derived neurotrophic factor. *J Neurosurg,* 2005; **102**: 216–222.

82 Patel NK, Bunnage M, Plaha P *et al.* Intraputamenal infusion of glial cell line-derived neurotrophic factor in PD: a two-year outcome study. *Ann Neurol,* 2005; **57**(2): 298–302.

83 Freed CR, Greene PE, Breeze RE *et al.* Transplantation of embryonic dopamine neurons for severe Parkinson's disease. *NEJM,* 2001; **344**(10): 710–719.

84 Olanow CW, Goetz CG, Kordower JH *et al.* A double-blind controlled trial of bilateral fetal nigral transplantation in Parkinson's disease. *Ann Neurol,* 2003; **54**: 403–414.

85 Folkerth RD and Durso R. Survival and proliferation of nonneural tissues, with obstruction of cerebral ventricles, in a parkinsonian patient treated with fetal allografts. *Neurology,* 1996; **46**: 1219–1225.

86 Schumacher JM, Ellias SA, Palmer EP *et al.* Transplantation of embryonic porcine mesencephalic tissue in patients with PD. *Neurology,* 2000; **54**: 1042–1050.

87 Dooneief G, Mirabello E, Bell K *et al.* An estimate of the incidence of depression in idiopathic Parkinson's disease. *Arch Neurol,* 1992; **49**: 305–307.

88 Jansen Steur ENH. Increase of Parkinson disability after fluoxetine medication. *Neurology,* 1993; **43**: 211–213.

89 Fernandez HH, Trieschmann ME, Burke MA *et al.* Quetiapine for psychosis in Parkinson's disease versus dementia with Lewy bodies. *J Clin Psych,* 2002; **63**: 513–515.

90 Friedman JH and Factor SA. Atypical antipsychotics in the treatment of drug-induced psychosis in Parkinson's disease. *Movement Disorders,* 2000; **15**(2): 201–211.

91 Emre M, Aarsland D, Albanese A *et al.* Rivastigmine for dementia associated with Parkinson's disease. *NEJM,* 2004; **351**: 2509–2518.

92 Wood BH, Bilclough JA, Bowron A *et al.* Incidence and prediction of falls in Parkinson's disease: a prospective multidisciplinary study. *J Neurol Neurosurg Psy,* 2002; **72**(6): 721–725.

93 Medcalf P. Good practice in the assessment and management of nocturnal Parkinson's disease symptoms. *Age Ageing,* 2005; **34**: 435–438.

94 Bhatia KP, Munchau A and Brown P. Botulinium toxin is a useful treatment in excessive drooling of saliva. *J Neurol Neurosurg Psy,* 1999; **67**: 697.

95 Hussain IF, Brady CM, Swinn MJ *et al.* Treatment of erectile dysfunction with sildenafil citrate (Viagra) in parkinsonism due to Parkinson's disease or multiple system atrophy with observations on orthostatic hypotension. *J Neurol Neurosurg Psy,* 2001; **71**: 371–374.

96 Jarman B, Hurwitz B, Cook A *et al.* Effects of community based nurses specialising in Parkinson's disease on health outcome and costs: randomised controlled trial. *BMJ,* 2002; **324**: 1072–1075.

97 Ramig LO, Countryman S, O'Brien C *et al.* Intensive speech treatment for patients with Parkinson's disease: short- and long-term comparison of two techniques. *Neurology,* 1996; **47**: 1496–1504.

98 Ramig LO, Sapir S, Fox C *et al*. Changes in vocal loudness following intensive voice treatment (LSVT) in individuals with Parkinson's disease: a comparison with untreated patients and normal age-matched controls. *Movement Disorders*, 2001; **16**(1): 79–83.

99 Comella CL, Stebbins GT, Brown-Toms N *et al*. Physical therapy and Parkinson's disease: a controlled clinical trial. *Neurology*, 1994; **44**: 376–378.

100 McKeith I, Mintzer J, Aarsland D *et al*. Dementia with Lewy bodies. *Lancet Neurology*, 2004; **3**(1): 19–28.

101 Litvan I, Campbell G, Mangone CA *et al*. Which clinical features differentiate progressive supranuclear palsy (Steel–Richardson–Olszewski syndrome) from related disorders? A clinicopathological study. *Brain*, 1997; **120**: 65–74.

102 McKeith IG, Galasko D, Kosaka K, *et al*. Consensus guidelines for the clinical and pathologic diagnosis of dementia with Lewy bodies (DLB): report of the consortium on DLB international workshop. *Neurology*, 1996; **47**: 1113–1124.

103 Ferman TJ, Smith GE, Boeve BF *et al*. DLB fluctuations: specific features that reliably differentiate ALD from AD and normal aging. *Neurology*, 2004; **62**: 181–187.

104 Kraybill ML, Larson EB, Tsuang W *et al*. Cognitive differences in dementia patients with autopsy-verified AD, Lewy body pathology or both. *Neurology*, 2005; **64**: 2069–2073.

105 McKeith I, Fairbairn A, Perry R *et al*. Neuroleptic sensitivity in patients with senile dementia of Lewy body type. *BMJ*, 1992; **305**: 673–678.

106 Schrag A, Ben-Shlomo Y and Quinn NP. Prevalence of progressive supranuclear palsy and multiple system atrophy; a cross-sectional study. *Lancet*, 1999; **354**: 1771–1775.

107 Nath U, Ben-Shlomo Y, Thomson RG *et al*. The prevalence of progressive supranuclear palsy (Steel–Richardson–Olszewski syndrome) in the UK. *Brain*, 2001; **124**: 1438–1449.

108 Litvan I, Mangone CA, McKee A *et al*. Natural history of progressive supranuclear palsy (Steele–Richardson–Olszewski syndrome) and clinical predictors of survival: a clinico-pathological study. *J Neurol Neurosurg Psy*, 1996; **61**: 615–620.

109 Maher ER and Lees AJ. The clinical features and natural history of the Steele–Richardson–Olszewski syndrome (progressive supranuclear palsy). *Neurology*, 1986; **36**: 1005–1008.

110 Conrad C, Andreadis A, Trojanowski JQ *et al*. Genetic evidence for the involvement of tau in progressive supranuclear palsy. *Ann Neurol*, 1997; **41**(2): 277–281.

111 Litvan I, Agid Y, Calne D *et al*. Clinical research criteria for the diagnosis of progressive supranuclear palsy (Steel–Richardson–Olszewski syndrome): report of the NINDS-SPSP International Workshop. *Neurology*, 1996; **47**: 1–9.

112 Wenning GR, Ebersbach G, Verny M, *et al*. Progression of falls in postmortem-confirmed parkinsonian disorders. *Movement Disorders*, 1999; **14**(6): 947–950.

113 Ghika J and Bogousslavsky J. Presymptomatic hypertension is a major feature in the diagnosis of progressive supranuclear palsy. *Arch Neurol*, 1997; **54**: 1104–1108.

114 Litvan I, Phipps M, Pharr VL *et al*. Randomized placebo-controlled trial of donepezil in patients with progressive supranuclear palsy. *Neurology*, 2001; **57**: 467–473.

115 Polo KB and Jabbari B. Botulinium toxin-A improves the rigidity of progressive supranuclear palsy. *Ann Neurol*, 1994; **35**(2): 237–239.

116 Wenning GK, Ben Shlomo Y, Magalhaes M *et al*. Clinical feature and natural history of multiple system atrophy: an analysis of 100 cases. *Brain*, 1994; **117**: 835–845.

117 Litvan I, Goetz CG, Jankovic J *et al*. What is the accuracy of clinical diagnosis of multiple system atrophy? A clinicopathologic study. *Arch Neurol*, 1997; **54**: 937–944.

118 Schrag A, Kingsley D, Phatouros C *et al*. Clinical usefulness of magnetic resonance imaging in multiple system atrophy. *J Neurol Neurosurg Psy*, 1998; **65**: 65–71.

119 Wenning GK, Litvan I, Jankovic J *et al*. Natural history and survival of 14 patients with corticobasal degeneration confirmed at postmortem examination. *J Neurol Neurosurg Psy*, 1998; **64**: 184–189.

120 Boeve BF, Lang AE and Litvan I. Corticobasal degeneration and its relationship to progressive supranuclear palsy and frontotemporal dementia. *Ann Neurol*, 2003; **54** (Suppl. 5): S15–19.

121 Schneider JA, Watts RL, Gearing M *et al*. Corticobasal degeneration: neuropathologic and clinical heterogeneity. *Neurology*, 1997; **48**: 959–969.

122 Morgante L, Rocca WA, Di Rossa AE *et al*. Prevalence of Parkinson's disease and other types of parkinsonism: a door-to-door survey in three Sicilian municipalities. *Neurology*, 1992; **42**: 1901–1907.

123 Jeste D, Lacro JP, Bailey A *et al*. Lower incidence of tardive dyskinesia with risperidone compared with haloperidol in older patients. *JAGS*, 1999; **47**: 716–719.

124 Jeste DV, Okamoto A, Napolitano J *et al*. Low incidence of persistent tardive dyskinesia in elderly patients with dementia treated with risperidone. *Am J Psychiatry*, 2000; **157**: 1150–1155.

125 Lee PE, Sykora K, Gill SS *et al*. Antipsychotic medications and drug-induced movement disorders other than parkinsonism: a population-based cohort study in older adults. *JAGS*, 2005; **53**(8): 1374–1379.

126 Rosenberg MR and Green M. Neuroleptic malignant syndrome: review of response to therapy. *Arch Intern Med*, 1989; **149**: 1927–1931.

127 Ebadi M and Srinivasan SK. Pathogenesis, prevention, and treatment of neuroleptic-induced movement disorders. *Pharmacological Rev*, 1995; **47**(4): 575–599.

128 Suh H, Bronson B and Martin R. Neuroleptic malignant syndrome and low-dose olanzapine. *Am J Psychiatry*, 2003; **160**(4): 796.

129 Goveas JS and Hermida A. Olanzapine induced "typical" neuroleptic malignant syndrome. *J Clin Psychopharmacology*, 2003; **23**(1): 101–102.

130 Hasan S and Buckley P. Novel antipsychotics and the neuroleptic malignant syndrome: a review and critique. *Am J Psychiatry*, 1998; **155**(8): 1113–1116.

131 Ueda M, Hamamoto M, Nagayama H *et al*. Susceptibility to neuroleptic malignant syndrome in Parkinson's disease. *Neurology*, 1999; **52**: 777–781.

132 Ohkoshi N, Satoh D, Nishi M *et al*. Neuroleptic malignant-like syndrome due to donepezil and maprotiline. *Neurology*, 2003; **60**(6):1050–1051.

133 Chandran GJ, Mikler JR and Keegan DL. Neuroleptic malignant syndrome: case report and discussion. *CMAJ*, 2003; **169**(5): 439–442.

134 Rosebush PI, Stewart T and Mazurek MF. The treatment of neuroleptic malignant syndrome: are dantrolene and bromocriptine useful adjuncts to supportive care? *Br J Psychiatry*, 1991; **159**: 709–712.

135 Velamoor VR. Neuroleptic malignant syndrome: recognition, prevention and management. *Drug Safety*, 1998; **19**(1): 73–82.

136 Thanvi B, Lo N and Robinson T. Vascular parkinsonism – an important cause of parkinsonism in older people. *Age Ageing*, 2005; **34**(2): 114–119.

137 Duinkerke A, Williams MA, Rigamonti D *et al*. Cognitive recovery in idiopathic normal pressure hydrocephalus after shunt. *Cognitive Behav Neurol*, 2004; **17**(3): 179–184.

138 Marmarou A, Young HF, Aygok GA *et al*. Diagnosis and management of idiopathic normal-pressure hydrocephalus: a prospective study in 151 patients. *J Neurosurg*, 2005; **102**: 987–997.

139 Esmonde T and Cooke S. Shunting for Normal Pressure Hydrocephalus (NPH). Cochrane Database Syst Rev 2002, Issue 3. Art. No.: CD003157. DOI: 10.1002/14651858.CD003157.

140 Hebb AO and Cusimano MD. Idiopathic normal pressure hydrocephalus: a systematic review of diagnosis and outcome. *Neurosurgery*, 2001; **49**(5): 1166–1186.

141 Iddon JL, Pickard JD, Cross JJL *et al*. Specific patterns of cognitive impairment in patients with idiopathic normal pressure hydrocephalus and Alzheimer's disease: a pilot study. *J Neurol Neurosurg Psy*, 1999; **67**: 723–732.

142 Elble RJ. Diagnostic criteria for essential tremor and differential diagnosis. *Neurology*, 2000; **54** (Suppl. 4): S2–6.

143 Koller WC, Hristova A and Brin M. Pharmacologic treatment of essential tremor. *Neurology*, 2000; **54** (Suppl. 4): S30–38.

144 Ondo W, Hunter C, Vuong KD *et al*. Gabapentin for essential tremor: a multiple-dose, double-blind, placebo-controlled trial. *Movement Disorders*, 2000; **15**(4): 678–682.

145 Connor GS. A double-blind placebo-controlled trial of topiramate treatment for essential tremor. *Neurology*, 2002; **59**: 132–134.

146 Brin MF, Lyons KE, Doucette J *et al*. A randomized, double masked, controlled trial of botulinium toxin type A in essential hand tremor. *Neurology*, 2001; **56**: 1523–1528.

147 Limousin P, Speelman JD, Gielen F *et al*. Multicentre European study of thalamic stimulation in parkinsonism and essential tremor. *J Neurol Neurosurg Psy*, 1999; **66**: 289–296.

148 Pahwa R, Lyons KL, Wilkinson SB *et al*. Bilateral thalamic stimulation for the treatment of essential tremor. *Neurology*, 1999; **53**: 1447–1450.

Chapter 5

Stroke

> **Box 5.1 CVA**
>
> Cerebrovascular accident (shortened to CVA) is a bizarre term. It is less well known to the public than the word 'stroke' and it implies to patients and relatives that some form of trauma has occurred. It contains more syllables than the word 'stroke' and is therefore an illogical 'abbreviation'. It is akin to calling a heart attack a 'myocardial accident'. It does not provide information regarding aetiology. Far more descriptive terms would be 'cerebrovascular embolus', 'infarct' or 'haemorrhage'. For these reasons it should be removed from the language of healthcare professionals.

Definitions

- *Stroke:* a sudden onset of a focal neurological deficit or reduced consciousness that is most likely caused by vascular aetiology and of duration greater than 24 hours (or resulting in death). However, conventionally, subarachnoid haemorrhage is also considered a form of stroke (usually presenting with a sudden onset of headache and meningism).
- *Transient ischaemic attack* (TIA): a sudden onset of a focal neurological deficit or monocular dysfunction that is most likely due to a vascular aetiology and of symptom duration less than 24 hours.
- *Reversible ischaemic neurological deficit* (RIND): a term for strokes of duration between one day and several weeks. It is of questionable additional clinical value and will not be used again in this text.

Epidemiology

Stroke is the most common acute vascular disorder, accounting for 45% of such events.[1] Its overall incidence is around 200–250 per 100 000 per year.[2] This figure for stroke, but not subarachnoid haemorrhage, increases with age. Eighty per cent of events occur in those over the age of 65 and 54% in those over the age of 75.[1] Currently the mean age of people having a cerebrovascular event in the UK is around 74 years.[1]

Subtypes of stroke

Strokes are divided into those caused by a blocked blood vessel and those caused by a bleed (haemorrhagic). The former of these is conventionally termed 'ischaemic', although this is a little imprecise as both types of stroke involve the death of brain cells due to hypoxia. Conventionally, subarachnoid haemorrhage (SAH) is also classified as a form of stroke. Approximately 85% of strokes are ischaemic and 15% are haemorrhagic (10% primary intracerebral haemorrhage and 5% SAH).[3]

Overall, the 30-day mortality rate for stroke has been found to be 19%. However, this varies according to stroke subtype, with better outcomes for those sustaining an ischaemic event (10%) than those with a haemorrhagic one (50%).[3] Prognosis is discussed further within the relevant sections for different stroke subtypes.

Assessment

The diagnosis of stroke is not always easy, especially for the non-specialist. One study has found that 20% of patients initially classified as having had a stroke by emergency physicians were subsequently shown to have an alternative pathology (e.g. post-ictal states, cerebral tumours, and toxic/metabolic disorders).[4] Common differential diagnoses are discussed on p 128. The clinical findings, rather than the results of imaging studies, are the key to achieving a successful diagnosis.

History

Onset

A history of a sudden onset of symptoms is crucial to the diagnosis of stroke. This is even more relevant with TIA, where neurological signs will usually have resolved prior to medical assessment. Activities at the time of symptom commencement may give clues to alternative explanations (e.g. postural change causing neurocardio-vascular symptoms) (*see* Chapter 10). The deficits of a stroke are usually maximal at the time of onset and will, characteristically, gradually improve after the event (albeit often over weeks to months), whereas with alternative diagnoses (e.g. tumours) deficits will tend to increase. Occasionally the symptoms of stroke will worsen over the first few days following onset (e.g. if cerebral oedema or haemorrhagic transform-ation develop). The presence of headache is not a good discriminator between ischaemia and haemorrhage, and commonly accompanies both. Severe headache at the onset could indicate SAH, giant cell arteritis or arterial dissection. Vomiting around the time of symptom onset is suggestive of a haemorrhagic aetiology.

Deficit

It is important to clarify the specific symptoms – patients may use vague terms such as 'my arm was dead' to mean either motor or sensory loss (or a combination). When available, a witness history is valuable. This is especially so if unconscious-ness is reported or seizures are suspected. Non-medical people's accounts of events may mistake dysphasia for confusion. Patients with significant neglect may be unaware of the degree of their deficit. Associated factors should be directly asked about. These include weakness or sensory disturbance in the face, arm and leg of each side of the body, changes in speech or vision, and the presence of headache. The greater eloquence of left-sided brain tissue in most individuals leads to a greater recognition of strokes on this side compared to those on the right.[5]

Risk factors

Vascular risk factors (e.g. smoking, hypertension, diabetes, other vascular disorders and atrial fibrillation) should be sought. A history of previous strokes is clearly important. The body parts or functions affected by any such prior events should be noted along with any residual deficits. Old impairments may be made more prominent under certain conditions – including during acute medical illnesses. This should be suspected when a very similar deficit to a previous stroke is provoked. A strong family history of stroke at a young age raises the possibility of an inherited vascular disorder (*see* p 128).

Social

An accurate social history will help to predict difficulties at the time of discharge (e.g. whether there are stairs within the property).

Examination

Clearly, a detailed neurological examination is crucial to assessment in those who have had a stroke. A thorough review of this is beyond the scope of this book but some of the aspects that are particularly relevant to stroke are discussed.

Motor deficit

A downward drift of an outstretched arm whilst the eyes are closed is suggestive of a subtle motor impairment, but this may also occur with proprioceptive sensory loss. Asking the patient to touch the tip of their nose with each finger in turn whilst the eyes remain closed can crudely assess this later problem. An evaluation of the functional impact of impairments is more informative than a numerical value (e.g. the MRC scale 0–5). Despite their (predominant) upper motor neuron aetiology, strokes often cause early flaccidity with later development of spasticity. Marked hypertonia at the onset may be due to a stroke affecting the basal ganglia.

Sensory deficit

The patient may describe a 'pins and needles' sensation in the absence of a discrete area of sensory loss on examination. Sensory inattention is a sign of a parietal lobe lesion. It is tested for by asking the patient to close their eyes with their hands placed in front of them. The patient is told to inform the examiner which hand if they feel one being touched. The hands are then touched individually, followed by both together. A patient with intact sensation but sensory inattention will correctly report the individual hands being touched but will only report the hand of the unaffected side when both are touched together.

Speech

Speech problems may have been identified whilst taking the history. When testing for speech problems it is important to ensure that the patient has the best chance of responding appropriately, for example their hearing aid is fitted and working. Asking the patient to obey commands tests comprehension of speech (i.e. identifies receptive dysphasia). These should initially be one-stage commands (e.g. 'Close your eyes'), but then can be more complex sequences (e.g. 'Point to the door, the window and then the ceiling'). Expressive dysphasia can be detected by asking the patient to name objects (e.g. pen and watch, then the smaller components of each, such as the nib, hands, etc.). Subtle dysarthria may be detected by asking the patient to repeat difficult phrases, for example 'West Register Street', 'baby hippopotamus' and 'biblical criticism'.

Swallowing

The assessment of swallowing is important in all patients who have sustained a stroke. It is discussed on p 261.

Visual fields

Some patients may be unaware of a homonymous hemianopia. Formal confrontation technique is not always possible, for example in patients with reduced consciousness levels or those with receptive dysphasia. An absence of a blink response to a threatening stimulus from the side (e.g. the examiner's finger brought rapidly towards the patient's eye) may detect a homonymous hemianopia. Visual inattention is similar to sensory inattention. Whilst standing in front of the patient with his or her arms outstretched, the examiner asks the patient to look directly at their nose and say if a hand is seen to move. The fingers of each outstretched hand are then wiggled in turn, followed by both hands together. The patient with visual inattention will correctly identify the individual movements but when both are moved together they will only report movement in the unaffected field.

Neglect

Neglect can occur in various forms. It can be neglect of own person (e.g. failing to use one side of the body) or of the environment (e.g. not appreciating obstacles on one side). It may be caused by lesions in the parietal lobe on either side of the brain, but is often more severe when it affects the non-dominant hemisphere. Functional impairment may be out of proportion with motor and sensory loss. A variety of techniques have been developed to aid its detection. These include clock-drawing (*see* p 7) and the star cancellation test.[6]

Gait

When a patient is capable of standing safely, gait should be examined. This may reveal subtle deficits in co-ordination or motor function not obvious when the patient is lying down.

Level of consciousness

In patients with a reduced consciousness level, the Glasgow Coma Scale score should be recorded (performed on the unaffected side of the body). Early unconsciousness suggests SAH or a brainstem haemorrhage. A very large cortical infarct may cause a reduced consciousness level that worsens over the following few days due to the development of oedema.

Vascular system

The examination of the vascular system is also relevant. Of particular note is the detection of atrial fibrillation (AF) (*see* Chapter 14) and hypertension (*see* Chapter 13). Auscultation over the carotid arteries for the detection of carotid bruits is an unreliable way to detect carotid stenosis.[7] It should not be used in place of a carotid Doppler and therefore has little value in the physical examination of a patient who has suffered a stroke or TIA.

Investigations

Blood tests

Basic blood tests should include a glucose level (to identify diabetes and exclude hypoglycaemia as a cause of symptoms), erythrocyte sedimentation rate (ESR) (to exclude vasculitis), and if the patient is on warfarin or in AF (when anticoagulation is likely to be considered in the near future) an international normalised ratio (INR). A high cholesterol level may identify a vascular risk factor, but in light of the Heart Protection Study (*see* p 112) patients even with normal levels should be considered for statin therapy and so its value at the time of an acute stroke is questionable.

In younger patients with no clear vascular risk factors, especially those with personal or family histories of thrombosis, a thrombophilia screen (e.g. factor V Leiden, antithrombin III, proteins C and S, and antiphospholipid antibodies) should be considered.

ECG

An electrocardiogram (ECG) should be performed to accurately identify the cardiac rhythm.

Brain imaging

Clinical criteria alone do not reliably distinguish between ischaemic and haemorrhagic strokes;[8] this is the primary aim of imaging the brain of patients who have sustained an acute stroke. On occasions it will have the additional benefit of detecting an alternative explanation for symptoms – such as a structural lesion. Guidelines recommend that this should occur as soon as possible and almost always within 24 hours.[9] Some clinical situations make more rapid brain imaging preferable. These are outlined below:

- current anticoagulant use or known bleeding disorder
- reduced level of consciousness

- progressive or fluctuating symptoms
- severe headache, neck stiffness, papilloedema, or fever
- consideration of thrombolysis
- symptom onset coincides with head trauma.

Computerised tomography (CT) scanning is widely available, quick to perform, and easy for patients to tolerate. However, it often does not show abnormalities immediately following an ischaemic stroke, especially with small infarcts and within the first six hours.[10] Changes may be subtle – such as loss of grey-white matter differentiation. Several days later, hypodense (dark grey or black) areas will develop with breakdown of the dead cells. CT scans are of most use in detecting bleeding straight after an event as blood appears hyperdense (white) and remains so for approximately 10 days (depending on the size of the bleed). After this time the blood is gradually broken down to intermediary products, which are isodense (grey like brain tissue) and then become hypodense. At this stage CT scanning cannot distinguish whether a haemorrhagic or ischaemic event has occurred.[11] Therefore, CT scans are ideally performed within one week of an event.

In general terms magnetic resonance imaging (MRI) scans give better definition than CT scans and so acute infarcts are more likely to be detected. This is particularly true for lesions within the posterior fossa (i.e. brainstem and cerebellum). However, acute haemorrhage is less distinct on MRI scans, but it can be made more apparent with the 'gradient echo' technique. This is also capable of detecting the breakdown products of blood, which allows MRI to distinguish haemorrhagic from ischaemic strokes well beyond one week after the event (up to several months). Another possibility is 'diffusion-weighted' MRI, with which acute infarcts appear hyperdense and are therefore more easily detected.[10] The efficacy of this has been demonstrated in a randomised trial setting,[12] although alternative pathologies may have a similar appearance (e.g. demyelination plaques). Approximately 20% of patients are unable to undergo MRI scanning either due to being unable to tolerate the noisy and claustrophobic procedure, or due to metallic implants (e.g. cerebral aneurysm clips or cardiac pacemakers).[10]

At the present time CT scanning of all patients with acute stroke to enable early detection of haemorrhage (and exclusion of some other pathology) seems the best option, MRI scanning being reserved for difficult cases where identifying an ischaemic lesion would be clinically helpful or those presenting beyond 10 days to exclude a haemorrhagic event.

Trans-oesophageal echocardiography

Trans-oesophageal echocardiography (TOE) has detected potential sources of embolism in around 60% of patients with cryptogenic stroke (strokes where there are no apparent causes). There is an 0.2% risk of serious complications with this procedure (including hypoxia, gastrointestinal bleeding and arrhythmias).[13] It is not a suitable routine test but may have a role in selected patients.

Subtypes of stroke

The Bamford classification is a clinical method of distinguishing strokes into four subtypes derived from the Oxfordshire Community Stroke Project.[14] The subtype of stroke sustained has prognostic significance (*see* p 115).

Lacunar stroke syndromes

Lacunar strokes syndromes (LACS) are usually caused by intrinsic thrombus within small penetrating cerebral blood vessels. The major risk factor for their development is hypertension. They are not associated with any cortical signs (e.g. dysphasia, inattention or hemianopia). The lenticulostriate arteries arise from the middle cerebral artery (MCA) and supply blood to the internal capsule. As the motor fibres are tightly packed together in this region, such a lesion will cause a deficit affecting a large body area (*see* Figure 5.1). This will either be the face and arm, arm and leg, or face, arm and leg. A more limited deficit is likely to have arisen from a cortical lesion (i.e. not LACS).

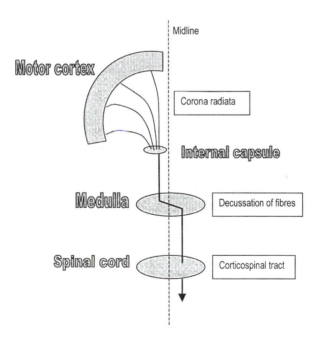

Figure 5.1 The motor pathways.

Lacunar events may also disturb the posterior circulation affecting the pons (causing an ataxic hemiparesis by affecting both motor and cerebellar fibres) or thalamus (where they may cause a pure sensory stroke) (*see* Figure 5.2). Mixed sensorimotor impairments have also been described. Many of these events are clinically silent.

The accumulation of multiple events can cause a subcortical dementia, small-stepping gait ('marche à petits pas') and/or pseudobulbar palsy. The small size of the lesions makes it common for them not to be seen on CT scanning.

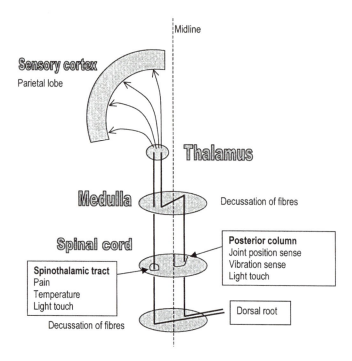

Figure 5.2 The sensory pathways.

Posterior circulation syndromes

Posterior circulation syndromes (POCS) involve lesions relating the vertebrobasilar system or posterior cerebral arteries. The clinical features of these are discussed on p 102.

Anterior circulation syndromes

Anterior circulation syndromes are subdivided into partial (PACS) and total (TACS) depending on the extent of the infarct. They are more likely than a lacunar stroke to be due to either a cardiac or large vessel embolus, or haemorrhage.

A TACS involves the combination of hemiplegia, hemianopia and at least one higher cognitive disturbance (e.g. dysphasia or inattention). A TACS is more likely than a PACS when there is an associated reduction in conscious level (indicating an extensive area of infarction).

A PACS causes a lesser combination of the features of a TACS or can cause a localised motor or sensory deficit (due to affecting a small area of either the motor or sensory cortex).

Infarcts

After a CT scan has been performed, if haemorrhage has been excluded, then the names of the Bamford subtypes are changed – the 'S' for syndrome is replaced by an 'I' for infarct, for example LACI, POCI, TACI and PACI.

Localisation of the event

Cerebral vascular supply

The basic anatomy of the circle of Willis is shown in Figure 5.3. The approximate cortical regions supplied by the major vessels are shown in Figure 5.4. The main functions of the cortical regions are shown in Figure 5.5.

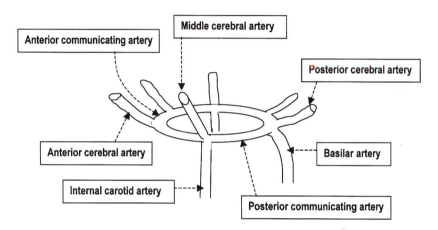

Figure 5.3   A three-dimensional representation of the circle of Willis.

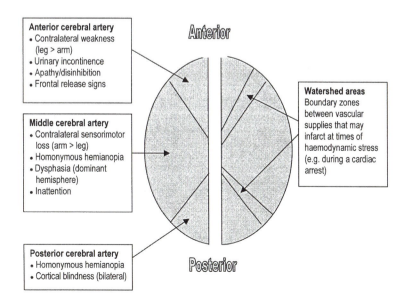

Figure 5.4   The approximate cortical areas supplied by the major blood vessels.

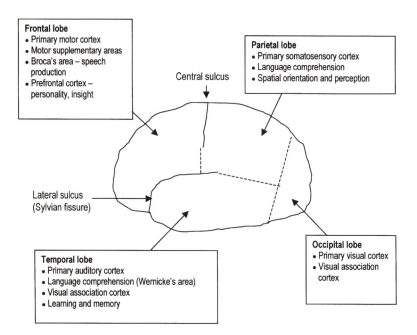

Figure 5.5 Functional areas of the brain.

Anterior circulation strokes

Anterior cerebral artery

The anterior cerebral artery (ACA) supplies a large portion of the frontal lobes. Infarction here may cause either apathy or disinhibition. There may also be emotional lability and urinary incontinence (due to loss of inhibitory reflexes and involvement of the nervous supply of the bladder). Examination may show frontal release signs (e.g. the grasp reflex (*see* p 10)). The medial aspect of the motor cortex is affected leading to a more marked motor deficit in the leg than that seen in the arm.

Middle cerebral artery

The middle cerebral artery (MCA) supplies the majority of the parietal and temporal lobes. Any motor deficit is usually more severe in the arm than in the leg. Due to the large representation of the hand in the motor cortex, it is possible to have a localised infarct that affects solely hand function. There will usually be associated cortical deficits, such as sensory inattention and dysphasia. Visual function may be affected with either a homonymous hemianopia or an upper or lower quadrantanopia (due to involvement of all or part of the optic radiation).

Posterior circulation strokes

The main components of the posterior circulation are shown in Figure 5.6. The subject is covered in greater detail elsewhere.[15]

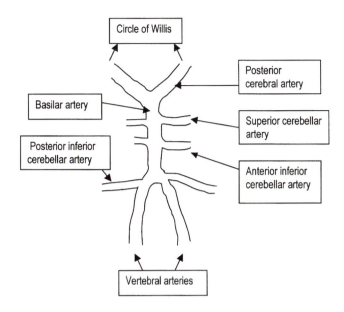

Figure 5.6 Simplified diagram of the posterior circulation of the brain.

Posterior cerebral artery

Lesions of the posterior cerebral artery (PCA) usually cause visual disturbances. This may be an isolated homonymous hemianopia (with macular sparing due to collateral supply from the MCA). Bilateral infarcts may lead to cortical blindness. This may be associated with confabulation of vision (Anton syndrome). Strokes within the visual association areas can provoke visual hallucinations. Visuospatial function is more likely to be affected with non-dominant hemisphere lesions.

Vertebrobasilar system

Cerebrovascular lesions of the vertebrobasilar system commonly present with lightheadedness or vertigo (*see* Chapter 8), double or lost vision, ataxia, and/or loss of power/sensation affecting one or both sides of the body.[16] However, the compact nature of structures in the region makes the occurrence of one symptom in isolation very unlikely. Signs of cerebellar involvement are listed in Table 5.1.

Brainstem lesions may also cause a disturbance of conjugate eye movements, Horner syndrome, or, rarely, a unilateral internuclear ophthalmoplegia. 'Top-of-the-basilar syndrome' is a term for patients with reduced conscious level, memory disturbance, small pupils and vertical gaze palsy secondary to infarction of the mid-brain and thalamus.[16] Basilar artery occlusion may cause bilateral limb signs or even the 'locked in' syndrome (the inability to move any part of the body except the eyes and eyelids in association with retained consciousness) due to bilateral pontine infarction. A diagram representing the anatomical levels of some structures within the brainstem to help localise a lesion is shown in Figure 5.7.

Table 5.1 Signs of cerebellar involvement

Vermis*	Hemispheres (ipsilateral signs)
Truncal ataxia	Nystagmus (fast phase towards affected side; *see* p 179)
	Dysarthria ('staccato speech')
	Past-pointing
	Intention tremor
	Dysdiadochokinesia
	Rebound phenomena (arms outstretched and eyes closed)
	Pendular reflexes
	Gait: ataxic, broad-based

*The vermis is the central part of the cerebellum, the two hemispheres lie laterally to this.

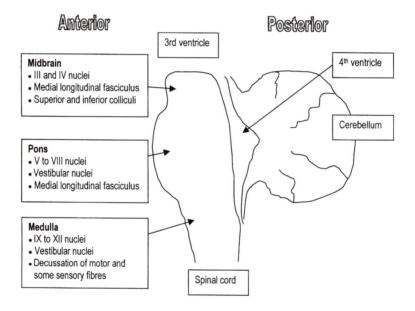

Figure 5.7 Anatomical location of key structures within the brainstem.

Various eponymous syndromes have been described relating to infarcts of the many small vessels supplying this region. They often result in ipsilateral cranial nerve palsies with contralateral limb signs (e.g. Weber syndrome – ipsilateral III nerve palsy plus contralateral limb weakness). Lateral medullary (or Wallenberg) syndrome is a rare but well-described combination of signs secondary to posterior inferior cerebellar artery territory infarction. The full features are listed in Table 5.2, but variants with only some features are equally likely (compare with Figures 5.1, 5.2 and 5.6 for an anatomical explanation of the make-up of deficits).

Thalamic infarction can cause a range of symptoms and signs. These include pure sensory strokes and some neuropsychological deficits. Amnesia can be caused by lesions affecting the limbic system (*see* Figure 1.6), but other neurological deficits would be expected to occur simultaneously. Lesions affecting the basal ganglia may induce movement disorders, such as hemiballismus or focal dystonia.

Table 5.2 The constellation of signs seen with lateral medullary syndrome

Ipsilateral	Contralateral
↓ facial sensation	↓ pain and temperature sensation trunk and limbs
Lower cranial nerve palsies	
Horner syndrome (miosis, ptosis, reduced facial sweating)	
Cerebellar signs	

Bilateral vertebrobasilar atheromatous disease can lead to symptoms due to hypoperfusion of the brainstem provoked by stimuli that further reduce blood flow (*see* p 181). These include increases in antihypertensive medication or rapid postural change.[17] Typically multiple brief, stereotyped episodes occur and common symptoms include lightheadedness, dysarthria, ataxia, blurred vision and diplopia.

Ischaemic strokes and TIAs

A blood vessel blockage may occur due to thrombus formation within the blood vessel itself or due to embolised thrombus from elsewhere. This is most commonly from clots formed on the walls of larger vessels (i.e. the carotid arteries or aorta) or within the left atrium of people in AF.

Risk factors

Hypertension

The SHEP trial randomised 4736 people over the age of 60 (mean age 72 years) with isolated systolic hypertension (systolic blood pressure (BP) >160 mmHg, diastolic BP <90 mmHg) to receive active treatment (a thiazide (chlorthalidone) plus a beta-blocker (atenolol) if required) or placebo.[18] The systolic BP readings averaged 143 mmHg in the treatment arm and 155 mmHg in the placebo group. The five-year stroke incidence rates were 5.2 per 100 people with treatment and 8.2 per 100 with placebo – a relative risk reduction of 36%.

Atrial fibrillation

Between 6% and 20% of people who sustain a stroke are found to be in AF, and these people have around a 15% risk of recurrence within the following year.[19] These patients have a worse prognosis than those in sinus rhythm, probably due to a greater tendency for large, cortical strokes to occur. People in AF who have not previously sustained a stroke have around a 4.5% risk of thromboembolism per year.[20]

Others

Smoking, diabetes and a history of vascular disease (including stroke) confer an increased risk of stroke. A positive family history is very occasionally relevant as there are some rare familial causes of stroke (*see* p 128). Obstructive sleep apnoea (OSA) has been found to carry around a doubling of the risk of stroke after correction for other variables.[21]

Transient ischaemic attacks

TIAs are defined by their symptom duration of less than 24 hours. However, 24 hours is an arbitrary figure and most TIAs are of duration less than three hours. They are almost always assumed to be caused by vessel blockages, as the symptoms from a haemorrhagic lesion are extremely unlikely to fully resolve within this time period. Symptoms lasting only seconds at a location other than the eye are unlikely to be due to a TIA. It was thought that TIAs represent a period of focal brain ischaemia rather than infarction (analogous to angina compared to a myocardial infarction (MI)). However, CT imaging of the brain reveals an area of cerebral infarction in 13% of TIA patients,[22] and a much higher proportion is revealed when MRI scanning is used.[23] The probability of an infarct being detected on scanning appears to increase linearly with duration of symptoms, being found in 35% of those with symptoms lasting days to weeks, and 49% of those with persistent symptoms following a minor stroke. TIAs share the same risk factors and secondary prevention strategies with ischaemic stroke. The risk of future stroke is similar in people who have had a TIA to those who have sustained a minor stroke (*see* p 115).

Migraine attacks and syncopal episodes are common causes of TIA misdiagnosis. Non-focal neurological symptoms (e.g. dizziness, confusion or loss of consciousness) occurring in isolation are not due to TIAs. The most frequent symptoms are unilateral weakness or sensory loss, dysarthria, dysphasia and transient visual problems.

Visual disturbances seen with TIAs include monocular vision loss, homonymous hemianopia and diplopia. Patients often are unable to distinguish between the loss of vision in one eye and the loss of one visual field (homonymous hemianopia). They may have tried covering each eye during the episode, which would provide more information, and so this should be asked about.

Transient monocular blindness (also known as 'amaurosis fugax') is a term for the sudden onset of visual loss in one eye. This may feel like a dark curtain coming across the visual field. There is no associated eye pain. Ophthalmoscopy should always be performed to detect abnormalities such as cholesterol emboli (yellow blobs within the retinal arterioles), haemorrhages, optic nerve pallor and papilloedema. In this way a primary ocular disorder that mimics a TIA may be detected. Eye pain, redness and pupillary changes suggest an alternative cause for the visual symptoms. ESR should be measured to exclude a vasculitic process.

Acute treatment of ischaemic stroke

Thrombolysis

Recombinant tissue plasminogen activator (rt-PA) has been found to be of benefit in some people following acute stroke. It works by converting plasminogen to plasmin, which breaks down the fibrin polymers that form clots – *see* Figure 5.8. Other thrombolytic agents have not been found to be similarly effective. To date, the worldwide number of patients who have received thrombolysis for acute stroke is very low, and even more so within the elderly.

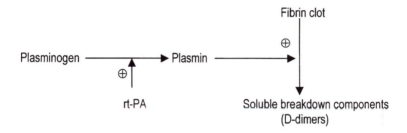

Figure 5.8   The mechanism of action of recombinant tissue plasminogen activator (rt-PA).

In one trial, 624 patients were randomised to either rt-PA or placebo within three hours of an acute ischaemic stroke (haemorrhage excluded by CT scanning).[24] A three-month assessment revealed that a higher proportion of patients had a favourable outcome (absence of death or severe disability) in the rt-PA group than placebo (odds ratio (OR) 1.7; 95% CI 1.2–2.6, $p = 0.008$). There were no significant differences in mortality between the groups. Symptomatic intracranial haemorrhage occurred in 20 patients (6.0%) with rt-PA compared to 2 (0.6%) with placebo.

A recent report of open-label cases thrombolysed within Canada has demonstrated similar outcomes to the above randomised controlled trial.[25] Over 2.5 years a total of 1135 patients (59% over the age of 70) had been treated, and 37% of these had a favourable outcome. There was a lower rate (4.6%) of symptomatic intracranial haemorrhage but 75% of these patients died whilst in hospital. Orolingual angio-oedema was seen in 1.3% of patients. The study suggests that the results of the randomised controlled trial may be realistically recreated in standard practice. However, the proportion of stroke patients treated with rt-PA in all of Canada over this period was <2%. Other analyses have estimated that overall, in the Western world, between 1% and 7% of acute ischaemic stroke patients currently receive thrombolysis.[26]

A Cochrane systematic review of the available trials demonstrated a large degree of heterogeneity in outcomes, partly due to differing protocols used.[27] Overall, thrombolysis with rt-PA was associated with a significant reduction in the combined end-point of death or dependency (OR 0.80; 95% CI 0.69–0.93), and a non-significant increase in deaths from all causes (OR 1.17; 95% CI 0.95–1.45). The use of thrombolysis significantly increased the risk of fatal intracranial haemorrhage (OR 3.60; 95% CI 2.28–5.68). Some signs seen on CT scanning may be able to detect those patients who are more likely to have haemorrhagic adverse events. There is evidence that it is more likely to occur when there is a marked early appearance of brain oedema, mass effect or a large area of hypodensity.[28]

The advent of rt-PA therapy presents logistical problems for many stroke centres, as a dedicated on-call rota involving at least four stroke consultants and ancillary staff is required. Also there has to be rapid transfer of patients from the community to hospital and rapid access to a 24-hour brain imaging service. Although a study comparing patients transferred from a peripheral hospital to a thrombolysis centre has suggested that the benefits can still be maintained,[29] in the UK acute ischaemic stroke is currently an unlicensed indication for rt-PA and only trained individuals can administer it on a named patient basis within registered specialist centres (UK Safe Implementation of Thrombolysis in Stroke Monitoring Study).[9]

In summary, there is evidence that some stroke patients benefit by reduced long-term disability from thrombolysis. However, the proportion of patients who are suitable candidates is likely to be less than 10% and it comes at a cost of increased intracranial haemorrhage (ICH) and early mortality. Barriers to treatment include access to hospital, CT scanning and a stroke specialist within three hours of symptom onset. Campaigns that raise patients' awareness of the need to seek rapid assessment are likely to be needed to improve the uptake.[30] Some of the outstanding uncertainties of this treatment may be answered by forthcoming trials (e.g. the Third International Stroke Trial (IST-3)).

Neuroprotective agents

There have been a number of trials testing the use of agents that may limit brain damage following a stroke (neuroprotective). Unfortunately they have all, so far, been unsuccessful.

Physiological parameters

The outcomes of stroke appear to be worse in those with pyrexia at the time of admission and better in those with low body temperature.[31,32] Paracetamol can reduce body temperature but its efficacy in this situation has not been proven. Forty per cent of patients admitted following acute stroke are hyperglycaemic, yet the optimal management of hyperglycaemia after stroke is unknown.[33] Given the benefits following acute MI, there is logic in thinking glucose control may be beneficial, and hyperglycaemia has been associated with worse post-stroke outcomes.[33] The GIST-UK trial is under way to try and answer this question.[34] It makes sense to correct any hypoxia. However, the routine use of high-flow oxygen in non-hypoxic acute stroke patients has not been shown to convey any advantage.[35] Dehydration at presentation appears to be associated with worse outcomes, but interventional studies showing a benefit of rigorous rehydration have not been performed.[36] Both very high and very low BP recordings at baseline have been associated with less favourable outcomes after stroke.[37]

The optimal management of early BP is unknown. Approximately 60% of patients have been found to have a systolic BP >160 mmHg following an acute stroke.[38] However, the BP will normalise spontaneously over a seven-day period in most of these people.[39] Some evidence suggests that early reductions in BP may be associated with a worse prognosis.[40] If a patient is already on BP-lowering medications, it is common practice to continue them (providing the patient can swallow) but the benefit or harm of this is unknown. The Royal College of Physicians (RCP) stroke guidelines recommend that an elevated BP should only be acutely lowered when hypertensive complications are likely, for example encephalopathy.[9] Another subgroup of patients has a low BP at presentation and whether steps to increase this parameter may be beneficial is also unclear. Trials are under way to try and solve such dilemmas.[41,42]

Secondary prevention of ischaemic stroke

Antiplatelet agents

Aspirin

Aspirin is absorbed in the stomach and upper small intestine. It has a half-life of just 20 minutes in the blood but has a much longer duration of action due to its irreversible binding with platelet enzymes.[43] Therefore, its effects last for the lifetime of the platelet (around 10 days). The platelets are replaced at around 10% per day, and so a single dose of aspirin still impairs the action of around 50% of circulating platelets after five days.[43] At low doses its main effect is to inhibit the enzyme cyclo-oxygenase 1 (COX 1). This results in the inability of platelets to produce thromboxane, which promotes platelet aggregation and induces vasoconstriction.[43] After one week of therapy, doses as low as 30 mg per day result in near complete inhibition of platelet thromboxane production.[44]

Low doses have little effect on either BP control or renal function but do increase the risk of gastrointestinal haemorrhage.[44] The risk of haemorrhage whilst taking aspirin is approximately doubled, resulting in around one to two major bleeding complications per 1000 patient-years. This is dose-dependent and so the lowest effective dose of aspirin should be used (probably 75–100 mg daily), higher doses do not appear to offer any additional vascular protection advantages.[43] The evidence for benefit below 75 mg per day is less clear.[45] There is also an increased risk of haemorrhagic stroke. A meta-analysis of aspirin trials involving over 50 000 patients found that the use of aspirin for three years resulted in 12 more haemorrhagic strokes per 10 000 population than placebo.[46]

In acute settings, where rapid and complete inhibition of platelets is required, a single higher loading dose of aspirin should be used (150–300 mg).[45] Gastric-coated formulations are associated with a reduced risk of gastrointestinal haemorrhage. However, this comes at the cost of a much-reduced bioavailability of the drug.[43] Occasionally, people may have a hypersensitivity reaction to aspirin.

The use of aspirin is associated with around a 25% reduction in the risk of serious vascular events (including a 33% reduction in non-fatal MI, 25% reduction in non-fatal stroke and a 17% reduction in vascular death).[45] The absolute size of the benefit is proportional to the baseline risk within an individual. Primary prevention in those at low baseline risk is unlikely to be effective.

There is evidence that early commencement of aspirin has a beneficial effect. When started within 48 hours of an acute stroke, at a dose of 160 mg per day, it is associated with a 14% reduction in four-week mortality compared to placebo (absolute risk 3.3% vs 3.9%).[47] Another study has confirmed this finding with a 300 mg daily dose of aspirin.[48] Here, recurrent stroke within 14 days was seen in 2.8% of those on aspirin compared to 3.9% in the placebo arm, without a significant increase in bleeding risk. So, in the immediate post-stroke period an aspirin dose of 160–300 mg is of proven value (RCP guidelines recommend an immediate dose of 300 mg).[9] In people unable to swallow it can be given rectally (300 mg PR daily) or in solution via a nasogastric (NG) tube.

See p 252 for the use of aspirin in AF.

Dipyridamole

Dipyridamole acts by blocking the breakdown of cyclic adenosine monophosphate (cAMP), which prevents the activation of second messengers in the pathway that leads to platelet aggregation. Clinically, the most significant side effect is headache, which leads to a number of patients discontinuing therapy.

A large randomised controlled trial (ESPS2) demonstrated a benefit of a modified release formulation of dipyridamole in combination with aspirin for the prevention of stroke.[49] Here 6602 patients who had had a recent stroke or TIA (within three months) were randomised to aspirin 25 mg bd, dipyridamole modified-release (MR) 200 mg bd, both, or placebo, and were followed up for a two-year period. The primary outcome of stroke or death showed a non-significant trend favouring aspirin and dipyridamole over aspirin alone (event rates 17% vs 20%, respectively). For the individual outcome of stroke there was a significant 23% relative risk (RR) reduction ($p = 0.006$) for the combination of agents compared to aspirin by itself.

This was not initially confirmed in other studies and a meta-analysis of anti-platelet trials did not demonstrate a benefit of this combination.[45] Proposed explanations for this discrepancy include the use of an unusual dose of aspirin (25 mg bd) within the positive trial or, possibly, an advantage of the MR formulation (taken bd) over standard-release (SR) versions (taken tds). More recently the ESPRIT study has supported a benefit of the combination of aspirin and dipyridamole.[50] Here 2763 patients (mean age 63 years) who had had a minor stroke or TIA within the last six months were randomised to aspirin (mean dose 75 mg) plus dipyridamole 200 mg bd (83% on MR preparation) or aspirin plus placebo over a mean follow-up period of 3.5 years. The primary outcome of vascular death, stroke, MI or major bleeding complication occurred in 16% of the aspirin group compared to 13% of those on combination therapy. The number needed to treat (NNT) for one year is around 100. There was no significant difference in bleeding rates between the groups. However, side effects were common with the combination of medications, especially headache – which resulted in 9% of patients discontinuing therapy. When the results of this trial are added to previous meta-analysis data, a significant benefit is seen in rates of vascular death, stroke and MI (RR 0.82; 95% CI 0.74–0.91). NICE has advised this combination for those who have had a stroke within the last two years.[51]

Clopidogrel

Clopidogrel prevents the aggregation of platelets by blocking the binding of adenosine diphosphate (ADP) to its receptor on their surface. This inhibits the binding of platelets to fibrin strands.

The CAPRIE study compared clopidogrel (75 mg) to aspirin (325 mg) in 19 185 patients (mean age 63 years) with a history of vascular disease (stroke, MI or peripheral vascular disease) over a mean follow-up of 1.9 years.[52] The primary outcome was combined rates of ischaemic stroke, MI or vascular death, for which there was a rate of 5.3% and 5.8% in the clopidogrel and aspirin groups, respectively. This just reached clinical significance ($p = 0.043$) and represents a relative risk reduction of 8.7% (95% CI 0.3–16.5%). Subgroup analysis suggests that this benefit is most marked for those with peripheral vascular disease and the results are not significant for either stroke or MI alone. Withdrawal rates were similar in both groups. Adverse effects seen more commonly with clopidogrel included rash and diarrhoea, those seen with aspirin included upper gastrointestinal (GI) discomfort, and GI and intracranial haemorrhage. The small benefit seen in the combined vascular end-points means that around 200 patients need to be treated with clopidogrel for a year to prevent one excess vascular event.

A more recent study has compared aspirin plus clopidogrel vs aspirin plus placebo in 15 603 patients (mean age 64, range 39–95 years) with vascular risk factors over a mean follow-up period of 28 months.[53] For the primary outcome of MI, stroke or vascular death there was no significant difference between the groups (6.8% with clopidogrel vs 7.3% with placebo; RR 0.93; 95% CI 0.83–1.05; $p = 0.22$). There was a higher rate of bleeding adverse events in the combination therapy group.

A meta-analysis of studies suggested that clopidogrel may have around an additional 10% relative risk reduction compared to aspirin.[45] The far higher cost of clopidogrel currently makes this a cost-ineffective strategy. It is usually reserved for the small percentage of people who have genuine aspirin allergy. Previously, it was believed that clopidogrel may be preferable to aspirin in those who had had an aspirin-induced peptic ulcer. However, a recent trial demonstrated a large benefit with the combination of aspirin and a proton pump inhibitor (PPI) over clopidogrel alone in recurrent bleeding rates in such people (0.7% per year vs 8.6%).[54] The combination of clopidogrel and a PPI was not tested, however, as the rate of recurrent bleeding was so low with aspirin and a PPI that if there is an additional benefit it is highly unlikely to be cost-effective.

Trials that have added clopidogrel to aspirin in the period immediately following unstable angina or myocardial infarction have demonstrated a clear benefit.[55,56] However, this combination has been found to have no additional benefit in secondary stroke prevention compared to clopidogrel alone and is associated with a significantly increased rate of bleeding complications.[57] So, this combination has no current role in the secondary prevention of stroke.

Anticoagulants

Warfarin

Warfarin is indicated for the prevention of stroke in those with AF who are at a moderate to high risk of recurrence. This is discussed on p 251. Due to the increased risk of bleeding into an area of infarct immediately following an ischaemic stroke, guidelines recommend that warfarin is not started in the initial two weeks (an antiplatelet agent may be used in the interim).[9] Its use has also been proposed in other groups at high risk of recurrent stroke (e.g. those with significant intracranial arterial stenosis[58]) but to date there is no randomised controlled trial evidence of superior efficacy to antiplatelet agents in people with sinus rhythm.[59] Therefore, the elevated risk of bleeding complications with warfarin means that its use cannot be justified outside those with AF unless there is an alternative clinical indication (e.g. a prosthetic heart valve).

Heparin

The use of subcutaneous heparin (various doses) has been compared to aspirin (300 mg) in over 19 000 acute stroke patients.[48] The study found a reduction in recurrent ischaemic events but this was offset by a similar increase in haemorrhagic complications, making heparin ineffective. When low-molecular-weight heparin was compared to aspirin in those with atrial fibrillation in the first two weeks from a stroke, no benefit was found.[19,60] Therefore, there is currently no role for heparin in the management of acute stroke.

Cholesterol reduction

A meta-analysis of trials involving over 90 000 patients on either a statin or placebo treatment found five-year reductions of around 20% for major vascular events (including stroke) per 1 mmol/l lowering of LDL cholesterol,[61] the absolute benefits clearly being greater in those at higher baseline vascular risk. This appears to be irrespective of baseline cholesterol level or agent used to produce the reduction.

The Heart Protection study randomised 20 536 people with vascular risk factors to receive simvastatin 40 mg daily or placebo over a five-year period.[62] They found a 25% relative risk reduction of stroke with active therapy (4.3% vs 5.7% absolute risk). There was also a reduction in those having TIAs or requiring carotid endarterectomy. The difference became significant after two years of therapy. LDL cholesterol was around 1.0 mmol/l lower with the statin therapy. The benefit appears to be present irrespective of starting cholesterol level. Statin use is recommended for most stroke patients.[9]

Blood pressure control

The control of hypertension is discussed in Chapter 13. The PROGRESS trial is of particular note to post-stroke patients.[63] In this study, 6105 patients who had sustained a previous stroke or TIA (mean age 64 years, median time of eight months since stroke event) were randomised to receive either a placebo or an angiotensin-converting enzyme inhibitor (ACEi) (perindopril) with a thiazide diuretic (indapamide), if required, over a four-year period. The active treatment was associated with a larger average reduction in BP of 9/4 mmHg (mean initial BP 147/86 mmHg), and a lower risk of recurrent stroke than placebo (10% vs 14%; relative risk reduction 28%; $p<0.0001$). The combination of therapeutic agents resulted in a greater mean fall in BP and subsequent larger positive effect. The benefit seen was irrespective of patients' starting BP.

Some physicians feel that this study demonstrates a specific benefit of ACEi therapy in this patient subgroup. However, most believe that is it the degree of control of BP, rather than the specific agent(s) used that is of most importance in the prevention of future stroke. Based mainly on the results of the PROGRESS study, the RCP guidelines recommend the use of thiazide diuretics and ACEi as first-line therapy for hypertensive people after a stroke.[9] According to the newly updated

Joint British Societies' Guidelines, the BP target following a stroke should be better than 130/80 mmHg for all patients (previously below 140/85 mmHg for non-diabetic individuals and 130/80 mmHg only for those with diabetes).[64]

Diabetes

In diabetic patients who have had a stroke tight blood sugar control is advised to reduce the risk of further events. The benefit of early control of abnormal sugar levels post-stroke is the subject of ongoing research.[34]

Smoking cessation

Smoking is a major modifiable risk factor for vascular disease, including stroke. However, even among younger smokers, only 22% have been noted to quit following a cerebrovascular event.[65] Up to half of all smokers die prematurely – on average 10 years earlier than non-smokers.[66] It is estimated that around 20% of all deaths in the developed world can currently be attributed to tobacco.[67] The main causes of death are cardiovascular, malignant and respiratory diseases. The prevalence of smoking is falling but is currently between 20% and 30% of the population in most developed countries. Smokers who manage to quit will see early benefits in respiratory function (possibly after a period of rebound increased mucus production) and later benefits in reduced cardiovascular risk. This increased risk falls to 50% after one year and approximates to the risk in non-smokers after 15 years.[67] The symptoms following quitting include anxiety, irritability, reduced concentration and weight gain.

To promote smoking cessation, doctors should enquire about smoking, advise on the benefits of stopping and offer referral to a specialist service. The mainstays of treatment are counselling and pharmacological treatments. Counselling should be performed by a trained person but this may be provided as a telephone service (e.g. NHS Smoking Helpline 0800 169 0 169). Pharmacological treatments include nicotine replacement (available in various preparations including patches and gum) and some atypical antidepressants (e.g. bupropion) that reduce cravings and withdrawal symptoms. They may be used alone or in combination.

Cochrane reviews on the efficacy of both nicotine and bupropion have suggested an approximate doubling of benefit compared to placebo (from around a 10% success rate to 20% with treatment).[68,69] A review of the efficacy of telephone quit lines also suggests a benefit.[70] Given the enormous number of smokers and the large detrimental effect on health, even a small positive effect may have profound public health benefits.

Carotid endarterectomy

Emboli from carotid artery plaques are thought to cause 15–20% of ischaemic strokes.[71] Carotid endarterectomy (CE) is a surgical technique that removes the inner layers of the carotid artery and any associated atheroma. The relative benefit of this procedure is proportional to the degree of vessel narrowing attributed to atheroma formation. The amount of internal carotid artery (ICA) stenosis can be estimated with carotid Doppler but is more accurately assessed by standard or magnetic resonance angiography. To complicate matters, there are differing systems for calculating the severity of any stenosis, which yield significantly different estimations.

The NASCET trial randomised 659 patients (mean age 66 years) who had sustained a TIA or non-disabling stroke in the relevant carotid territory within the last 120 days, and had a stenosis of 70–99%, to surgical intervention or usual medical care.[72] After two years the stroke rate was 26% in the medical arm compared to 9% in those who underwent surgery. However, the peri-operative stroke or death rate was 5.8% despite using only highly skilled surgeons.

A further component of the NASCET trial randomised 2226 patients with stenoses less than 70% to surgery or control groups.[73] No benefit of surgery was found compared to control subjects with stenoses less than 50% (death or stroke occurred in 15% vs 19%; $p = 0.16$) and only a small benefit in those with stenoses between 50% and 69% (16% vs 22%; $p = 0.045$).

In the ECST trial 3024 patients (mean age 62 years) with carotid territory symptoms within the last six months were randomised to early surgery or a control group and followed up for a period of six years.[74] The participants had a range of degrees of carotid stenosis. Overall there was no benefit of surgery for the primary outcome measure of death or major stroke (37% in both groups). However, the subgroup that had stenosis of 80% or more did benefit (primary outcome reached in 15% of the surgery group compared to 27% of control subjects). There was a 7% risk of death or major stroke within 30 days of undergoing surgery.

In summary, CE is of proven benefit in patients with a stenosis of 70–99% who have sustained a stroke or TIA in that territory within the last six months.[71] It is of borderline benefit in those with stenoses of 50–70%, depending on the surgical complication rate, and of no benefit in those with a symptomatic stenosis below 50%.[71]

CE for asymptomatic stenosis may have a small benefit for patients with stenoses of 60–99%, an expected survival of more than five years and when operated on by a surgeon with a peri-operative stroke or death rate of less than 3%.[71]

The timing of the surgery is also critical. Analysis of data from the major carotid surgery trials has shown a large benefit for having surgery within two weeks of a symptomatic event compared to a delay of over 12 weeks (the NNT to prevent one stroke is five with early surgery vs 125 when delayed).[75]

Having a surgeon with a very low complication rate is crucial. As medical therapy for the secondary prevention of stroke improves, the risk versus benefit profile of carotid surgery may change. In the ECST trial fewer than 10% of participants were on lipid-lowering medications, in the NASCET trial around 15% of participants were initially on lipid-lowering therapy and this rose to around 40% by the end of the trial.[73,74] It is not recommended for patients with a probable cardio-embolic source (e.g. those in AF) – these patients were excluded from the major trials.

Studies so far have not distinguished between different subtypes of anterior circulation stroke. Logic would suggest that the benefits of CE would be greatest in those whose stroke's mechanism was most likely due to an embolus from the relevant carotid artery (i.e. not LACIs (*see* p 99)) and who have significant brain remaining in that territory to protect (i.e. not TACIs). Also, pure sensory strokes are likely to be due to posterior circulation aetiology and, therefore, be uninfluenced by carotid atheroma. This would suggest that PACI strokes are the group most likely to benefit from CE.

Carotid stenting

Arterial stenting is a less invasive revascularisation option for the carotids. However, initial studies found a high rate of emboli formation during the procedure. This has been lessened by the use of emboli-prevention devices. When the technique was compared to endarterectomy in a randomised controlled trial recruiting patients who were deemed to be at high risk to undergo surgical intervention, the results suggested it was at least as effective for these patients.[76] However, a more recent trial comparing stenting to CE has shown a higher 30-day stroke or death rate with stenting (9.6% vs 3.9%).[77] Its use is currently restricted to specialist centres.[9]

Prognosis of ischaemic stroke

It is difficult to predict individual patients' outcomes after a stroke. Overall, 10% of people who sustain ischaemic strokes are dead after one month, and this figure rises to 23% after one year.[14] A breakdown of the prognosis with specific stroke subtypes is shown in Table 5.3. The risk of recurrence over a five-year period is estimated to be 15–40%.[2] The highest risk of recurrent stroke is seen with those of the PACI subtype.[14] The risk of future stroke in those who have sustained a TIA has been found to be 8% after one week, 12% after one month and 17% after three months.[78] Equivalent figures for those who have sustained a minor stroke are very similar (12%, 15% and 19%, respectively). After 10 years, 54% of those who have had a TIA or minor stroke will have had at least one further vascular event and 60% will be dead.[79]

Table 5.3 A comparison of the composition and prognosis of stroke subtypes in the Bamford classification scheme[14]

Stroke subtype	Percentage of all ischaemic strokes	Independent at one year (%)	Dead at 30 days from stroke (%)	Dead at one year from stroke (%)
Lacunar circulation infarct	25	60	2	11
Posterior circulation infarct	24	62	7	19
Partial anterior circulation infarct	34	55	4	16
Total anterior circulation infarct	17	4	39	60

A scoring tool has been developed to try to stratify those patients at highest risk of stroke following a TIA in order to more rapidly assess them and address modifiable risk factors. This is called the 'ABCD', standing for Age (one point scored if aged 60 or above), Blood pressure (one point if either systolic >140 mmHg or diastolic >90 mmHg), Clinical features (two points if unilateral weakness, one point if only speech affected, anything else doesn't score) and Duration of symptoms (two points if lasted 60 minutes or longer, one point if 10–59 minutes, 0 if <10 minutes). It has been found that the risk of stroke within seven days of a TIA is very low (<5%) in those with an ABCD score of four or less, but around 12% in those with a score of five and around 30% in those with a score of six.[80] One criticism of this scoring system is that the clinical features component will fail to detect posterior circulation symptoms, but such patients would, of course, not be candidates for carotid surgery.

Intracerebral haemorrhage

Epidemiology

Approximately 15% of all strokes are haemorrhagic. They are subdivided into intracerebral haemorrhage (ICH) and subarachnoid haemorrhage (SAH) (see later). ICH is classified into primary and secondary causations. Primary events account for around 80% and are related to vascular damage to perforating arteries caused by hypertension or cerebral amyloid angiopathy (CAA).[81] Secondary events are caused by an alternative underlying abnormality. These include arteriovenous malformations, aneurysms, tumours and coagulopathies. ICH is further subdivided according to anatomical location, into deep (at the basal ganglia, brainstem or cerebellum) and lobar (cortical). The incidence of ICH is around 10–20 per 100 000 population per year, but it is more common in the elderly, males and certain ethnic groups (especially Black and Japanese).[81]

Pathophysiology

Hypertension causes damage to the walls of small vessels. This mechanism is most commonly associated with deep haemorrhages. In the elderly, lobar bleeds are associated with CAA, whereas deep bleeds are associated with hypertension.[20] CAA is especially likely when two or more bleeds have occurred (together or at separate times).[82] Older bleeds may be detected by gradient-echo MRI scanning.[36] The bleeds associated with CAA are usually at the grey-white matter border, but occasionally they may affect the cerebellum. The increased bleeding tendency is caused by beta-amyloid deposition in the vessel walls.

Arteriovenous malformations are the most common cause of ICH in those aged below 45 years (see p 127). Intracranial aneurysms and cerebral venous thrombosis (see p 129) are infrequent causes of ICH. Anticoagulant (see p 252) and, to a lesser extent, antiplatelet (see p 109) use may also be causative. There may be genetic factors that play a role in haemorrhage as a positive family history conveys an elevated risk. Lobar haemorrhage is more common in those who possess an apolipoprotein E4 or E2 allele.[83]

Clinical features

Like other strokes types, the presentation may be an abrupt onset of a focal neurological deficit. However, ICH is a more common cause of reduced conscious-ness due to the haematoma's mass effect causing compression of the brainstem structures (i.e. the reticular activating system).[81] A low Glasgow Coma Scale score at presentation carries a worse prognosis. Headache and vomiting may be due to either raised intracranial pressure or meningism secondary to leakage of blood into the ventricular system. When seizures are associated, they are most likely in the first 24 hours after onset.

Early clinical deterioration (within 24 hours) due to an increase in the size of the haematoma is seen in around 40% of patients (increase in size of >33%).[84] In the majority of these cases this enlargement occurs in the first hour from onset. It has been shown that worsening within the first 48 hours can also occur secondary to vasogenic oedema.[81] Corticosteroids have not been found to be beneficial in this form of cerebral oedema. Osmotic diuretics such as mannitol may have a role, but randomised controlled trial evidence of benefit is lacking.

Haemorrhagic stroke treatment

Blood pressure control

The control of BP in the acute phase, as with ischaemic stroke (*see* p 108), is a controversial area and the best management will not be known until further trials have been completed. After the acute phase, BP guidance is as for the secondary prevention of ischaemic strokes (*see* p 112).

Recombinant activated factor VII

Early haematoma enlargement (mainly within the first four hours) is thought to be a significant factor associated with poor outcomes following ICH.[85] A randomised trial compared the use of various doses of recombinant activated factor VII to placebo in 399 people (median age 66 years) with acute intracerebral haemorrhage (within four hours of onset).[86] It was found that the active therapy was associated with less early haematoma enlargement. This led to a lower 90-day mortality rate with the active treatment compared to placebo (18% vs 29%; $p = 0.02$). However, there was a higher rate of serious thrombo-embolic complications (mainly MI and ischaemic stroke) with active treatment (7% vs 2%). Overall this is a promising result but further studies are required before this can become standard therapy.

Reversal of anticoagulation

When ICH is associated with oral anticoagulant use (most commonly warfarin), early haematoma expansion may continue for up to 48 hours after the onset.[85] For this reason it is felt that rapid reversal of anticoagulation is of key importance. Studies have found that prothrombin complex concentrate (PCC) is more effective at achieving this than vitamin K and/or fresh frozen plasma (FFP).[87] PCC contains concentrated amounts of the vitamin K-dependent clotting factors II (prothrombin), VII, IX and X. The interaction of these factors with vitamin K and warfarin is shown in Figure 5.9. FFP contains clotting factors but in a non-concentrated form and with variable amounts of each component. It is usually fast acting but short-lived. Vitamin K has the disadvantage of a slow onset of action. Current guidelines recommend the use of PCC (dose calculated by weight) plus vitamin K (usually 5 mg intravenously (IV)).[88] When PCC is unavailable, FFP is an alternative.

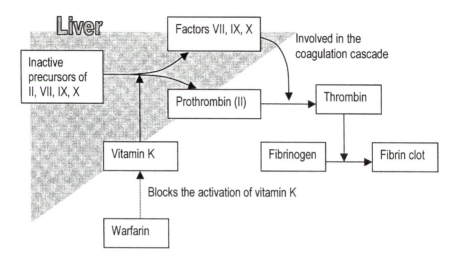

Figure 5.9   The roles of vitamin K, warfarin and the vitamin K-dependent clotting factors in thrombus formation.

Anticoagulation or antiplatelets after intracerebral haemorrhage

Generally speaking, people who have survived ICH are at a greater future risk of ICH rather than ischaemic stroke.[89] However, there is a subgroup of patients who have sustained an intracerebral bleed who are at an increased risk of ischaemic stroke (e.g. those who have prosthetic heart valves or are in AF). The question as to whether these patients should receive some form of blood-thinning therapy has not been well answered by current evidence.[90] Extrapolating from available data, it is usual practice that anticoagulant or antiplatelet therapy is avoided in patients in atrial fibrillation alone.[8,20] Overall, patients with prosthetic heart valves have been calculated to have a 4% per year risk of thrombo-embolism while off warfarin, compared to a 1% annual risk on warfarin (2% per year on antiplatelet agents).[91] It is generally accepted that a two-week period off warfarin carries a low (but not zero[92]) risk of embolus whilst the bleeding source repairs itself. Typically, such patients are then re-anticoagulated. The treatment of deep vein thrombosis (DVT) after ICH is discussed on p 123.

Surgery

The STICH trial randomised 1033 patients (mean age 62 years) with acute ICH to either early surgery (within 24 hours) or initial conservative management.[93] Eligible patients had a haematoma seen on CT scanning of at least 2 cm diameter and a Glasgow Coma Scale score of five or more. The responsible neurosurgeon was also to be uncertain about the benefits of either treatment. The surgical technique was left to the choosing of the surgical team. Those in the conservative arm were allowed later surgery if the treating team felt it would be beneficial. This occurred in 26% of these patients at a mean time interval of 31 hours from randomisation. The results did not show a significant benefit of early surgery. A favourable outcome (absence of death or significant disability) was reported in 26% of those with early surgery compared to 24% of the conservative treatment group (OR 0.89; 95% CI 0.66–1.19; p = 0.4). Those patients presenting with a Glasgow Coma Scale score of eight or less almost universally had a poor outcome. So, where surgical uncertainty exists, patients do not appear to benefit from early surgical intervention. Of course, there may be subgroups, such as posterior fossa haematomas or following the development of hydrocephalus, where surgical intervention is beneficial. For this reason, obtaining neurosurgical advice is usually still appropriate for cases of ICH.

Prognosis

ICH carries a high early mortality rate of between 30% and 50% in the first 30 days.[84] Coupled to this, only 20% of those afflicted manage to regain functional independence. Factors associated with worse prognosis include low Glasgow Coma Scale score at admission, advanced age, large bleed volume and the presence of blood within the ventricular system. When the ICH is associated with oral anticoagulant use, the mortality rate is around 70%.[85] Overall the recurrence rate has been estimated at around 2.4% per year.[89] However, the risk in the elderly is higher[94] and figures of 15% per year for lobar bleeds, but only 2% per year for deep hemispheric bleeds have been found.[20] The association with CAA may explain why lobar bleeds are more likely to recur. The control of hypertension after the acute phase is associated with a reduction in recurrence rates.[81] If an underlying secondary cause is suspected, and the patient would be a surgical candidate, then a conventional or MR angiogram should be performed.

Subarachnoid haemorrhage

Subarachnoid haemorrhage (SAH) accounts for around 2–5% of all strokes, and ruptured intracranial aneurysms cause around 80% of SAH.[95] It is more common in women than men, and the mean age of onset is 55 years.[95] Risk factors for bleeding include hypertension, smoking, excessive alcohol intake and cocaine use.[95] The occurrence of intracranial aneurysms has a familial component due to the association with some genetic conditions (e.g. polycystic kidney disease and some connective tissue disorders).[95] The aneurysms are most likely to occur at arterial branching sites at, or close to, the circle of Willis (see Figure 5.3).

SAH should be suspected in patients with a sudden onset of severe headache ('worst ever'). The pain may be diffuse or localised. Additional suggestive features that may be present include neck pain, photophobia, nausea/vomiting and reduced consciousness. Sudden loss of consciousness may be the presenting feature. Focal neurological signs are occasionally present. A third nerve palsy can be caused by compression by an expanding, or bleeding, posterior communicating artery aneurysm.

When SAH is clinically suspected it is recommended that urgent CT scanning is obtained. When performed within 12 hours, this will detect around 95% of SAH. If the CT is negative, a lumbar puncture (LP) should be performed.[9] A period of at least 12 hours should have passed since the symptom onset to the time of the LP and spectrophotometry should be used to maximise the chance of detecting xanthochromia (the result of breakdown of blood cells in the cerebrospinal fluid (CSF) to form yellow bilirubin, which cannot be caused by a traumatic tap).[9]

Treatment

Acute BP control following SAH is often recommended in those with markedly elevated blood pressures, but this approach lacks randomised controlled trial evidence of benefit, and a target value has not been defined. RCP guidelines recommend the use of the anti-vasospastic agent nimodipine (a calcium channel blocker), in cases of SAH.[9] A Cochrane review suggested evidence of a benefit with 60 mg of nimodipine four-hourly.[96] A neurosurgical opinion should be sought and most patients will be transferred to a neurosurgical unit. When SAH is secondary to the rupture of an intracranial aneurysm, treatment of the aneurysm can reduce the probability of recurrent bleeding. A recent trial that compared open surgery with vessel clipping to endovascular embolisation with coiling for intracranial aneurysms that were anatomically suitable for either technique, found a survival benefit with the less invasive technique of coiling (death or dependency at one year: 24% vs 31%).[97] When there is a strong family history of SAH, or with a history of polycystic kidney disease, screening family members for aneurysms is probably indicated.

Prognosis

Aneurysmal SAH has a poor prognosis with a 50% fatality rate, and around one-third of survivors require long-term care.[95] Non-aneurysmal SAH has a better prognosis. Adverse prognostic indicators include a reduced Glasgow Coma Scale score at the time of admission, large volume of bleed and older age.[95] Common complications in the first two weeks after SAH, which worsen outcomes, include vasospasm, hydrocephalus and rebleeding.[95] Vasospasm has a peak incidence between five and 14 days after SAH and is usually only seen following aneurysmal bleeds. Hydrocephalus is more likely to develop in patients who have intra-ventricular extravasation of the bleed.

Subacute treatment of stroke

Stroke units

The nature of stroke units varies but the basic components are similar, being multidisciplinary rehabilitation delivered by specialist staff in a ward that is geo-graphically discrete from the rest of the hospital. In comparison to usual care, stroke units have been found to be associated with a reduction in one-year mortality (OR 0.83; 95% CI 0.69–0.98; $p<0.05$) and the combined outcome of death and institutionalisation (OR 0.75; 95% CI 0.65–0.87; $p<0.0001$) with no net increase in length of stay.[98] The benefits are still apparent in patients followed-up 10 years after their stroke.[99]

Rehabilitation

Stroke is a major cause of disability. Fortunately, almost always some, and oc-casionally complete, functional recovery is expected. After one year around two-thirds of the survivors of strokes will be functionally independent.[3] Rehabilitation is, clearly, a very important aspect of post-stroke recovery. It is discussed in Chapter 15.

Post-stroke nutrition

Malnutrition is a real concern for any elderly person admitted to hospital for a prolonged period. When this is complicated by dysphagia secondary to stroke, the risks are further elevated. The normal swallowing process and treatment methods are discussed on p 261. The recent publication of the FOOD trials (three separate randomised controlled trials evaluating post-stroke nutrition) has increased our understanding of this area.[100,101] They are discussed below under the relevant subheadings.

Nutritional supplements

In the FOOD trial of patients who were hospitalised following an acute stroke, but who were able to swallow normally, 4023 patients (mean age 71 years) were randomised to receive standard hospital meals either alone or with additional nutritional supplements.[100] No significant benefit was found in death or poor outcome with this intervention. However, only 8% of patients were deemed to be under-nourished at the start of the trial. This suggests that nutritional supplements should not be used routinely, but they may have a role in selected undernourished individuals.

Enteral tube feeding

The two common methods of enteral tube feeding are discussed below, followed by a review of the components of the FOOD trials that recruited dysphagic patients, which may guide clinical practice in this area.

- *Nasogastric* (NG) *tubes*: are usually easily inserted on hospital wards. They can be irritating to the patient's nasopharynx, and are prone to becoming dislodged (accidentally or deliberately). The maintenance of such tubes is more difficult in the significant number of individuals with associated acute confusional states.
- *Percutaneous endoscopic gastrostomy* (PEG) *tubes*: feeding tubes that are inserted through the stomach wall under endoscopic guidance (although alternative methods involving either radiologically guided or surgically placed tubes are occasionally used).[102] They have the advantage over NG tubes of not being irritating to the nasopharynx and generally being more comfortable for longer-term usage. The disadvantage is that they are invasive and need a minor surgical procedure to insert them. The most common reason for PEG insertion in the UK is for dysphagia following a stroke.

The insertion procedure itself is usually well tolerated and has a low complication rate (less than 2%).[103] However, in the hospitalised elderly there is a 30-day mortality rate of 24–28%, rising to 63% at one year.[104,105] Studies looking at patients admitted for elective PEG insertion have found lower mortality rates;[106] however, this is not applicable to those who are hospitalised following an acute stroke. Those at highest risk include patients with a history of aspiration pneumonia or an age over 75 years.[107] The presence of dementia is also an adverse predictive factor (*see* p 30). Complications related to the PEG tube commonly occurring in the year after insertion include obstruction of the tube (11%), infection (9%) and bleeding (7%) at the insertion site, leakage around the tube (4%) and peritonitis (2%).[106]

PEG tubes do not exclude the development of an aspiration pneumonia.[108] Patients continue to be at risk of aspirating oral secretions or regurgitated stomach contents. The best patient position for feeding and the optimal duration and frequency of feeds are unknown. Logic suggests that being upright during feeds may reduce the regurgitation risk compared to being recumbent. If so, feeds at discrete times when sitting upright out of bed may be better than prolonged slow feeds when reclining, especially overnight.

The FOOD trials for dysphagic patients

The FOOD trials had two further components that enrolled patients who were dysphagic following an acute stroke.[101] In both arms the patients were allowed to commence oral feeding if their swallow improved during the study period.

The first of these randomised 859 patients (mean age 76 years) to receive enteral tube feeding (PEG or NG) as soon as possible or to avoid enteral feeding for at least seven days (these patients received IV or subcutaneous (SC) fluids alone). Tube feeding was associated with a non-significant trend towards a reduction in absolute mortality of 5.8% (95% CI −0.8 to 12.5; $p = 0.09$) with a non-significant reduction in death or poor outcome (severe disability) of 1.2% (95% CI −4.2 to 6.6; $p = 0.7$). This suggests that early feeding may have a modest effect on improvement in mortality but is likely to increase the number of patients who survive with severe disability. The authors recommend that early tube feeding should be offered to dysphagic acute stroke patients.

The second FOOD trial in dysphagic acute stroke patients randomised 321 people (mean age 76 years) who were judged appropriate for enteral feeding to receive either a PEG or NG tube within three days of randomisation and continued for as long as practical. They found that PEG tubes were associated with a borderline significant increase in death or poor outcome, compared to NG feeding, of 7.8% (95% CI 0.0–15.8; $p = 0.05$). This suggests that, at least within the first few weeks of an acute stroke, NG feeding is preferable to PEG feeding. Of course, there may be patients in whom PEG insertion is a better option, for example due to intolerance of NG tubes.

Complications following stroke

Complicating conditions occurring whilst in hospital after an acute stroke are common. One study found a rate of 59%,[109] the most common being falls (22%), skin breaks (18%), urinary tract infections (UTI) (16%) and chest infections (12%). Depression and shoulder subluxation tend to occur later in the course of recovery.

Some degree of haemorrhagic transformation may be detected on follow-up brain imaging in around one-third of ischaemic strokes, but a far smaller number are symptomatic. It is thought to be more common after large-sized infarcts than smaller ones.

Thrombo-embolism

Estimates of the incidence of DVT and pulmonary embolus (PE) after stroke vary widely, perhaps reflecting differing diagnostic criteria. A UK hospital-based study reported a DVT rate of 3% when identified by case note review.[109] PEs may account for up to 20% of early deaths following stroke.[110]

Prophylaxis

When heparin was given following acute stroke, the increased rate of haemorrhagic complications negated any anti-thrombotic benefits.[48] Routine use of prophylactic anticoagulation is not recommended in post-stroke patients.[9]

Compression hosiery has been found to be beneficial in preventing thrombo-embolic complications after surgical intervention.[111] However, there are very few data regarding their use in the post-stroke population. Despite this, they are recommended in most stroke patients with reduced motor function of the legs.[9]

Treatment of DVT after intracerebral haemorrhage

An alternative approach in the prevention of a PE following a DVT is the use of a caval filter. Here a device is percutaneously inserted into the inferior vena cava to act as a filter preventing emboli travelling from the deep leg veins to the lungs. It is proposed that they may have a role in patients with contraindications to anticoagulation therapy (e.g. ICH). However, randomised controlled trial evidence of benefit is lacking. When they were assessed in conjunction with heparin for those at high risk of thrombo-embolic events, an early lower incidence of PE (1% vs 5% after 12 days) was offset by a higher late incidence of DVT (21% vs 12% after two years) compared to those without filters.[112] Thrombus formation on the filter is a recognised complication that may increase the risk of emboli. Some physicians advocate the use of anticoagulation, rather than filters, in those with DVT following ICH when the risk of re-bleeding is lowest (i.e. with non-lobar ICH (see p 116)).[113]

Post-stroke depression

Depression after stroke is common. Screening for it may be made difficult by cognitive changes such as dysphasia. Some alternative rating scales have been developed for such patients.[114] The selective serotonin reuptake inhibitor (SSRI) citalopram has been found to be effective in the management of post-stroke depression.[115] However, a significant number of cases will spontaneously resolve in the first two months. Depression is discussed in more detail in Chapter 3.

Pain

Central post-stroke pain is a form of neuropathic pain occurring in the affected side of the body. It should be treated in the same way as other neuropathic pains (see p 285). Shoulder pain is also seen following stroke. Shoulder–hand syndrome is autonomically mediated (reflex sympathetic dystrophy). Here the pain may be associated with swelling and changes in colour or temperature of the affected arm. An alternative cause is shoulder subluxation related to motor weakness. This can largely be prevented by appropriate patient positioning/support and careful use of handling techniques to avoid strain on the shoulder joint.

Other problems

Falls, incontinence, pressure ulcers, dementia and delirium are all common problems following a stroke. They are discussed in detail within the relevant chapters.

Driving

Currently, in the UK, drivers of standard vehicles are required to stop driving for one month after a stroke. They may resume driving after this time if a satisfactory recovery has been made. They only need to inform the DVLA if there is a persisting deficit beyond one month. An exception to this rule is if recurrent TIAs have occurred within a short time interval, in which case the DVLA should be informed. Full guidance is available at the DVLA website (www.dvla.gov.uk/at_a_glance/ch1_neurological.htm). As with any change in health status, the driver should inform his or her insurance company of their diagnosis. Links to driving regulation resources in countries other than the UK are shown in Box 1.2.

Less common causes of stroke

The following text discusses some of the less common causes of stroke. Most are very rare in the elderly but more frequently a cause of stroke in younger people.

Approximately 1% of strokes occur in people aged 15–45 years.[65] The term 'cryptogenic stroke' is used to describe stroke where there is no obvious underlying cause. Relatively, this is a much more common occurrence in younger people (up to 40% of such patients).[65]

A review of the causes of stroke in the young found that the most common definite causes were: carotid or vertebrobasilar artery dissection (19%) or atheroma (8%); cardio-embolic sources (5% – mainly AF or bacterial endocarditis); vascular inflammation (2%); and cerebral autosomal dominant arteriopathy with sub-cortical infarcts and leukoencephalopathy (CADASIL) (1%, *see below*).[65] These strokes had a mortality rate of 4.5% in the first year. The stroke recurrence rate was around 1% per year.

Arterial dissection

Arterial dissection is, essentially, a tear in the artery wall. It can cause a stroke by two mechanisms. First, blood can accumulate between the arterial layers resulting in stenosis; second, the tear may expose the circulating blood to thrombogenic underlying tissues, resulting in clot formation and/or subsequent embolisation. Usually it is triggered by some form of mild trauma, although the actual incident may not be recalled. This may vary from major accidents to trivial occurrences such as a violent cough or sneeze. Spontaneous events are more likely in those with underlying connective tissue disorders. Dissection may account for around 2% of strokes overall and perhaps 20% of those in younger age groups.[116]

It should be suspected when pain at the side (carotid) or back of the head (vertebrobasilar) is a major feature just before the onset of focal symptoms. Other clues are a history of trauma and the occurrence in younger people without clear vascular risk factors. A partial Horner syndrome (miosis and ptosis only) is a clinical feature of carotid dissection due to the close anatomical association of sympathetic fibres with the internal carotid artery. Dissection here may also result in lower cranial nerve palsies.

Currently, diagnosis is most frequently confirmed by MR angiography.

It is believed that embolisation of thrombus is the most common mechanism leading to cerebral ischaemia. For this reason some physicians advocate the use of anticoagulation with an INR of 2–3 for three to six months, although there are no randomised trials demonstrating a benefit with this approach.[116] An alternative option is the use of antiplatelet agents.

Patent foramen ovale

A patent foramen ovale (PFO) occurs in around 27% of the adult population.[117] Essentially, it is a hole between the right and left atria (*see* Figure 5.10) and is a normal component of the fetal circulation that usually closes at the time of birth. It is speculated that a PFO could allow a venous embolism to pass from the right to the left side of the heart and cause a stroke (a paradoxical embolism). This may be more likely to occur at times when right atrial pressure is elevated and the pressure gradient with the left atrium is reversed, for example during straining.[118] The role of PFO in the genesis of stroke remains controversial.

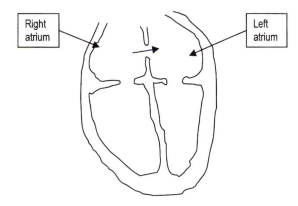

Figure 5.10   Patent foramen ovale.

Retrospective reviews of echocardiography results have found an elevated detection of PFO among those under the age of 55 who have sustained a stroke compared to control subjects (40% vs 10%).[119] However, the investigators were not blinded to the patients' past histories and indications for performing the scans varied between groups. Against PFO being a risk factor for stroke is the fact that patients with a cryptogenic stroke are rarely found to have a venous source of embolism. However, this has been seen with confirmed cases of pulmonary embolism.

One meta-analysis of case–control studies supported the idea that the presence of a PFO increases the risk of stroke in patients below the age of 55 but an association was less clear in older subjects.[120] However, a more recent meta-analysis did not find an increased stroke risk associated with PFO status.[121] Some studies have suggested that the combination of a PFO with an atrial septal aneurysm confers a particularly high risk,[122] but other studies have not supported this idea.[123]

Even if a PFO is thought to be causative in stroke, there is little trial evidence to define the best management strategy and so it remains a matter of some debate.[124] The results of studies of the use of aspirin or warfarin are conflicting. Perhaps the best currently available evidence comes from a subgroup of the Warfarin–Aspirin Recurrent Stroke Study (WARSS) who underwent TOE.[123] Patients in this study were randomly allocated to warfarin or aspirin. The subgroup contained 630 patients (mean age 59, range 30–85 years), 34% of whom were found to have a PFO. After two years there was no significant difference in stroke or TIA rates between the group with and that without a PFO. Nor was there any difference in events between those allocated to warfarin or aspirin. A recent meta-analysis of trials also found no difference in efficacy with aspirin or warfarin, but increased rates of bleeding complications in those allocated to anticoagulation.[121]

A percutaneous technique of mechanical PFO closure has been developed, but there are no randomised controlled trials demonstrating its efficacy at reducing the risk of stroke.[124] The risk of recurrent stroke or TIA in patients with a PFO treated with warfarin or aspirin has been found to be between 3.4% and 3.8% per year.[125] One series found a similar annual recurrence rate of 3.4% following percutaneous closure.[125] Serious complications occur in around 1.5% of people undergoing the procedure. They include major haemorrhage, cardiac tamponade, pulmonary embolism and death. The recruitment of sufficient patients to perform suitably powered randomised controlled trials in this area is in part hampered by the trend for the open-label insertion of devices.[126]

Until better evidence becomes available, based on the risks of causing harm with the proposed therapies, aspirin seems to be the current safest option. If a paradoxical embolism is suspected, a source should be searched for; clearly, if identified a course of warfarin may then be appropriate. Risk factors for thrombo-embolism (e.g. oral contraceptive use and the thrombophilias) should be addressed. The role of percutaneous closure will remain unclear until randomised controlled trial evidence becomes available.

Other cardiac sources of emboli

AF is by far the most common cardiac source of emboli. Less common alternatives include thrombus formed on a less mobile ventricle wall following an acute MI, valvular vegetations secondary to infective endocarditis, and thrombus formed on the surface of atrial myxomas.

Vasculitis

The most common vasculitis causing cerebral ischaemia in the UK is giant cell arteritis (GCA). This is seen only in those over the age of 50 years. It is usually associated with non-specific symptoms, such as fatigue, myalgia and weight loss. Less common alternative vasculitides include systemic lupus erythematosus (SLE). When suspected, an ESR and auto-antibody studies should be performed. In the case of GCA, a temporal artery biopsy may confirm the diagnosis. Characteristically it responds very rapidly to high-dose steroids.

Arteriovenous malformations

Arteriovenous malformations (AVMs) are congenital abnormalities of blood vessels that result in the formation of an abnormal coil of arteries and veins. The basic anatomy of an AVM is shown in Figure 5.11. There are no capillaries between the larger vessels, resulting in direct shunting of blood from the arterial to the venous system. They are estimated to have a prevalence of less than 0.01% of the total population.[127]

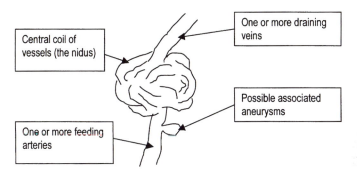

Figure 5.11   The basic anatomy of an ateriovenous malformation (AVM).

AVMs may be asymptomatic or produce symptoms. Over half present with haemorrhagic stroke, and around a quarter with seizures.[128] Headache and progressive neurological deficit are less common presentations. They appear to be more likely to cause symptoms in the young with a mean age of onset of 31 years.[127] They may account for around 3% of strokes, and around one-third of ICH in people below the age of 45 years.[129]

The annual risk of haemorrhage has been estimated to be around 2–3%.[128] The presence of associated aneurysms and a history of hypertension are thought to increase bleeding risk. The mortality with such events is between 10% and 20%.[127] However, the natural history is poorly understood, in part due to the trend toward early intervention.

Occasionally there are clinical signs of AVMs. These include overlying skin pigmentation (the Sturge–Weber syndrome), a cranial bruit or evidence of associated hereditary haemorrhagic telangiectasia. They may be seen on CT scanning (especially with contrast) but are more readily detected on MRI images. Arteriography may provide more anatomical and functional information.

Intervention is usually undertaken on the premise that it will reduce future bleeding risk. Alternative indications include the treatment of intractable seizures and progressive neurological impairment. Due to the lower cumulative lifetime risk in the elderly, intervention is rarely undertaken. Treatment options include microsurgical techniques, endovascular embolisation and radiosurgery.[127] The larger and deeper the AVM, the higher the complication rate. There are no randomised controlled trials to evaluate the benefits of interventional techniques compared to a conservative approach.

Mitochondrial disorders

Mitochondria were originally symbiotic bacteria that migrated into animal cells with the advantage of being able to perform aerobic metabolism. They possess their own DNA and are inherited by division of the mitochondria contained within the maternal egg cell. Various disorders have been described relating to mutations in the mitochondrial DNA.[130] One of these is 'mitochondrial encephalomyopathy, lactic acidosis and stroke-like episodes' (MELAS).

This disorder is very rare and usually presents in children or young adults with focal neurological deficits, seizures and progressive cognitive impairment. There may be an associated history of exercise intolerance, deafness, diabetes, migraine and/or learning disability. Fasting plasma and CSF lactate levels are elevated. Muscle biopsy may demonstrate ragged red fibres or abnormal mitochondria. There is no treatment for this condition.

CADASIL

Cerebral autosomal dominant arteriopathy with subcortical infarcts and leuko-encephalopathy (CADASIL) is a very rare (autosomal-dominantly) inherited disorder. It presents with migraine attacks and cerebrovascular events in early adulthood, and leads to a progressive cognitive impairment. Death usually occurs prior to the age of 60 years. It is caused by mutations in the notch 3 gene located on chromosome 19, which lead to abnormalities in the structure of small blood vessels. Vascular lesions will be seen on brain imaging. Blood vessel abnormalities can sometimes be detected in tissue samples from skin or muscle biopsies.

Differential diagnoses of stroke

Migraine

The classic presentation of migraine (an aura, particularly flashing/zigzag lights, followed by headache) is easily distinguished from stroke. The onset of symptoms is also more gradual, worsening over several minutes. There may be associated nausea and photophobia. Occasionally atypical migraines without headache can occur. Rarely a migraine may be followed by prolonged neurological symptoms due to cerebral infarction thought to be secondary to vascular spasm.

Seizures

Seizures may cause symptoms that are mistaken for stroke. Following an ictal episode there may be poor recollection of the event and there may also be an associated transient weakness in the affected limbs (Todd paresis). A further complicating factor is that some strokes will provoke seizures at their onset. In patients with no history of stroke, the onset of seizures after the age of 60 is associated with an increased risk of cerebrovascular disease.[131]

Symptoms of seizures tend to be 'positive' – resulting in additional phenomena such as jerking movements or hallucinations, compared to stroke, that tends to cause 'negative' symptoms – loss of functions such as sensation or power. An MRI scan should be performed in patients with suspected seizures to exclude a structural lesion that may not be detected on CT scanning.

Brain tumours

Classically, brain tumours cause slowly progressive neurological deficits that can be easily distinguished from strokes by careful history. It is reported that transient neurological symptoms can occur. Possible explanations for these include partial seizures, vascular 'steal' phenomena or haemorrhage into the tumour with compression of surrounding tissues. The clinical finding of papilloedema makes the diagnosis more likely to be a tumour than a stroke. They are usually detected on CT scanning – especially when contrast is used and peripheral enhancement is seen. MRI scans may provide more information if the diagnosis is in doubt.

Subdural haematoma

Occasionally, subdural haematomas can cause focal neurological symptoms. They are more common in those who take warfarin, the elderly and alcoholics (probably due to brain shrinkage). There may be no history of head trauma. The onset is usually subacute. Headache is commonly associated. There may also be impaired consciousness, confusion and/or a fluctuating course. The haemorrhage is usually seen on CT scanning, but difficulty may arise between one and three weeks from the onset when the blood may appear isodense to surrounding brain tissue.

Cerebral venous thrombosis

Venous thrombosis can occur in the intracranial veins or venous sinuses. This can result in venous infarction and associated haemorrhage. The annual incidence has been estimated to be between three and four cases per million, and the majority of cases occur in women of child-bearing age.[132] There is a spectrum of clinical presentations, ranging from a rapidly declining conscious level to slowly progressive lesions that mimic cerebral tumours or abscesses.[133] The majority of patients will have headache and 40% develop seizures.[132] Intracranial hypertension may be present with papilloedema and associated brief visual disturbances. Risk factors include the use of oral contraceptives and pregnancy (especially the third trimester and immediately post-birth). Minor cranial or venous trauma (including central venous cannulation and lumbar punctures) can precipitate events.[132]

Cavernous sinus thrombosis is usually precipitated by infections in the paranasal sinuses or orbit.[132] It is associated with proptosis, chemosis and oculomotor palsies.

Central venous thrombosis should be considered in younger patients with atypical headache or stroke-like symptoms in the absence of vascular risk factors.[132] Lesions may be seen on CT scanning (haemorrhagic infarcts that may be multiple and not confined to arterial territories), but the advent of MRI and MR venography has improved its recognition.[132]

Anticoagulant treatment, initially with heparin and then warfarin (INR 2–3) for at least six months, is usually advised. This is based on data from several small randomised trials and larger non-randomised series.[132] Over 80% of patients will have a favourable outcome.[132]

Transient global amnesia

Transient global amnesia (TGA) is a condition in which there is a loss of memory lasting less than 24 hours. During the event subjects are able to function normally and show no other evidence of abnormality. The mechanism is unknown. The idea that it could be a variant of cerebrovascular disease has been suggested but vascular risk factors are not strongly associated and prognosis is far better than that of individuals who have sustained a TIA.[134] Alternative explanations include a form of migraine or epilepsy.

Other differentials

Metabolic disorders are occasionally mistaken for stroke, for example hypo/hyper-glycaemia and hyponatraemia. They are likely to have a subacute onset and be associated with cognitive impairment. Cerebral abscesses may cause a focal neuro-logical deficit, but would usually be of subacute onset and associated with delirium and fever. Psychiatric disorders (e.g. conversion reactions) may have a presentation mimicking stroke. Clues to the diagnosis include a past psychiatric history, young age at onset, inconsistent history, no hard neurological signs and normal brain imaging.

Further reading

Warlow CP, Dennis MS, van Gijn J et al. Stroke: a practical guide to management, 2nd ed. Oxford: Blackwell Science, 2001.

References

1 Rothwell PM, Coull AJ, Fairhead JF et al. Population-based study of event-rate, incidence, case fatality, and mortality for all acute vascular events in all arterial territories (Oxford Vascular Study). Lancet, 2005; 366: 1773–1783.
2 Wolfe CDA. The impact of stroke. Br Med Bulletin, 2000; 56(2): 275–286.
3 Bamford J, Sandercock P, Dennis M et al. A prospective study of acute cerebrovascular disease in the community: the Oxfordshire Community Stroke Project –1981–86. J Neurol Neurosurg Psy, 1990; 53: 16–22.
4 Libman RB, Wirkowski E, Alvir J et al. Conditions that mimic stroke in the emergency department: implications for acute stroke trials. Arch Neurol, 1995; 52: 1119–1122.
5 Foerch C, Misselwitz B, Sitzer M et al. Difference in recognition of right and left hemispheric stroke. Lancet, 2005; 366: 392–393.
6 Halligan PW, Marshall JC and Wade DT. Visuospatial neglect: underlying factors and test sensitivity. Lancet, 1989; 2(8668): 908–911.
7 Hankey GJ and Warlow CP. Symptomatic carotid ischaemic events: safest and most cost effective way of selecting patients for angiography, before carotid endarterectomy. BMJ, 1990; 300: 1485–1491.
8 Keir S, Wardlaw JM, Sandercock PAG et al. Antithrombotic therapy for patients with any form of intracranial haemorrhage: a systematic review of the available controlled studies. Cerebrovasc Dis, 2002; 14: 197–206.
9 Intercollegiate Stroke Working Party. National Clinical Guidelines for Stroke, 2nd ed. (Available at: www.rcplondon.ac.uk/pubs/books/stroke/stroke_guidelines_2ed.pdf)
10 Wardlaw JM and Farrall AJ. Diagnosis of stroke on neuroimaging: 'scan all immediately' strategy improves outcomes and reduces cost. BMJ, 2004; 328: 655–656.

11 Wardlaw JM, Keir SL and Dennis MS. The impact of delays in computed tomography of the brain on the accuracy of diagnosis and subsequent management in patients with minor stroke. *J Neurol Neurosurg Psy,* 2003; **74**: 77–81.

12 Fiebach JB, Schellinger PD, Jansen O *et al.* CT and diffusion-weighted MR imaging in randomized order: diffusion-weighted imaging results in higher accuracy and lower inter-rater variability in the diagnosis of hyperacute ischemic stroke. *Stroke,* 2002; **33**: 2206–2210.

13 Daniel WG, Erbel R, Kasper W *et al.* Safety of transesophageal echocardiography: a multi-center survey of 10,419 examinations. *Circulation,* 1991; **83**: 817–821.

14 Bamford J, Sandercock P, Dennis M *et al.* Classification and natural history of clinically identifiable subtypes of cerebral infarction. *Lancet,* 1991; **337**: 1521–1526.

15 Tatu L, Moulin T, Bogousslavsky J *et al.* Arterial territories of human brain: brainstem and cerebellum. *Neurology,* 1996; **47**: 1125–1135.

16 Savitz SI and Caplan LR. Vertebrobasilar disease. *NEJM,* 2005; **352**(25): 2618–2626.

17 Shin H, Yoo K, Chang HM *et al.* Bilateral intracranial vertebral artery disease in the New England Medical Center Posterior Circulation Registry. *Arch Neurol,* 1999; **56**: 1353–1358.

18 SHEP Cooperative Research Group. Prevention of stroke by antihypertensive drug treatment in older persons with isolated systolic hypertension. *JAMA,* 1991; **265**(24): 3255–3264.

19 Saxena R, Lewis S, Berge E *et al.* Risk of early death and recurrent stroke and effect of heparin in 3169 patients with acute ischemic stroke and atrial fibrillation in the international stroke trial. *Stroke,* 2001; **32**: 2333–2337.

20 Eckman MH, Rosand J, Knudsen KA *et al.* Can patients be anticoagulated after intracerebral haemorrhage? A decision analysis. *Stroke,* 2003; **34**: 1710–1716.

21 Yaggi HK, Concato J, Kernan WN *et al.* Obstructive sleep apnea as a risk factor for stroke and death. *NEJM,* 2005; **353**(19): 2034–2041.

22 Koudstaal PJ, van Gijn J, Frenken CWGM *et al.* TIA, RIND, minor stroke: a continuum, or different subgroups? *J Neurol Neurosurg Psy,* 1992; **55**: 95–97.

23 Awad I, Modic M, Little JR *et al.* Focal parenchymal lesions in transient ischemic attacks: correlation of computed tomography and magnetic resonance imaging. *Stroke,* 1986; **17**(3): 399–403.

24 National Institute of Neurological Disorders and Stroke rt-PA Stroke Study Group. Tissue plasminogen activator for acute ischaemic stroke. *NEJM,* 1995; **333**(24): 1581–1587.

25 Hill MD and Buchan AM. Thrombolysis for acute ischaemic stroke: results of the Canadian Alteplase for Stroke Effectiveness Study. *Canadian Med Assoc J,* 2005; **172**(10): 1307–1312.

26 Cocho D, Belvis R, Marti-Fabregas J *et al.* Reasons for exclusion from thrombolytic therapy following acute ischemic stroke. *Neurology,* 2005; **64**(4): 719–720.

27 Wardlaw JM, del Zoppo G, Yamaguchi T *et al.* Thrombolysis for acute ischaemic stroke. Cochrane Database Syst Rev 2003, Issue 3. Art. No.: CD000213. DOI: 10.1002/14651858. CD000213.

28 Albers GW, Amarenco P, Easton JD *et al.* Antithrombotic and thrombolytic therapy for ischemic stroke: the Seventh ACCP Conference on Antithrombotic and Thrombolytic Therapy. *Chest,* 2004; **126**(Suppl.): 483S–512S.

29 Merino JG, Silver B, Wong E *et al.* Extending tissue plasminogen activator use to community and rural stroke patients. *Stroke,* 2002; **33**(1): 141–146.

30 California Acute Stroke Pilot Registry (CASPR) Investigators. Prioritizing interventions to improve rates of thrombolysis for ischemic stroke. *Neurology,* 2005; **64**(4): 654–659.

31 Wang Y, Lim LL, Levi C *et al.* Influence of admission body temperature on stroke mortality. *Stroke,* 2000; **31**(2): 404–409.

32 Kammersgaard LP, Jorgensen HS, Rungby JA *et al.* Admission body temperature predicts long-term mortality after acute stroke: the Copenhagen Stroke Study. *Stroke,* 2002; **33**(7): 1759–1762.

33 Williams LS, Rotich J, Qi R *et al.* Effects of admission hyperglycemia on mortality and costs in acute ischemic stroke. *Neurology,* 2002; **59**: 67–71.

34 Gray CS, Hildreth AJ, Alberti GKMM *et al.* Poststroke hyperglycemia: natural history and immediate management. *Stroke,* 2004; **35**(1): 122–126.

35 Ronning OM and Guldvog B. Should stroke victims routinely receive supplemental oxygen? A quasi-randomized controlled trial. *Stroke,* 1999; **30**(10): 2033–2037.

36 Bhalla A, Sankaralingam S, Dundas R *et al.* Influence of raised plasma osmolality on clinical outcome after acute stroke. *Stroke,* 2000; **31**(9): 2043–2048.

37 Leonardi-Bee J, Bath P, Phillips SJ *et al.* Blood pressure and clinical outcomes in the International Stroke Trial. *Stroke,* 2002; **33**(5): 1315–1320.

38 Robinson TG and Potter JF. Blood pressure in acute stroke. *Age Ageing,* 2004; **33**(1): 6–12.

39 Morfis L, Schwartz RS, Poulos R *et al.* Blood pressure changes in acute cerebral infarction and hemorrhage. *Stroke,* 1997; **28**(7): 1401–1405.

40 Castillo J, Leira R, Garcia MM *et al.* Blood pressure decrease during the acute phase of ischemic stroke is associated with brain injury and poor stroke outcome. *Stroke,* 2004; **35**(2): 520–526.

41 The COSSACS Trial Group. COSSACS (Continue or Stop post-Stroke Antihypertensives Collaborative Study): rationale and design. *J Hypertension,* 2005; **23**(2): 455–458.

42 The CHHIPS Trial Group. CHHIPS (Controlling Hypertension and Hypotension Immediately Post-Stroke) Pilot Trial: rationale and design. *J Hypertension,* 2005; **23**(3): 649–655.

43 Patrono C, Coller B, Fitzgerald GA *et al.* Platelet-active drugs: the relationships among dose, effectiveness, and side effects. *Chest,* 2004; **126**(3 Suppl.): 234–264S.

44 Patrono C, Garcia Rodriguez LA, Landolfi R *et al.* Low-dose aspirin for the prevention of atherothrombosis. *NEJM,* 2005; **353**(22): 2373–2383.

45 Antithrombotic Trialists' Collaboration. Collaborative meta-analysis of randomised trials of antiplatelet therapy for prevention of death, myocardial infarction, and stroke in high risk patients. *BMJ,* 2002; **324**: 71–86.

46 He J, Whelton PK, Vu B *et al.* Aspirin and risk of hemorrhagic stroke: a meta-analysis of randomized controlled trials. *JAMA,* 1998; **280**(22): 1930–1935.

47 CAST (Chinese Acute Stroke Trial) Collaborative Group. CAST: randomised placebo-controlled trial of early aspirin use in 20,000 patients with acute ischaemic stroke. *Lancet,* 1997; **349**: 1641–1649.

48 International Stroke Trial Collaborative Group. The International Stroke Trial (IST): a randomised trial of aspirin, subcutaneous heparin, both, or neither among 19,435 patients with acute ischaemic stroke. *Lancet,* 1997; **349**: 1569–1581.

49 Diener H, Cunha L, Forbes C *et al.* European Stroke Prevention Study 2. Dipyridamole and acetylsalicylic acid in the secondary prevention of stroke. *J Neurological Sciences,* 1996; **143**: 1–13.

50 The ESPRIT Study Group. Aspirin plus dipyridamole versus aspirin alone after cerebral ischaemia of arterial origin (ESPRIT): randomised controlled trial. *Lancet,* 2006; **367**(9523): 1665–1673.

51 National Institute for Clinical Excellence. Clopidogrel and modified release dipyridamole in the prevention of occlusive vascular events. May 2005. (Available at: www.nice.org.uk/pdf/TA090guidance.pdf)

52 CAPRIE Steering Committee. A randomised, blinded, trial of clopidogrel versus aspirin in patients at risk of ischaemic events (CAPRIE). *Lancet,* 1996; **348**: 1329–1339.

53 Bhatt DL, Fox KAA, Hacke W *et al.* Clopidogrel and aspirin versus aspirin alone for prevention of atherothrombotic events. *NEJM,* 2006; **354**(16): 1706–1717.

54 Chan FKL, Ching JYL, Hung LCT *et al.* Clopidogrel versus aspirin and esomeprazole to prevent recurrent ulcer bleeding. *NEJM,* 2005; **352**(3): 238–244.

55 The Clopidogrel in Unstable Angina to Prevent Recurrent Events Trial Investigators. Effects of clopidogrel in addition to aspirin in patients with acute coronary syndromes without ST-segment elevation. *NEJM,* 2001; **345**(7): 494–502.

56 COMMIT (ClOpidogrel and Metoprolol in Myocardial Infarction Trial) collaborative group. Addition of clopidogrel to aspirin in 45,852 patients with acute myocardial infarction: randomised placebo-controlled trial. *Lancet,* 2005; **366**: 1607–1621.

57 Diener H, Bogousslavsky J, Brass LM *et al.* Aspirin and clopidogrel compared with clopidogrel alone after recent ischaemic stroke or transient ischaemic attack in high-risk patients (MATCH): randomised, double-blind, placebo-controlled trial. *Lancet,* 2004; **364**: 331–337.

58 Chimowitz MI, Lynn MJ, Howlett-Smith H *et al.* Comparison of warfarin and aspirin for symptomatic intracranial arterial stenosis. *NEJM,* 2005; **352**(13): 1305–1316.

59 Mohr JP, Thompson JLP, Lazar RM *et al.* A comparison of warfarin and aspirin for the prevention of recurrent ischemic stroke. *NEJM,* 2001; **345**(20): 1444–1451.

60 Berge E, Abdelnoor M, Nakstad PH *et al.* Low molecular weight heparin versus aspirin in patients with acute ischaemic stroke and atrial fibrillation: a double-blind randomised study. *Lancet*, 2000; **355**: 1205–1210.

61 Cholesterol Treatment Trialists' (CTT) Collaborators. Efficacy and safety of cholesterol-lowering treatment: prospective meta-analysis of data from 90,056 participants in 14 randomised trials of statins. *Lancet*, 2005; **366**: 1267–1278.

62 Heart Protection Study Collaborative Group. Effects of cholesterol-lowering with simvastatin on stroke and other major vascular events in 20,536 people with cerebrovascular disease or other high-risk conditions. *Lancet*, 2004; **363**: 757–767.

63 PROGRESS Collaborative Group. Randomised trial of a perindopril-based blood-pressure-lowering regimen among 6105 individuals with previous stroke or transient ischaemic attack. *Lancet*, 2001; **358**: 1033–1041.

64 Joint British Societies' guidelines on prevention of cardiovascular disease in clinical practice. *Heart*, 2005; **91**(Suppl. V): v1–v52.

65 Leys D, Bandu L, Henon H *et al.* Clinical outcome in 287 consecutive young adults (15 to 45 years) with ischemic stroke. *Neurology*, 2002; **59**: 26–33.

66 Schroeder SA. What to do with a patient who smokes. *JAMA*, 2005; **294**(4): 482–487.

67 Peto R, Boreham J, Lopez AD *et al.* Mortality from tobacco in developed countries: indirect estimation from national vital statistics. *Lancet*, 1992; **339**: 1268–1278.

68 Hughes JR, Stead LF and Lancaster T. Antidepressants for smoking cessation. Cochrane Database Syst Rev 2004, Issue 4. Art. No.: CD000031. DOI: 10.1002/14651858.CD000031.pub2.

69 Silagy C, Lancaster T, Stead L *et al.* Nicotine replacement therapy for smoking cessation. Cochrane Database Syst Rev 2004, Issue 3. Art. No.: CD000146. DOI: 10.1002/14651858.CD000146.pub2.

70 Stead LF, Lancaster T and Perera R. Telephone counselling for smoking cessation. Cochrane Database Syst Rev 2003, Issue 1. Art. No.: CD002850. DOI: 10.1002/14651858.CD002850.

71 Chaturvedi S, Bruno A, Feasby T *et al.* Carotid endarterectomy – an evidence-based review: report of the Therapeutics and Technology Assessment Subcommittee of the American Academy of Neurology. *Neurology*, 2005; **65**: 794–801.

72 North American Symptomatic Carotid Endarterectomy Trial Collaborators. Beneficial effect of carotid endarterectomy in symptomatic patients with high-grade carotid stenosis. *NEJM*, 1991; **325**(7): 445–453.

73 Barnett HJM, Taylor DW, Eliasziw M *et al.* Benefit of carotid endarterectomy in patients with symptomatic moderate or severe stenosis. *NEJM*, 1998; **339**(20): 1415–1425.

74 European Carotid Surgery Trialists' Collaborative Group. Randomised trial of endarterectomy for recently symptomatic carotid stenosis: final results of the MRC European Carotid Surgery Trial (ECST). *Lancet*, 1998; **351**: 1379–1387.

75 Rothwell PM, Eliasziw M, Gutnikov SA *et al.* Endarterectomy for symptomatic carotid stenosis in relation to clinical subgroups and timing of surgery. *Lancet*, 2004; **363**: 915–924.

76 Yadav JS, Wholey MH, Kuntz RE *et al.* Protected carotid-artery stenting versus endarterectomy in high-risk patients. *NEJM*, 2004; **351**(15): 1493–1501.

77 Mas J, Chatellier G, Beyssen B *et al.* Endarterectomy versus stenting in patients with symptomatic severe carotid stenosis. *NEJM*, 2006; **355**(16): 1660–1671.

78 Coull AJ, Lovett JK and Rothwell PM. Population based study of early risk of stroke after transient ischaemic attack or minor stroke: implications for public education and organisation of services. *BMJ*, 2004; **328**: 326.

79 van Wijk I, Kapple LJ, van Gijn J *et al.* Long-term survival and vascular event risk after transient ischaemic attack or minor ischaemic stroke: a cohort study. *Lancet*, 2005; **365**: 2098–2104.

80 Rothwell PM, Giles MF, Flossmann E *et al.* A simple score (ABCD) to identify individuals at high early risk of stroke after transient ischaemic attack. *Lancet*, 2005; **366**: 29–36.

81 Qureshi AI, Tuhrim S, Broderick JP *et al.* Spontaneous intracerebral hemorrhage. *NEJM*, 2001; **344**(19): 1450–1460.

82 Knudsen KA, Rosand J, Karluk D *et al.* Clinical diagnosis of cerebral amyloid angiopathy: validation of the Boston criteria. *Neurology*, 2001; **56**: 537–539.

83 Woo D, Sauerbeck LR, Kissela BM *et al.* Genetic and environmental risk factors for intra-cerebral hemorrhage: preliminary results of a population-based study. *Stroke,* 2002; **33**(5): 1190–1196.

84 Brott T, Broderick J, Kothari R *et al.* Early hemorrhage growth in patients with intracerebral hemorrhage. *Stroke,* 1997; **28**: 1–5.

85 Steiner T, Rosand J and Diringer M. Intracerebral hemorrhage associated with oral antico-agulant therapy: current practices and unresolved questions. *Stroke,* 2006; **37**(1): 256–262.

86 Mayer SA, Brun NC, Bergtrup K *et al.* Recombinant activated factor VII for acute intracer-ebral hemorrhage. *NEJM,* 2005; **352**(8): 777–785.

87 Cartmill M, Dolan G, Byrne JL *et al.* Prothrombin complex concentrate for oral anticoagulant reversal in neurosurgical emergencies. *Br J Neurosurg,* 2000; **14**(5): 458–461.

88 Hankey JP. Warfarin reversal. *J Clin Pathology,* 2004; **57**: 1132–1139.

89 Bailey RD, Hart RG, Benavente O *et al.* Recurrent brain hemorrhage is more frequent than ischemic stroke after intracranial hemorrhage. *Neurology,* 2001; **56**: 773–777.

90 Wani M, Nga E and Navaratnasingham R. Should a patient with primary intracerebral haemorrhage receive antiplatelets or anticoagulant therapy? *BMJ,* 2005; **331**: 439–442.

91 Ananthasubramaniam K, Beattie JN, Rosman HS *et al.* How safely and for how long can warfarin therapy be withheld in prosthetic valve patients hospitalized with a major hemorrhage? *Chest,* 2001; **119**(2): 478–484.

92 Shah N and Dawson SL. Intracerebral haemorrhage, prosthetic heart valve and anti-coagulation. *J R Soc Med,* 2004; **97**(3): 129–130.

93 Mendelow AD, Gregson BA, Fernandes HM *et al.* Early surgery versus initial conservative treatment in patients with spontaneous supratentorial intracerebral haematomas in the International Surgical Trial in Intracerebral Haemorrhage (STICH): a randomised trial. *Lancet,* 2005; **365**: 387–397.

94 Vermeer SE, Algra A, Franke CL *et al.* Long-term prognosis after recovery from primary intracerebral hemorrhage. *Neurology,* 2002; **59**: 205–209.

95 Suarez JI, Tarr RW and Selman WR. Aneurysmal subarachnoid haemorrhage. *NEJM,* 2006; **354**: 387–396.

96 Rinkel GJE, Feigin VL, Algra A *et al.* Calcium antagonists for aneurysmal subarachnoid haemorrhage. Cochrane Database Syst Rev 2005, Issue 1. Art. No.: CD000277. DOI: 10.1002/14651858.CD000277.pub2.

97 Molyneux AJ, Kerr RSC, Yu L *et al.* International subarachnoid aneurysm trial (ISAT) of neurosurgical clipping versus endovascular coiling of 2143 patients with ruptured intra-cranial aneurysm: a randomised comparison of effects on survival, dependency, seizures, rebleeding, subgroups, and aneurysm occlusion. *Lancet,* 2005; **366**: 807–819.

98 Stroke Trialists' Collaboration. Collaborative systematic review of the randomised trials of organised inpatient (stroke unit) care after stroke. *BMJ,* 1997; **314**: 1151–1159.

99 Drummond AER, Pearson B, Lincoln NB *et al.* Ten year follow-up of a randomised controlled trial of care in a stroke rehabilitation unit. *BMJ,* 2005; **331**: 491–492.

100 The FOOD Trial Collaboration. Routine oral nutritional supplementation for stroke patients in hospital (FOOD): a multicentre randomised controlled trial. *Lancet,* 2005; **365**: 755–763.

101 The FOOD Trial Collaboration. Effect of timing and method of enteral tube feeding for dysphagic stroke patients (FOOD): a multicentre randomised controlled trial. *Lancet,* 2005; **365**: 764–772.

102 Pennington C. To PEG or not to PEG. *Clin Med,* 2002; **2**(3): 250–255.

103 Dharmarajan TS, Unnikrishnan D and Pitchumoni CS. Percutaneous endoscopic gas-trostomy and outcome in dementia. *Am J Gastroent,* 2001; **96**(9): 2256–2263.

104 Sanders DS, Carter MJ, D'Silva J *et al.* Survival analysis in percutaneous endoscopic gastrostomy: a worse outcome in patients with dementia. *Am J Gatroent,* 2000; **95**: 1472–1475.

105 Grant MD, Rudberg MA and Brody JA. Gastrostomy placement and mortality among hospitalized Medicare beneficiaries. *JAMA,* 1998; **279**(24): 1973–1976.

106 Callaghan CM, Haag KM, Weinberger M *et al.* Outcomes of percutaneous endoscopic gastrostomy among older adults in a community setting. *JAGS,* 2000; **48**(9): 1048–1054.

107 Light VL, Slezak FA, Porter JA *et al.* Predictive factors for early mortality after percutaneous endoscopic gastrostomy. *Gastroint Endosc,* 1995; **42**(4): 330–335.

108 Finucane TE and Bynum JPW. Use of tube feeding to prevent aspiration pneumonia. *Lancet*, 1996; **348**: 1421–1424.

109 Davenport RJ, Dennis MS, Wellwood I *et al.* Complications after acute stroke. *Stroke*, 1996; **27**(3): 415–420.

110 Kelly J, Rudd A, Lewis R *et al.* Venous thromboembolism after acute stroke. *Stroke*, 2001; **32**: 262–267.

111 Wells PS, Lensing AWA and Hirsh J. Graduated compression stockings in the prevention of postoperative venous thromboembolism: a meta-analysis. *Arch Int Med*, 1994; **154**: 67–72.

112 Decousus H, Leizorovicz A, Parent F *et al.* A clinical trial of vena caval filters in the prevention of pulmonary embolism in patients with proximal deep-vein thrombosis. *NEJM*, 1998; **338**(7): 409–415.

113 Barton AL and Dudley NJ. Caval filter placement for pulmonary embolism in a patient with a deep vein thrombosis and primary intracerebral haemorrhage. *Age Ageing*, 2002; **31**: 144–146.

114 Turner-Stokes L and MacWalter R. Use of antidepressant medication following acquired brain injury: concise guidance. *Clinical Med*, 2005; **5**: 268–274.

115 Anderson G, Vestergaard K and Lauritzen L. Effective treatment of poststroke depression with the selective serotonin reuptake inhibitor citalopram. *Stroke*, 1994; **25**: 1099–1104.

116 Schievink WI. Spontaneous dissection of the carotid and vertebral arteries. *NEJM*, 2001; **344**(12): 898–906.

117 Hagen PT, Scholz DG and Edwards WD. Incidence and size of patent foramen ovale during the first 10 decades of life: an autopsy study of 965 normal hearts. *Mayo Clin Proc*, 1984; **59**: 17–20.

118 Falk RH. PFO or UFO? The role of a patent foramen ovale in cryptogenic stroke. *Am Heart J*, 1991; **121**(4): 1264–1266.

119 Lechat P, Mas JL, Lascault G *et al.* Prevalence of patent foramen ovale in patients with stroke. *NEJM*, 1988; **318**(18): 1148–1152.

120 Overell JR, Bone I and Lees KR. Interatrial septal abnormalities and stroke: a meta-analysis of case-control studies. *Neurology*, 2000; **55**: 1172–1179.

121 Messe SR, Silverman IE, Kizer JR *et al.* Practice parameter: recurrent stroke with patent foramen ovale and atrial septal aneurysm: report of the Quality Standards Subcommittee of the American Academy of Neurology. *Neurology*, 2004; **62**: 1042–1050.

122 Mas J, Arquizan C, Lamy C *et al.* Recurrent cerebrovascular events associated with patent foramen ovale, atrial septal aneurysm, or both. *NEJM*, 2001; **345**(24): 1740–1746.

123 Homma S, Sacco RL, Di Tullio MR *et al.* Effect of medical treatment in stroke patients with patent foramen ovale: patent foramen ovale in cryptogenic stroke study. *Circulation*, 2002; **105**: 2625–2631.

124 Kizer JR and Devereux RB. Patent foramen ovale in young adults with unexplained stroke. *NEJM*, 2005; **353**(22): 2361–2372.

125 Windecker S, Wahl A, Chatterjee T *et al.* Percutaneous closure of patent foramen ovale in patients with paradoxical embolism: long-term risk of recurrent thromboembolic events. *Circulation*, 2000; **101**: 893–898.

126 Maisel WH and Laskey WK. Patent foramen ovale closure devices: moving beyond equipoise. *JAMA*, 2005; **294**(3): 366–369.

127 Fleetwood IG and Steinberg GK. Arteriovenous malformations. *Lancet*, 2002; **359**: 863–873.

128 Ogilvy CS, Stieg PE, Awad I *et al.* Recommendations for the management of intracranial arteriovenous malformations: a statement for healthcare professionals from a special writing group of the Stroke Council, American Stroke Association. *Circulation*, 2001; **103**: 2644–2657.

129 Al-Shahi R and Warlow C. A systematic review of the frequency and prognosis of arteriovenous malformations of the brain in adults. *Brain*, 2001; **124**: 1900–1926.

130 DiMauro S and Schon EA. Mechanisms of disease: mitochondrial respiratory-chain diseases. *NEJM*, 2003; **348**(26): 2656–2668.

131 Cleary P, Shorvon S and Tallis R. Late-onset seizures as a predictor of subsequent stroke. *Lancet*, 2004; **363**: 1184–1186.

132 Stam J. Thrombosis of the cerebral veins and sinuses. *NEJM*, 2005; **352**(17): 1791–1798.

133 van den Bergh WM, van der Schaaf I and van Gijn J. The spectrum of presentations of venous infarction caused by deep cerebral vein thrombosis. *Neurology*, 2005; **65**: 192–196.

134 Lewis SL. Aetiology of transient global amnesia. *Lancet*, 1998; **352**: 397–399.

Bladder and bowel

Chapter 6

Urinary incontinence

Urinary incontinence (UI) is a major cause of morbidity and frequently a factor in residential care placement. Estimations of its prevalence vary according to the definition used. In a recent study of post-menopausal women aged over 50 years, 64% had had symptoms of UI within the past year.[1] Seventeen per cent of men aged over 60 report having suffered UI, with 4% reporting daily episodes.[2] UI is common after stroke and has been found in 53% of patients at presentation, falling to 32% at one year.[3] The prevalence of UI in general nursing homes has been found to be 70%.[4] UI is associated with dementia, and it afflicts around 84% of institutionalised demented people.[5] The presence of UI carries an increased risk of hospitalisation and nursing home placement.[6] The cause of incontinence is usually multi-factorial in older people and a multi-directional approach rather than a single curative procedure is frequently required. With appropriate, often simple, interventions, cure or improvement is commonly possible.

Causes of urinary incontinence

The appropriate passage of urine is dependent not only on adequate bladder and sphincter function, but also on cognitive, mobility, dexterity and environmental factors. The normal control of bladder action requires frontal cortical input in the control of external sphincter contraction/relaxation and also learned behavioural factors that can be affected by frontal lobe pathology (e.g. inappropriate passage of urine due to disinhibition). There is also a need for an intact motor cortex for both mobility and bladder motor control. The bladder motor neurons lie inferomedially and may be affected by such lesions as anterior cerebral artery infraction (see p 102) or normal pressure hydrocephalus (see p 84). Other cortical processes are also necessary; for example, a patient with a parietal lobe lesion may have difficulty finding the toilet due to geographical apraxia. Lesions affecting the spinal cord or peripheral nerves can impair bladder and sphincter action. A review of the nervous supply to the bladder is shown in Figure 6.1.

Getting to the toilet requires adequate mobility, which is dependent on many different sensory and motor elements (see p 184). A certain amount of dexterity is then necessary to remove clothing. All of these processes may be affected by intercurrent illness, including urinary tract infection (UTI), and medications. There may be additional environmental obstructions to overcome, such as a flight of stairs between the patient and the toilet.

Factors relating to both quality and quantity of urine may also predispose to UI. This may be excessive urine production due to associated medical conditions (diabetes or hypercalcaemia) or diuretic therapy. Or it may be related to the irritant nature of highly concentrated or infected urine in the bladder. The role of the volume of daily fluid drunk in the aetiology of UI is unclear. A study comparing

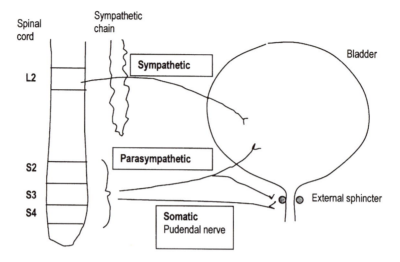

Figure 6.1 The nervous supply of the bladder.

intake to number of micturitions per day in incontinent women did not demonstrate a clear relationship.[7]

On top of all of the above, a number of conditions can affect the bladder and sphincter directly and indirectly (such as a loaded rectum). Bladder activity may be overactive (detrusor instability) or underactive (neurogenic bladder). The bladder sphincter or outlet may be incompetent (stress incontinence) or blocked (e.g. benign prostatic hyperplasia (BPH)) (*see* Figure 6.2).

Further, ageing alone may make things more difficult. Bladder functional capacity appears to decrease whilst residual capacity increases. Also, healthy older adults produce a larger proportion of their urine at night than younger people.[8] The nocturnal production of urine may be further increased in the presence of peripheral oedema that can re-enter the circulation whilst supine at night.

Specific subtypes

Urge

Urge UI is also referred to as detrusor instability, overactivity or hyper-reflexia. It is caused by intermittent inappropriate strong contractions of the bladder. It tends to produce symptoms of a sudden sensation of bladder fullness and the need to pass urine causing the patient to rush to the toilet. When incontinence occurs it is characteristically an infrequent, large-volume loss. It is the most common cause of UI in the institutionalised elderly.[9] 'Overactive bladder' is a term for the occurrence of urgency with or without UI, which is usually associated with frequency and nocturia.[10]

It is caused either by an upper motor neuron (UMN) lesion affecting the bladder nerves or a detrusor muscle disorder. In the elderly, it is often precipitated by cerebrovascular or neurodegenerative disease.

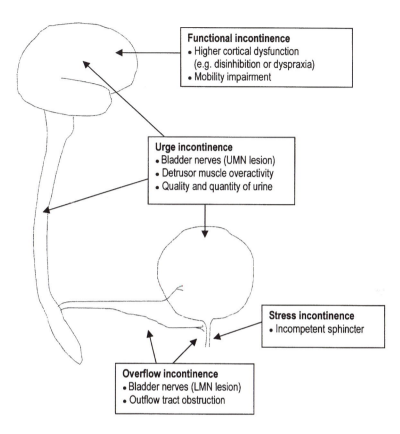

Functional incontinence
- Higher cortical dysfunction
  (e.g. disinhibition or dyspraxia)
- Mobility impairment

Urge incontinence
- Bladder nerves (UMN lesion)
- Detrusor muscle overactivity
- Quality and quantity of urine

Stress incontinence
- Incompetent sphincter

Overflow incontinence
- Bladder nerves (LMN lesion)
- Outflow tract obstruction

Figure 6.2 Intrinsic factors that are associated with urinary incontinence (UI). UMN = upper motor neuron; LMN = lower motor neuron.

Stress

Stress UI is due to an inadequate sphincter. This is almost exclusively seen in women and is associated with parity, obesity and previous hysterectomy. Rarely, it occurs in males, for example after prostatic surgery. Characteristically a small amount of urine is leaked following increased intra-abdominal pressure, such as after coughing, sneezing or exercising.

It may also be provoked by alpha-adrenergic blocking medication (e.g. prazosin) that affects the sympathetic innervation of the bladder neck and urethral smooth muscle.[11]

Overflow

Overflow UI is usually due to an under-active bladder or a blocked bladder outlet. This can occur with lesions affecting the spinal cord (e.g. multiple sclerosis) or peripheral nerves (e.g. diabetic neuropathy). It is a common cause of incontinence in older men due to blockage secondary to BPH. It may also be induced by constipation. The incontinence tends to be a continuous loss of small amounts of urine.

Functional

Functional UI is a rather loose term to group together factors outside the bladder and sphincter that lead to incontinence. It includes mobility and environmental contributors.

Mixed

Mixed UI is when more than one cause of incontinence is present. This is commonly the case in the elderly.

Assessment

History

The history, although imprecise, may give clues to the type of incontinence. It should be remembered that several different mechanisms might coexist. The duration of symptoms may give clues as to the likelihood of an acute causation, such as a UTI or the relative timing to the commencement of medications. Questions should try to look for specific UI subtypes, for example:

- Do you get a sudden desire to pass water and have to rush to the toilet?
- Do you ever leak urine when you cough or sneeze?
- What's the flow of your urine like?

The frequency and amount of urine lost should be established as well as the distress caused and current coping strategy. The use of a bladder diary to record the timing, frequency and approximate amounts of urine lost may be beneficial. Easily reversible causes should be sought:

- UTI (e.g. dysuria and haematuria)
- medication-related
- constipation.

Medications that may induce incontinence include those with anticholinergic properties (e.g. tricyclic antidepressants (TCAs)) that may result in bladder underactivity, and those that may cause increased urine formation (i.e. diuretics). Any sedating medication may reduce either the awareness of the need to pass water or the ability to safely access the toilet. There is some evidence that cholinesterase inhibitors may also induce UI, although this is usually only transient.[12]

Past medical history may indicate contributory conditions. A social and functional history may identify likely environmental barriers. Enquire about the amount and type of fluids taken, especially caffeine and alcohol.

Examination

Palpation of the abdomen may reveal a distended bladder or faecally loaded colon. Rectal examination may detect faecal impaction and give an (inaccurate) impression of prostatic size. Neurological examination is necessary to identify any of the many potential contributory factors discussed previously. Mobility should be assessed (*see* p 186). A formal cognitive assessment including tests for dyspraxia may be indicated (*see* Chapter 1).

Investigations

Urinalysis can help to exclude a precipitating infection. Haematuria in the absence of infection should raise the suspicion of either bladder calculi or malignancy. An abnormal urinalysis should prompt a mid-stream urine (MSU) sample to be sent. Baseline blood tests should exclude diabetes and hypercalcaemia. A post-voiding bladder scan can identify incomplete bladder emptying. A residual urine volume of more than 100 ml is abnormal in a younger person. In older people the residual volume of the bladder becomes increased and a value of up to 200 ml may not indicate urinary retention.

Urodynamic studies are sometimes useful in determining the cause of UI. They usually involve the insertion of tubes into the bladder and rectum. The patient requires reasonable cognitive capacity to comply with the tests. Their value is not well-defined in the elderly. They are probably most helpful when surgical intervention is being planned. A number of different tests come under the heading of urodynamics. The most frequently performed are cystometry and uroflowmetry. Other tests include those that utilise ultrasound or X-ray imaging (with the aid of radio-opaque fluids) and provide more structural information. These investigations are discussed more thoroughly elsewhere.[13]

Cystometry

Cystometry is performed with a pressure-sensing probe in the rectum and a catheter in the bladder that can be used to instil fluid and also measure bladder pressure. Fluid is slowly run into the bladder (up to 100 ml/min). Bladder pressure should only rise slowly with filling. In normal people the first desire to pass urine should not occur until after 200 ml have been put into the bladder and a strong desire should only occur after at least 300 ml. This information gives an idea of bladder capacity. The rectal (abdominal) pressure reading is subtracted from the bladder reading to give an estimate of the pressure being generated by the detrusor muscle. In this way, abnormal detrusor contractions (overactivity) can be detected. During the process the patient is also asked to cough and perform the Valsalva manoeuvre. Leakage of urine in the absence of an increase in detrusor pressure indicates stress incontinence (*see* Figure 6.3).

Uroflowmetry

Uroflowmetry is the measurement of rate and volume of urine passed during micturition. This is achieved by passing urine into a special measurement device. It may be performed following cystometry with the bladder and rectal pressure transducers still in place. In this way the bladder pressure generated can be matched with urine flow. An under-active bladder or a high pressure required to overcome outflow tract obstruction may be observed (*see* Figure 6.4).

Treatment

In this section general management issues are discussed followed by specific interventions for subtypes of incontinence, and finally the use of catheters and

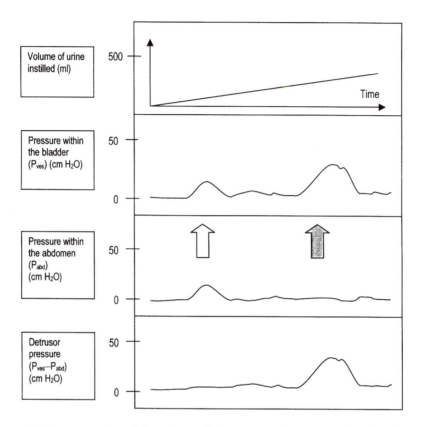

Figure 6.3 Representation of data obtained during a urodynamic study. The light arrow represents the patient coughing – the rise in intra-abdominal pressure is seen in both P_{ves} and P_{abd}, but the subtracted values ($P_{ves} - P_{abd}$) show that there is no increase in detrusor muscle tone. The shaded arrow represents an abnormal strong bladder contraction (triggered by increasing fluid volume within the bladder), which was associated with leakage of urine, indicating an overactive bladder.

pads. A flow diagram to show an overview of the assessment and management of UI is shown in Figure 6.5.

General management strategies

UI is not always curable, but there is almost always at least some improvement that can be made to the life of the individual. Given the multi-factorial nature of most incontinence in elderly people, it is often best managed by a multi-faceted approach incorporating different members of a multi-disciplinary team. Whilst in hospital this can be helped by goal-setting, careful bladder charting and regular review.

Clinics led by nurse continence advisers are becoming increasingly common. They are able to combine lifestyle advice with education and treatment strategies tailored for individuals. A study randomised 421 cognitively unimpaired people (approximately half of whom were aged over 65 years) with UI to either four-weekly clinic visits or a control group for a 25-week period.[14] The most often-used

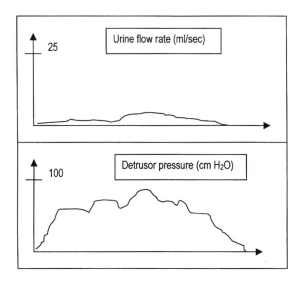

Figure 6.4 Example of uroflowmetry: obstructed outflow. Low urine volumes are passed despite high detrusor pressures ($P_{ves} - P_{abd}$).

interventions were advice on fluid and caffeine intake, pelvic muscle exercises and bladder training. The results showed an improvement in daily incontinent episodes from a mean of 2.1 to 1.0 in the intervention arm compared with 2.4 to 2.2 in the control subjects ($p = 0.001$). A limitation of this study is the absence of a sham intervention for the control group.

In patients with urinary incontinence of mixed aetiology, it appears that treating the individual components is an effective strategy. For example, anticholinergic agents appear to be effective in reducing urge incontinent episodes even in women with mixed urge–stress UI.[15]

Environmental modifications

Sometimes, environmental modifications that reduce the time to access toileting facilities are sufficient to prevent UI. Possible solutions include bedside commodes, anti-spill bottles (that contain a one-way valve for those with reduced manual dexterity) and elasticated or Velcro clothing fasteners to enable rapid removal.

Pelvic floor exercises

Pelvic floor muscle training may be used for stress, urge or mixed stress–urge incontinence. It tends to show promising early results but these do not appear to be maintained. A study found significant initial success rates with an intensive exercise regime compared to a home exercise programme but this benefit had disappeared at a 15 year follow-up.[16]

A group of 204 women (mean age 61 years) with stress, urge or mixed incontinence, were randomised to either bladder training, pelvic muscle exercises or a combined treatment group.[17] The results showed that bladder training and pelvic muscle exercises had similar outcomes irrespective of the urodynamic diagnosis. There was a small initial additional benefit with a combination of both of these therapies but this was not apparent after three months.

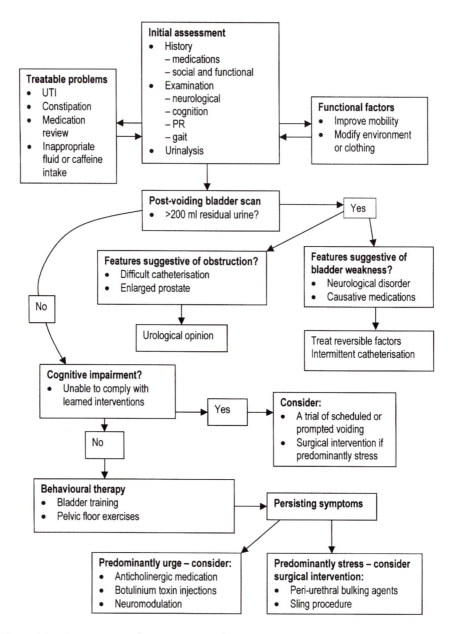

Figure 6.5   Assessment and management of urinary incontinence (UI) in an older person.

Bladder training

Bladder training is a technique whereby individuals are taught to control their bladder activity and then gradually increase the time interval between micturitions. Depending on initial frequency, intervals are commenced at 30–60-minute gaps and then extended by 30 minutes each week. The aim is to be able to have three-hour gaps between toilet visits without the occurrence of UI.

A study compared a six-week bladder training programme to a control group in 123 community-dwelling women (mean age 68, range 55–90 years) who had either stress or urge UI without marked cognitive impairment (Mini Mental State Examination (MMSE) score >23).[18] The treatment group had a significant reduction in the number of incontinent episodes per week compared to the controls (mean 21 pre-treatment falling to nine post-treatment (a 57% reduction), vs 22 falling to 19 episodes (a 14% reduction), respectively, $p = 0.0001$). The benefits appeared to be maintained at a six-month follow-up assessment.

Urge incontinence

Behavioural treatment

The term 'behavioural treatment' (BT) incorporates several different techniques that share common features. They require patient education on the physiology and anatomy of the urogenital tract. They use patient bladder diaries for initial assessment and subsequent monitoring. There is also some form of intervention that enables the patient to improve control. This may incorporate biofeedback assistance, which helps teach patients how to control their bladder and sphincter muscle tone.

Box 6.1   Hormone replacement therapy

Hormone replacement therapy (HRT) has previously been advocated as a treatment for female UI, the logic behind this practice being that HRT could reverse the age-related changes in the female urinary tract, for example atrophic vaginitis. Oestrogen receptors have been found within genitourinary tissues, including the bladder wall. Trial results had been mixed, but some small studies had suggested a possible benefit.[19] Recently, a subgroup analysis of the Women's Health Initiative study looked at the effect of HRT on urinary symptoms in 23 296 post-menopausal women over a one-year period.[1] They found that UI was more likely to develop in women on HRT who were continent at baseline than with placebo. Also, those with incontinence at baseline were more likely to become worse following HRT treatment compared to placebo. Therefore, the best available evidence shows that HRT may cause or worsen incontinence and so it has no role in its treatment.

A study that recruited 197 cognitively unimpaired women (mean age 68, range 55–92 years) with urge UI, compared a biofeedback-assisted behavioural strategy to daily anticholinergic medication or a placebo group over an eight-week period.[20] They found an 81% reduction in the incidence of incontinent episodes in the behavioural intervention group compared to 69% and 39% in the drug and placebo arms, respectively ($p = 0.04$ and $p < 0.001$ for comparison to drug and placebo). There was also a small additional benefit in a subgroup of patients from this study who subsequently combined treatments.[21] However, a number of subjects within this study also had stress UI symptoms that may have responded better to behavioural therapy, biasing the study in its favour.[22]

BT with biofeedback has been compared to BT without feedback or self-administered BT (self-help booklet) in 222 cognitively unimpaired women with urge UI (mean age 65, range 55–92 years) over an eight-week period.[23] No significant differences in efficacy were demonstrated between the groups. This finding suggests that the use of biofeedback is not necessary for a beneficial effect with BT.

Prompted voiding

In those patients who do not have the cognitive capacity to comply with behavioural therapies, prompted voiding is an alternative. This technique involves asking the patient (up to three times) if they would like to go to the toilet at regular intervals, for example two-hourly. When this was tried with nursing home residents (mean age 85, mean MMSE score 13), around 40% of incontinent individuals had a significant improvement in continence (defined as being wet on less than 20% of checks).[24] The same study proposed that a three-day trial of intervention may adequately identify all of those individuals who would benefit.

In a trial of 133 incontinent women (mean age 85 years, mean MMSE score 13/30) who resided in nursing home care, women randomised to a 13-week programme of prompted voiding demonstrated a reduction in UI frequency compared to baseline and a control group.[25] This was seen as a fall in incontinence episodes from an average of 2.22 to 1.65 per day, compared to a reduction from 2.07 to 1.90 in the control group, that is, a reduction of 26% vs 8%. The actual clinical relevance of this reduction is unclear. Presumably the residents in the treatment group continued to use pads after the intervention period. Also, this was achieved by the use of additional staff within the nursing homes and the practicality of such a scheme outside a clinical trial is unknown. When a prompted-voiding strategy was attempted to prevent nocturnal incontinence, no significant benefit was demonstrated.[26]

Scheduled toileting

In scheduled toileting, a pattern of toileting is developed with regular, pre-specified timing, for example at two-hourly intervals or planned to coincide with an individual's toileting habit. Small trials have suggested a mild benefit but the associated increased workload often leads to poor staff compliance.[5,27]

Anticholinergic medication

Anticholinergic drugs used in the treatment of UI act at muscarinic receptors. Five subtypes of muscarinic receptor have been identified (M1 to M5).[28] The main subtypes found on smooth muscle are M2 and M3, whereas the other subtypes are more commonly found in brain tissue. The most often prescribed agents are oxybutynin and tolterodine. Tropsium is a newer agent with a similar mechanism of action.

Anticholinergic medications have many potential adverse effects in the elderly (*see* Table 3.2). They have been associated with cognitive deterioration and delirium in elderly patients, particularly those with neurodegenerative disorders.[29–32] They may actually predispose to the development of Alzheimer-type pathology within these patients,[33] and oxybutynin has also been shown to adversely affect cognition in normal individuals.[34] They should only be used with caution in older people and avoided all together in those with baseline cognitive impairment (also, there is little to suggest any efficacy within this group[5]). Other common side effects include constipation, dry mouth, blurred vision, orthostatic hypotension, drowsiness and urinary retention. These often result in discontinuation of the drug.

In animal models, tolterodine appears to have a more marked affect on bladder contraction than salivary gland inhibition. It is less lipophilic and so it is postulated that it may not cross the blood–brain barrier as much as oxybutynin and so it may cause fewer central nervous system (CNS) adverse effects.[35] However, clinical trials have not detected such a difference.[36] Initial studies comparing these two agents have found a similar efficacy with a reduced incidence of dry mouth in the tolterodine group.[28,37,38]

The majority of trials have enrolled younger individuals. However, tolterodine has been compared to placebo in 177 ambulant, cognitively unimpaired elderly people (mean age 75, range 62–92 years) with urge UI.[39] Over a four-week period there was a small reduction in frequency of incontinent episodes with 2 mg bd of tolterodine compared to placebo (by a mean of 0.7 episodes per day from a baseline mean of 2.8 episodes per day vs no reduction from 5.1 episodes per day in the control group, $p = 0.007$, compared to placebo). It is unclear whether such a change is of clinical significance. A 1 mg bd dose did not significantly reduce incontinent episodes. It should be noted that there were significant differences between the groups at baseline. The main adverse event reported was dry mouth; however, there was only a short study period and detailed cognitive evaluation was not undertaken.

Extended-release (ER) preparations (taken once daily) are available for oxybutynin and tolterodine. They appear to be similarly effective as standard formulations but may have a lower incidence of dry mouth.[40] This finding is probably due to less marked fluctuation in drug levels. Tolterodine ER appears to have similar effects in older and younger cohorts with an incidence of dry mouth of 24% in those over the age of 65 (compared to 7% in the placebo arm).[41]

Several trials have compared oxybutynin and tolterodine. A study of 332 men and women (mean age 58, range 21–87 years) without significant comorbidities, were randomised to either oxybutynin ER 10 mg daily or tolterodine 2 mg bd for a 12-week period.[42] There was a significantly bigger improvement in weekly UI events in the oxybutynin group compared to tolterodine (28.6 at baseline falling to 7.1 vs 27.0 and 9.3, respectively, $p = 0.02$). There were no significant differences in the incidence of adverse events. The most common side effect was dry mouth, occurring in approximately 30% of participants in both groups.

A study of 790 women with overactive bladder (mean age 60, range 18–92 years) compared the ER preparations of oxybutynin (10 mg) and tolterodine (4 mg) over a 12-week period.[43] The baseline mean UI episodes per week was 37 in both groups and this fell to 11 episodes per week after 12 weeks of treatment in both groups (a 70% reduction). The only significant difference in adverse events was the incidence of dry mouth, which was 30% in the oxybutynin group and 22% in the tolterodine group.

A transdermal preparation of oxybutynin has also been compared to tolterodine ER.[44] Both drugs appeared to have similar efficacy, with less dry mouth in the transdermal oxybutynin group at the cost of application-site pruritis (14% of recipients).

Tropsium chloride is another anti-muscarinic agent. It has been shown to be more effective than placebo at reducing urge incontinence in 523 men and women (mean age 62) with the most common adverse event being dry mouth.[45] It has no obvious advantage over other available agents.

So, it seems that anticholinergic medications may be beneficial in some individuals who have urge UI without cognitive impairment. Unfortunately, urge UI is often associated with cognitive impairment in the elderly. They appear to be less effective than behavioural strategies[20] and carry significant side effects. For these reasons they should be reserved for patients who fail to respond to non-pharmacological measures. ER or transdermal formulations are more expensive but could be tried in those who have significant dry mouth with standard preparations.

Intravesical therapy

Botulinium toxin has been used to treat urge incontinence. It is injected directly into the detrusor muscle under cystoscopic guidance. In a study recruiting 59 patients (mean age 41, range 20–72 years) with neurogenic urge UI (due to a spinal cord lesion or multiple sclerosis) who currently used intermittent catheterisation, a single botulinium toxin injection was compared to placebo over a 24-week period.[46] There was a significant reduction in incontinent episodes (around 50%) in the treatment group compared to the placebo. Around 25% of the subjects developed a UTI during the study period. Injection site pain was reported by a small number of people. There were no significant differences in adverse effects noted between the two groups.

A non-randomised series of 30 patients found an improvement in symptoms in 73% of subjects.[47] The effects lasted an average of five months. Side effects included transient urinary dysfunction, difficulty initiating micturition, and an increased residual urine volume.

There have also been studies using this treatment in non-neurogenic urge incontinence. Results suggest that it may be effective and have only a small incidence of inducing urinary retention.[48] It seems likely that botulinium toxin will be used more frequently in the management of UI in the future.

Neuromodulation

Neuromodulation, or sacral nerve stimulation, involves the use of an implantable electrical stimulation device that acts on the sacral nerve roots to inhibit bladder contractility. It has been trialled in the treatment of refractory urge UI in younger patients (mean age 47, range 20–79) with some success.[49] Disadvantages include cost, the need for an invasive procedure and associated complications (including pain, lead migration and the need for surgical revision).

Acupuncture

A study compared weekly acupuncture sessions to a placebo acupuncture technique in 74 women (median age 51, range 22–82 years) with overactive bladder over a four-week period.[50] They found a 59% reduction in incontinent episodes in the acupuncture group compared to a 40% reduction in the placebo arm but this did not achieve statistical significance. The role of acupuncture in UI, if any, is not yet defined.

Stress incontinence

Pelvic muscle exercises

The theory with pelvic muscle exercises is that the pubococcygeous muscle's action can be increased, resulting in an increased closing force on the urethra.[51] They are suitable for cognitively unimpaired, highly motivated women. Exercises need to be repeated 30–200 times per day. They appear to be more effective than no treatment or a placebo treatment but their actual effect size is hard to judge on available evidence.[52] Such exercises must be continued indefinitely. When an exercise programme was compared to a biofeedback technique, there were no significant differences in outcome between the groups (but both did better than a control group).[53]

Vaginal cones

Vaginal cones are a series of objects of varying weight that the incontinent woman holds within the vaginal cavity for around 20 minutes a day. The weight is gradually increased with the aim of strengthening the pelvic floor. When compared to pelvic floor exercises, vaginal cones were less effective.[54] They are occasionally associated with vaginitis or bleeding and patient concordance is poor. Their use can no longer be recommended.

Electrical stimulation

External electrical stimulators have been used to try to improve pelvic floor musculature. This technique appears to be less effective than standard pelvic muscle exercises and is associated with some discomfort and motivational problems.[54] When it was combined with a behavioural training programme, there was no additional benefit compared to BT alone.[55] Its use can no longer be recommended.

Drugs

An alpha agonist agent (phenylpropanolamine hydrochloride) has been found to be as effective as pelvic floor muscle exercises for stress UI in 157 women (mean age 68, range 55–90 years) over a six-month period.[51] Side effects limit the clinical use of such agents, the most important being hypertension. A Cochrane review concluded that there was 'weak evidence' of efficacy of a variety of adrenergic compounds in women with stress UI but a number of associated side effects.[56]

More recently, a combined serotonin and norepinephrine reuptake inhibitor (duloxetine) has been proposed for stress incontinence, the theory being that serotinergic neurons may suppress bladder parasympathetic actions. A trial recruited 494 women (mean age 51, range 24–83 years) with predominant stress UI and randomised them to duloxetine or placebo over a 12-week period.[57] There was a reduction in the *median* frequency of UI (50% vs 29% for placebo, $p = 0.002$).

The trialists report use of a median (rather than a mean) due to a few extreme outlier values. However, there was no associated improvement in quality of life scores and there were significant adverse events reported. 22% of the duloxetine group discontinued treatment due to adverse events, compared to 5% of the placebo group ($p<0.001$). Adverse events seen significantly more often were nausea, dry mouth, constipation, fatigue, insomnia, dizziness, increased sweating, vomiting, somnolence and tremor. It may well be that the positive effects of this medication were mediated either by alpha-agonist properties or by an anticholinergic effect in those with mixed incontinence given the high incidence of anticholinergic type side effects. It seems hard to justify the use of duloxetine on the current evidence for such a small beneficial effect, particularly in the elderly who are more likely to have adverse reactions.

Surgery

A variety of surgical procedures have been developed for the treatment of stress incontinence. Early reports suggest high rates of improvement or cure. Trials of open retropubic colposuspension have found a 69–88% cure rate.[58] However, the longer-term results may be less impressive. In a survey of community-dwelling women, 73% who had previously undergone surgery had had at least one incontinent episode in the past month and 53% were currently using absorbent pads.[59] Colposuspension aims to elevate the tissues that surround the lower bladder and upper urethra. Laparoscopic colposuspension has the advantage of quicker recovery times due to the absence of a major abdominal incision but possibly at the expense of poorer long-term outcomes.[60]

Anterior vaginal repair uses an approach through the vaginal wall. Bladder neck needle suspension employs sutures to attach the vaginal to the abdominal wall. Available evidence suggests that both of these methods are less successful than open abdominal retropubic colposuspension.[61,62]

More recent work has focused on less invasive surgical procedures, leading to the pubovaginal sling becoming more popular. Even less invasive methods of this procedure include tension-free vaginal tape. The tape supports the mid-urethra and it is thought that this prevents incontinence by inducing some urethral kinking.[63] A follow-up study of 692 women who had undergone a tension-free tape procedure between two and eight years previously showed that those with pure stress incontinence had an 85% chance of cure even after four to eight years, whereas those with mixed incontinence had only a 30% chance of cure after this amount of time.[64]

Peri-urethral bulking agents

Injectable peri-urethral bulking agents have become increasingly popular as a minimally invasive treatment for female stress UI. The initial substance injected was collagen; however, there are now various alternative agents.[65] It may be performed under local anaesthesia and endoscopic guidance. The injectable material is placed submucosally, adjacent to the proximal urethra. This appears to increase urethral closing pressure and prevent urine leakage. Early results from small series are mixed, showing improvement in 11–85% and cure in 7–95%.[65] Randomised controlled trial data are lacking.

Overflow incontinence

Prostatic hyperplasia

Finasteride is a 5-alpha-reductase inhibitor that blocks the conversion of testosterone to dihydrotestosterone (*see* Figure 11.2). It has been found to cause a reduction in prostatic size with subsequent improvement in urine flow and reduced obstructive symptoms.[66] The main side effects reported are loss of libido and impotence. Symptoms may also be improved with alpha-adrenergic blocking agents (e.g. prazosin). These drugs may induce orthostatic hypotension (OH) (*see* Chapter 10). Transurethral resection of the prostate (TURP) is a successful surgical intervention and can be performed under local anaesthesia.

Catheters

Indwelling catheters

In some circumstances catheters will be the most appropriate intervention for the patient. However, they are associated with a number of problems, including blockage, infection and interference with sexual activity. They have also been associated with chronic pyelonephritis and renal inflammation.[67] Recurrent blockage of catheters can be minimised by using silicone-coated devices and maintaining a high fluid intake. Bypassing of catheters can be reduced by using a catheter with a smaller lumen (larger bore tubes can hamper the efficacy of sphincter closure around them) and, if this fails, the concomitant use of bladder relaxing medication.[68] Mobile patients will use a 300 ml portable leg bag. They, or their carers, need to be educated on the appropriate use of this.

Intermittent catheterisation

Intermittently passing a catheter to drain a full bladder is an alternative to a permanent indwelling catheter. This can either be self-administered or performed by a carer. It may be associated with a lower infection rate than indwelling devices and has other advantages such as preservation of sexual function. Evidence suggests that it is well-tolerated by the elderly.[69]

External catheters

Condom-like external catheters are sometimes appropriate. Their main disadvantage is difficulty retaining them. They are also prone to increased infection rates and skin breakdown.

Pads

There is a variety of pads available for use in incontinent individuals. They can be divided into body-worn pads and flat bed pads. The body-worn pads can be either disposable or machine washable. Flat bed pads are a form of absorbent sheet that can be placed beneath a patient in bed. The body-worn pads are almost always preferable as they are able to absorb more fluid, may have a gel lining that keeps urine away from the skin, do not affect the pressure distribution properties of specialised mattresses and do not become wrinkled under the patient, causing increased pressure damage.[70] There is some evidence that disposable pads are associated with fewer skin adverse events than their washable equivalents.[71]

References

1 Hendrix SL, Cochrane BB, Nygaard IE *et al.* Effects of estrogen with and without progestin on urinary incontinence. *JAMA,* 2005; **293**(8): 935–948.

2 Stothers L, Thom D and Calhoun E. Urologic diseases in America project: urinary incontinence in males – demographics and economic burden. *J Urology,* 2005; **173**(4): 1302–1308.

3 Kolominsky-Rabas PL, Hilz M, Neundoerfer B *et al.* Impact of urinary incontinence after stroke: results from a prospective population-based stroke register. *Neurourol Urodyn,* 2003; **22**: 322–327.

4 Chiang L, Ouslander J, Schnelle J *et al.* Dually incontinent nursing home residents: clinical characteristics and treatment differences. *JAGS,* 2000; **48**(6): 673–676.

5 Skelly J and Flint AJ. Urinary incontinence associated with dementia. *JAGS,* 1995; **43**(3): 286–294.

6 Thom DH, Haan MN and Van Den Eeden SK. Medically recognized urinary incontinence and risks of hospitalization, nursing home admission and mortality. *Age Ageing,* 1997; **26**: 367–374.

7 Wyman JF, Elswick RK, Wilson MS *et al.* Relationship of fluid intake to voluntary micturitions and urinary incontinence in women. *Neurourol Urodyn,* 1991; **10**: 463–473.

8 Kirkland JL, Lye M, Levy DW *et al.* Patterns of urine flow and electrolyte excretion in healthy elderly people. *BMJ,* 1983; **287**: 1665–1667.

9 Resnick NM, Yalla SV and Laurino E. The pathophysiology of urinary incontinence among institutionalized elderly persons. *NEJM,* 1989; **320**(1): 1–7.

10 Tubaro A. Defining overactive bladder: epidemiology and burden of disease. *Urology,* 2004; **64** (Suppl. 6A): 2–6.

11 Mathew TH, McEwen J and Rohan A. Urinary incontinence secondary to prazosin. *Med J Aust,* 1988; **148**: 305–306.

12 Hashimoto M, Imamura T, Tanimukai S *et al.* Urinary incontinence: an unrecognised adverse effect with donepezil. *Lancet,* 2000; **356**: 568.

13 Stanton S and Morgan AK. *Clinical Urogynaecology,* 2nd ed. London: Churchill Livingston, 2000.

14 Borrie MJ, Bawden M, Speechley M *et al.* Interventions led by nurse continence advisers in the management of urinary incontinence: a randomized controlled trial. *CMAJ,* 2002; **166**(10): 1267–1273.

15 Khullar V, Hill S, Laval K *et al.* Treatment of urge-predominant mixed urinary incontinence with tolterodine extended release: a randomized, placebo-controlled trial. *Urology,* 2004; **64**(2): 269–275.

16 Bo K, Kvarstein B and Nygaard I. Lower urinary tract symptoms and pelvic floor muscle exercise adherence after 15 years. *Obstet Gynecol,* 2005; **105**(5): 999–1005.

17 Wyman JF, Fantl JA, McClish DK *et al.* Comparative efficacy of behavioral interventions in the management of female urinary incontinence. *Am J Obstet Gynecol,* 1998; **179**(4): 999–1007.

18 Fantl JA, Wyman JF, McClish DK *et al.* Efficacy of bladder training in older women with urinary incontinence. *JAMA,* 1991; **265**(5): 609–613.

19 Moehrer B, Hextall A and Jackson S. Oestrogens for urinary incontinence in women. Cochrane Database of Syst Rev 2003; issue 2.

20 Burgio KL, Locher JL, Goode PS *et al.* Behavioral vs drug treatment for urge urinary incontinence in older women: a randomized controlled trial. *JAMA,* 1998; **280**(23): 1995–2000.

21 Burgio KL, Locher JL and Goode PS. Combined behavioural and drug therapy for urge incontinence in older women. *JAGS,* 2000; **48**: 370–374.

22 Payne CK. Behavioral therapy for overactive bladder. *Urology,* 2000; **55** (Suppl. 5A): 3–6.

23   Burgio KL, Goode PS, Locher JL *et al.* Behavioral training with and without biofeedback in the treatment of urge incontinence in older women: a randomized controlled trial. *JAMA*, 2002; **288**(18): 2293–2299.

24   Ouslander JG, Schnelle JF, Uman G *et al.* Predictors of successful prompted voiding among incontinent nursing home residents. *JAMA*, 1995; **273**(17): 1366–1370.

25   Hu T, Igou JF, Kaltreider DL *et al.* A clinical trial of a behavioral therapy to reduce urinary incontinence in nursing homes: outcome and implications. *JAMA*, 1989; **261**(18): 2656–2662.

26   Ouslander JG, Al-Samarrai N and Schnelle JF. Prompted voiding for nighttime incontinence in nursing homes: is it effective? *JAGS*, 2001; **49**(6): 706–709.

27   Ostaszkiewicz J, Johnston L and Roe B. Habit retraining for the management of urinary incontinence in adults. Cochrane Database Syst Rev 2004, Issue 2. Art. No.: CD002801. DOI: 10.1002/14651858.CD002801.pub2.

28   Chapple CR. Muscarinic receptor antagonists in the treatment of overactive bladder. *Urology*, 2000; **55** (Suppl. 5A): 33–46.

29   Donnellan CA, Fook L, McDonald P *et al.* Oxybutynin and cognitive dysfunction. *BMJ*, 1997; **315**: 1363–1364.

30   Edwards KR and O'Connor JT. Risk of delirium with concomitant use of tolterodine and acetylcholinesterase inhibitors. *JAGS*, 2002; **50**(6): 1165–1166.

31   Williams SG and Staudenmeier J. Hallucinations with tolterodine. *Psych Services*, 2004; **55**(11): 1318–1319.

32   Tsao JW and Heilman KM. Transient memory impairment and hallucinations associated with tolterodine use. *NEJM*, 2003; **349**(23): 2274–2275.

33   Perry EK, Kilford L, Lees AJ *et al.* Increased Alzheimer pathology in Parkinson's disease related to antimuscarinic drugs. *Ann Neurol*, 2003; **54**: 235–238.

34   Katz IR, Sands LP, Bilker W *et al.* Identification of medications that cause cognitive impairment in older people: the case of oxybutynin chloride. *JAGS*, 1998; **46**(1): 8–13.

35   Scheife R and Takeda M. Central nervous system safety of anticholinergic drugs for the treatment of overactive bladder in the elderly. *Clin Therap*, 2005; **27**(2): 144–153.

36   Chu FM, Dmochowski RR, Lama DJ *et al.* Extended-release formulations of oxybutynin and tolterodine exhibit similar central nervous system tolerability profiles: a subanalysis of data from the OPERA trial. *Am J Obstet Gynecol*, 2005; **192**(6): 1849–1854.

37   Abrams RF, Anderstrom C and Mattiasson A. Tolterodine, a new antimuscarinic agent: as effective but better tolerated than oxybutynin in patients with an overactive bladder. *Br J Urol*, 1998; **81**: 801–810.

38   Appell RA. Clinical efficacy and safety of tolterodine in the treatment of overactive bladder: a pooled analysis. *Urology*, 1997; **50** (Suppl. 6A): 90–96.

39   Malone-Lee JG, Walsh JB, Maugourd M *et al.* Tolterodine: a safe and effective treatment for older patients with overactive bladder. *JAGS*, 2001; **49**(6): 700–705.

40   Van Kerrebroeck P, Kreder K, Jonas U *et al.* Tolterodine once-daily: superior efficacy and tolerability in the treatment of the overactive bladder. *Urology*, 2001; **57**(3): 414–421.

41   Zinner NR, Mattiasson A and Stanton SL. Efficacy, safety, and tolerability of extended-release once-daily tolterodine treatment for overactive bladder in older versus younger patients. *JAGS*, 2002; **50**: 799–802.

42   Appell RA, Sand P, Dmochowski R *et al.* Prospective randomized controlled trial of extended-release oxybutynin chloride and tolterodine tartrate in the treatment of overactive bladder: results of the OBJECT study. *Mayo Clin Proc*, 2001; **76**: 358–363.

43   Diokno AC, Appell RA and Sand PK. Prospective, randomized, double-blind study of the efficacy and tolerability of the extended-release formulations of oxybutynin and tolterodine for overactive bladder: results of the OPERA trial. *Mayo Clin Proc*, 2003; **78**: 687–695.

44   Dmochowski RR, Sand PK, Zinner NR *et al.* Comparative efficacy and safety of transdermal oxybutynin and oral tolterodine versus placebo in previously treated patients with urge and mixed urinary incontinence. *Urology*, 2003; **62**(2): 237–242.

45   Zinner N, Gittelman M, Harris R *et al.* Tropsium chloride improves overactive bladder symptoms: a multicenter phase III trial. *J Urology*, 2004; **171**: 2311–2315.

46   Schurch B, de Sèze M, Denys P *et al.* Botulinum toxin type a is a safe and effective treatment for neurogenic urinary incontinence: results of a single treatment, randomized, placebo controlled 6-month study. *J Urology*, 2005; **174**(1): 196–200.

47 Kuo H. Urodynamic evidence of effectiveness of botulinium A toxin injection in treatment of detrusor overactivity refractory to anticholinergic agents. *Urology*, 2004; **63**(5): 868–872.

48 Cruz F and Silva C. Botulinum toxin in the management of lower urinary tract dysfunction: contemporary update. *Curr Opin Urol*, 2004; **14**(6): 329–334.

49 Schmidt RA, Jonas U, Oleson KA *et al*. Sacral nerve stimulation for treatment of refractory urinary urge incontinence. *J Urology*, 1999; **162**(2): 352–357.

50 Emmons SL and Otto L. Acupuncture for overactive bladder: a randomized controlled trial. *Obstet Gynecol*, 2005; **106**(1): 138–143.

51 Wells TJ, Brink CA, Diokno AC *et al*. Pelvic muscle exercise for stress urinary incontinence in elderly women. *JAGS*, 1991; **39**(8): 785–791.

52 Hay-Smith EJC, Bo K, Berghmans LCM *et al*. Pelvic floor muscle training for urinary incontinence in women. Cochrane Database Syst Rev 2001, Issue 1. Art. No.: CD001407. DOI: 10.1002/14651858.CD001407.

53 Burns PA, Pranikoff K, Nochajski TH *et al*. A comparison of effectiveness of biofeedback and pelvic muscle exercise treatment of stress incontinence in older community-dwelling women. *J Gerontol* 1993; **48**(4): M167–174.

54 Bo K, Talseth T and Holme I. Single blind, randomised controlled trial of pelvic floor exercises, electrical stimulation, vaginal cones and no treatment in management of genuine stress incontinence in women. *BMJ*, 1999; **318**: 487–493.

55 Goode PS, Burgio KL, Locher JL *et al*. Effect of behavioural training with or without pelvic floor electrical stimulation on stress incontinence in women: a randomized controlled trial. *JAMA*, 2003; **290**(3): 345–352.

56 Alhasso A, Glazener CMA, Pickard R *et al*. Adrenergic drugs for urinary incontinence in adults. Cochrane Database Syst Rev 2005 Issue 3. Art. No.: CD001842. DOI: 10.1002/14651858.CD001842.pub2.

57 Van Kerrebroeck P, Abrams P, Lange R *et al*. Duloxetine versus placebo in the treatment of European and Canadian women with stress urinary incontinence. *BJOG*, 2004; **111**: 249–257.

58 Lapitan MC, Cody DJ andGrant AM. Open retropubic colposuspension for urinary incontinence in women. Cochrane Database Syst Rev 2005, Issue 3. Art. No.: CD002912. DOI: 10.1002/14651858.CD002912.pub2.

59 Diokno AC, Burgio K, Fultz NH *et al*. Prevalence and outcomes of continence surgery in community dwelling women. *J Urol*, 2003; **170**: 507–511.

60 Moehrer B, Ellis G, Carey M *et al*. Laparoscopic colposuspension for urinary incontinence in women. Cochrane Database Syst Rev 2000, Issue 3. Art. No.: CD002239. DOI: 10.1002/14651858.CD002239.

61 Glazener CMA and Cooper K. Anterior vaginal repair for urinary incontinence in women. Cochrane Database Syst Rev 2001, Issue 1. Art. No.: CD001755. DOI: 10.1002/14651858.CD001755.

62 Glazener CMA and Cooper K. Bladder neck needle suspension for urinary incontinence in women. Cochrane Database Syst Rev 2004, Issue 2. Art. No.: CD003636. DOI: 10.1002/14651858.CD003636.pub2.

63 Atherton MJ and Stanton SL. The tension-free vaginal tape reviewed: an evidence-based review from inception to current status. *BJOG*, 2005; **112**: 534–546.

64 Holmgren C, Nilsson S, Lanner L *et al*. Long-term results with tension-free vaginal tape on mixed and stress urinary incontinence. *Obstet Gynecol*, 2005; **106**(1): 38–43.

65 Kershen RT, Dmochowski RR and Appell RA. Beyond collagen: injectable therapies for the treatment of female stress urinary incontinence in the new millennium. *Urol Clin N Am*, 2002; **29**: 559–574.

66 Gormley GJ, Stoner E, Bruskewitz RC *et al*. The effect of finasteride in men with benign prostatic hyperplasia. *NEJM*, 1992; **327**: 1185–1191.

67 Warren JW, Muncie HL, Hebel JR *et al*. Long-term urethral catheterization increases risk of chronic pyelonephritis and renal inflammation. *JAGS*, 1994; **42**(12): 1286–1290.

68 Resnick NM. Geriatric incontinence. *Urol Clin N Am*, 1996; **23**(1): 55–74.

69 Pilloni S, Krhut J, Mair D *et al*. Intermittent catheterisation in older people: a valuable alternative to the indwelling catheter? *Age Ageing*, 2005; **34**: 57–60.

70 Hampton S. Importance of the appropriate selection and use of continence pads. *Br J Nursing*, 2005; **14**(5): 265–269.

71 Brazzelli M, Shirran E and Vale L. Absorbent products for containing urinary and/or faecal incontinence in adults. Cochrane Database Syst Rev 1999, Issue 3. Art. No.: CD001406. DOI: 10.1002/14651858.CD001406.

Chapter 7

Bowel disorders

This chapter does not cover every aspect of the health of the ageing bowel. Instead, three topics of high relevance to geriatric practice have been reviewed: constipation, *Clostridium difficile* diarrhoea and faecal incontinence.

Constipation

Constipation is classically defined as passing stools less often than once every three days. It may alternatively be described as difficulty passing stools (dyschezia) due to their hard or pebble-like nature or difficulty in initiating evacuation despite regular bowel motions.[1] A distinction of subtypes of constipation into either slow transit time or difficult stool expulsion has been proposed but some overlap does exist.[2] Constipation is more common in older than younger people, but its incidence and prevalence are hard to establish accurately as people's perception of constipation often differs from the clinical definition. A survey of older people found that around 30% reported constipation but only 3% actually opened their bowels less than three times per week.[3] A study of the community-dwelling elderly (aged 65–93 years) found a prevalence of chronic constipation of 24% (defined as straining at stool or less than three motions per week more than 25% of the time).[4] Changes in the bowel associated with ageing that may increase the likelihood of developing constipation include reduced neuronal function and anal sphincter fibrosis.

A number of factors are necessary to maintain normal bowel function (*see* Figure 7.1). These include adequate hydration, dietary fibre and mobility. The colon usually removes 90% of water from its contents. Despite this, the normal composition of faeces is approximately three-quarters water with the rest being mainly fibre, bacteria and inorganic matter (e.g. calcium and phosphate). The percentage of absorbed water is increased in the presence of dehydration or a prolonged bowel transit time. Dietary fibre helps retain stool water by assisting peristalsis due to its bulk and by an osmotic effect. Moving around appears to have an additive effect to bowel peristalsis in reducing the transit time. The gastrocolic reflex is a normal hormonally mediated physiological occurrence whereby colonic contraction is stimulated 20–30 minutes after gastric distension. Hence, bowel evacuation is more likely after eating. Defaecation is also more likely to occur first thing in the morning.[5]

Parasympathetic activity and the effects of various hormone agents are important in maintaining bowel propulsion.[6] The surrounding striated muscle structures of the diaphragm, abdominal wall and pelvic floor are important in the normal defaecation process.

Pathological conditions of the bowel, including diverticulosis, irritable bowel syndrome, colonic carcinoma and painful anal disorders (e.g. fissures), are additional factors in constipation in some individuals. The normal process is often disturbed by illness due to immobility, dehydration, change in dietary intake and medications that reduce bowel motility (*see* Table 7.1). Some comorbidities

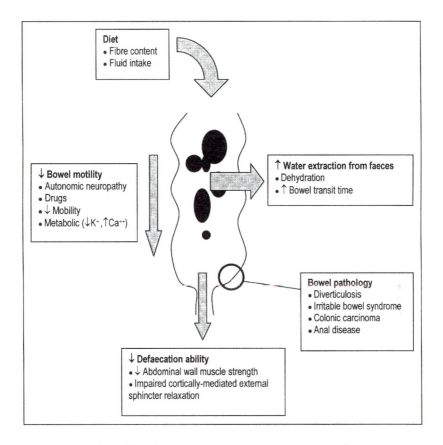

Figure 7.1   Factors that affect the development of constipation.

Table 7.1   Medications that commonly cause constipation in the elderly

---

Opiates
Metallic ions (e.g. iron, calcium and aluminium)
Calcium channel-blockers (especially verapamil)
Antispasmodics
Anticholinergics (e.g. tricyclic antidepressants (TCAs), oxybutynin and tolterodine) – a two to three times increased risk of constipation is noted with the use of these agents in nursing home residents[7]
Dopamine agonists
Diuretics (via dehydration)

---

predispose to constipation, for example autonomic neuropathy (e.g. Parkinson's disease and diabetes) and hypothyroidism. Metabolic disturbances, including hypercalcaemia and hypokalaemia, can cause constipation. Defaecation requires abdominal muscle contraction, which can be disturbed by conditions such as herniation of the abdominal wall. Raised toilet seats that help immobile patients to access toilets may be counterproductive as they can disrupt the normal abdominal wall actions during defaecation.[6]

If untreated constipation can cause urinary retention, overflow diarrhoea, bowel obstruction and, rarely, perforation. Faecal impaction is discussed on p 167.

Assessment

History

A history of recent change in bowel habit should always raise the concern that there may be an underlying bowel malignancy. Red flags include weight loss and rectal bleeding. It is important to qualify what the patient actually means by constipation; this may be aided by the use of a stool diary. For patients in hospital, a stool chart can be utilised. The accuracy of stool description may be increased by use of the Bristol Stool Scale.[8] This is a seven-point descriptive scale ranging from hard lumps of stool (1) to watery motions (7) that correlates with bowel transit time. The timing of symptom onset may coincide with potential precipitants, such as the commencement of medications.

Examination

Abdominal examination may demonstrate faecal loading in the colon. Rectal examination can detect faecal loading, assess stool consistency and detect contributory lesions such as a rectal carcinoma, anal fissure or thrombosed haemorrhoid.

Investigations

Blood tests should exclude hypothyroidism, hypokalaemia and hypercalcaemia. A full blood count (FBC) showing a microcytic anaemia increases the likelihood of a gastrointestinal malignancy. Abdominal X-ray can detect bowel obstruction or high faecal impaction if clinically suspected. Colonoscopy is useful for detecting colonic neoplasia when indicated. Barium enemas are usually less well tolerated than colonoscopy and may provide less information, including the inability to take biopsies of suspicious lesions. In studies looking at colonoscopy in the over-75s, there is around a 10% pick-up rate for colonic neoplasia.[9,10] These patients may go on to have surgical treatment or, possibly, endoscopic palliative stenting. Serious complications are rare (<1%) but there are high rates of incompletion (around 40%) due to either poor bowel preparation or procedural intolerance. Further testing, including transit studies, manometry and defaecography, may be considered in specialist clinics for resistant, unexplained constipation.

Treatment

If an underlying cause can be identified then this should be addressed. Contributory factors such as dehydration and immobility should be improved when possible. If the patient's diet is believed to contain insufficient fibre, then dietary advice is appropriate (aiming for 20–40 g of fibre per day[11]). When constipation is opiate-induced, there is some evidence from studies in younger people that inhibitors of opiate receptors may be beneficial.[12]

Laxatives

In general there is very little evidence for the treatment of constipation.[13] When considering the subgroup that is elderly people, the evidence is even more scarce. Trials tend to be small and of low quality.[14] A systematic review of the efficacy of various constipation treatments found a pooled effect of bulk laxatives of an increase of 1.4 bowel movements per week (95% CI 0.6–2.2) compared to 1.5 for all other laxative agents combined (95% CI 1.1–1.8).[15] There were insufficient data to adequately compare individual agents. The main available agents are discussed below. As there is little to choose between the agents in terms of evidence of efficacy, their use is usually driven by potential adverse effects and cost.

Bulking agents

- *Natural fibres*: bran, psyllium (the ground husk of the psyllium seed), ispaghula.
- *Synthetic agents*: e.g. methylcellulose, polycarbophil.

Bulking agents cause an increased stool mass due to unabsorbed fibre and increased stool water retention attributed to an associated osmotic effect, which leads to a reduced bowel transit time by peristalsis assistance and softer stools.

Bacterial metabolism of these substances within the gut can lead to abdominal bloating and excessive flatus production. Major problems in the elderly include cases of intestinal obstruction both of the lower bowel and oesophagus.[16] In the most extreme case bowel perforation has been reported.[17] These may be related to excessive dietary fibre or insufficient water intake. Oesophageal problems may be more likely in association with an impaired swallowing reflex or reduced oeso-phageal motility. Therefore, these agents should be avoided in individuals who cannot drink adequate amounts of fluid. They play an important role in the treatment of diverticular disease and irritable bowel syndrome – both of which may cause constipation.

Osmotic laxatives

Osmotic laxatives increase stool water content by preventing water absorption by the bowel endothelium and thus make them easier to pass. The disadvantage of this is the potential to cause dehydration, especially in the elderly.

Poorly absorbed ions, such as magnesium and phosphate, may cause hyper-magnesaemia, hyperphosphataemia and subsequent hypercalcaemia. The risk of side effects is increased in the elderly, those with renal impairment and with prolonged exposure of the large bowel to the ions, for example when there is faecal impaction.[16]

Lactulose (a disaccharide) and sorbitol (a sugar alcohol) are partially metabolised by bacteria in the large bowel, which may cause flatulence and abdominal pain due to CO_2 production. When these two agents were compared in a clinical trial, no significant difference in efficacy was detected.[18] Lactulose was compared to a senna-fibre (ispaghula) combination in 77 older people (mean age 83 years) in long-stay hospital wards or nursing homes in a crossover design study.[19] There was a significantly higher mean daily stool frequency with the senna-fibre combination (0.8 stools per day vs 0.6; $p = 0.001$). No significant side-effect differences were reported.

Polyethylene glycol (PEG) is a mixture of polymers that increase stool water content due to an osmotic effect. Molecules with a molecular weight of 3350 or above are used as they cannot be absorbed by the gut.[11] PEG has been shown to be effective in the treatment of faecal impaction (*see* p 167). It comes in a sachet that is added to sufficient water so as to remove the risk of dehydration. It is not metabolised by bowel bacteria and is not absorbed.

In a study of 70 patients with constipation (mean age 42 years), PEG was compared to placebo over a six-month period.[20] A significantly higher rate of remission was seen in the treatment group (77% vs 22% in the placebo arm; $p<0.01$). There were no significant differences in adverse-event rates between the two groups. It has been compared to lactulose in 115 patients (mean age 55 years but 37% between the ages of 65 and 89) with chronic constipation over a four-week period.[21] There was a small but significant increase in mean daily stool frequency with PEG compared to lactulose (1.3 vs 0.9; $p = 0.005$). Adverse-event rates were similar for both groups; there was an increased incidence of diarrhoea in the PEG group early in the treatment regimen but it appeared to be associated with less flatus production.

PEG appears to be a safe and effective agent for use in the elderly. Its higher cost than other agents means that it should be reserved for those who are unresponsive to initial, cheaper therapy.

Stimulant laxatives

Senna is derived from plants of the genus *Cassia*, it passes to the large bowel where it is converted by bacteria to its active compound.[11] It may have a toxic effect on the colonic mucosa leading to melanosis coli (pigment deposition in bowel epithelial macrophage cells). This was previously thought to be associated with colonic neoplasia following long-term usage but a recent study challenges this association.[22] Its effects commence when it arrives in the colon which, depending on transit time, usually takes around six to eight hours. Therefore, if taken at bedtime its effects should coincide with the post-breakfast gastrocolic reflex.

Bisacodyl has similar actions and speed of onset to senna.[11]

Danthron is associated with carcinoma formation in animal studies.

Stool softeners

Docusate sodium is a synthetic detergent that is thought to allow greater penetration of water and fat into the faeces and thereby softens them. It may also have a mild stimulatory effect. It was compared to psyllium in 170 people (mean age 37, range 20–74 years) with chronic constipation over a two-week period.[23] The make-up of this study group was heterogeneous with 73% of participants having a definition of constipation based on passing fewer than three stools per week and 27% being included on the basis of passing hard, small volume stools. After two weeks, the stool frequency of the psyllium group had increased from 3.1 motions per week to 3.5, compared to a fall in the docusate group from 3.4 at baseline to 2.9 per week ($p = 0.02$). There was an associated, non-significant difference in stool weights. The psyllium group increased from 261 g/week to 354 g/week compared to a rise from 282 g/week to 312 g/week in the docusate arm after two weeks. This study suggests that psyllium may be more effective than docusate. However, given the young and heterogeneous nature of the study population, it is hard to know whether these results are applicable to older people with constipation. There is no evidence of a benefit of stool softeners in preventing constipation in the chronically ill or immobile elderly.[11,24]

Lubricating agents

Mineral oils have been used previously in the management of constipation. Due to the associated problems of anal seepage, fat-soluble vitamin deficiency and aspiration lipoid pneumonia, they should no longer be used in older people.

Enemas
Phosphate enemas

Phosphate enemas contain sodium acid phosphate and sodium phosphate, which have an osmotic effect resulting in increased stool water. They usually induce defaecation within 10 minutes of administration. There is no available evidence of efficacy in the treatment of constipation.[25] They have, rarely, been associated with significant side effects. These include hyperphosphataemia and hypernatraemia, which appear to be more likely in patients with either renal impairment or significant dehydration. They have been associated with rectal bleeding and perforation and should be avoided in people with rectal or anal disease. Patients who are subsequently incontinent are at risk of skin lesions from the solution. Given the lack of evidence of efficacy and the potential harms, they should only be used with caution in the frail elderly.

Other enemas

Simple water or osmotically active agents (such as sorbitol) have been used as enemas in people with constipation. They are associated with fewer adverse effects than phosphate enemas.

Suppositories

Glycerin and bisacodyl suppositories are available. Bisacodyl has a local stimulatory effect on bowel contractions. The suppositories have an effect in around 10–15 minutes.[11] Glycerin has an osmotic action, drawing water into the stools.

Therapeutic recommendations

A suggested protocol for the management of constipation is shown in Figure 7.2. In constipated elderly people who are otherwise well and ambulant, a wide range of oral agents could be tried. These include bulking agents, osmotic agents (lactulose, sorbitol and PEG), stimulants (bisacodyl and senna) and docusate. All of these agents have few side effects and there is little evidence of variance in efficacy. The choice of agent tried first should be based on cost. Suppositories and enemas are an alternative but evidence of benefit is lacking and patient acceptance is likely to be lower.

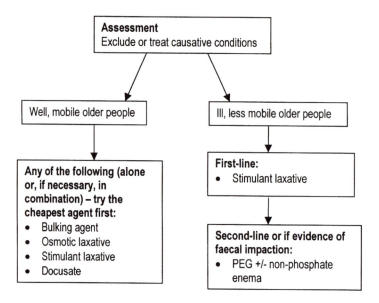

Figure 7.2 A suggested protocol for the management of constipation.

In the constipated elderly who are unwell, hospitalised and less mobile, there are fewer appropriate treatments. Osmotic agents that may lead to dehydration should be avoided in those with reduced fluid intake. Bulking agents should also be avoided in this group and those with impaired swallowing due to a risk of bowel obstruction. Docusate has little evidence of efficacy in this situation. So, a stimulant laxative may be appropriate as a first-line agent. If this fails or if there is evidence of faecal impaction, then PEG should be tried. Non-phosphate enemas may also be useful in cases of faecal impaction. If pharmacotherapy fails to resolve faecal impaction, then manual evacuation may be necessary (*see* p 167).

Clostridium difficile diarrhoea

Clostridium difficile is a spore-forming Gram-positive rod bacterium that is some-times present as a normal commensal organism in the gut (2–3% of healthy, non-hospitalised adults). It is more commonly found in older, hospitalised patients, who have an asymptomatic carriage rate of about 20%.[26] It is the major cause of antibiotic-associated diarrhoea, and in the frail elderly it is a significant disease with a mortality rate of up to 25%.[26] Although traditionally associated with hospitalised patients, the community prevalence is rising.[27]

Characteristically, clinical features start between four and nine days after anti-biotic exposure. The most frequently causative antibiotics are third-generation cephalosporins and clindamycin, but other agents, including penicillins and fluoro-quinolones, have also been implicated. The risk of developing diarrhoea increases with age, which may be due to both an increased colonisation prior to antibiotics and an increased susceptibility to developing disease. Transmission is by the faecal–

oral route. Hospital environments harbour the organism and its spores. Around three-quarters of patients with *C. difficile* isolated have contracted it while in hospital – usually through the ingestion of spores. Sites from which the organism has been isolated, not surprisingly, include toilets and bedpans, but also hospital floors and the hands of medical staff. Bedpan washers may not kill the spores and therefore bedpans of infected patients should be autoclaved. The spores are also resistant to some disinfectant agents.

Factors other than advanced age and antibiotic use that increase the risk of *C. difficile* infection include the use of proton pump inhibitors (PPI), nasogastric (NG) tube insertion, shared toilet facilities and long duration of hospitalisation.[26] The PPIs appear to reduce a gastric acid-mediated natural protection from the organism.[28] Other implicated drugs include H_2 blockers (presumably for a similar reason), and non-steroidal anti-inflammatory drugs (NSAIDs), although the mechanism of action of the latter class is unknown.[27]

C. difficile can produce two toxins (named 'A' and 'B'). The toxins may be produced in varying amounts by different strains of bacteria and both probably cause a disruption in the mucosal layer leading to fluid and protein loss with or without frank haemorrhage. At least one form that produces toxin B, but not toxin A, has been isolated, which has implications when testing for the organism.

Clinical features

In the elderly the most common presentation is watery diarrhoea that may have a characteristic greenish appearance. Vomiting, abdominal pain and fever are sometimes associated. It is a recognised cause of delirium. A form of disease without diarrhoea also exists. It should be considered in the differential diagnosis of a non-specifically unwell, hospitalised, elderly patient with a very high white cell count (WCC) (20 000–30 000 cells/mm³). It may present as a severe colitis or an acute abdomen and lead to toxic megacolon.[29] Pseudomembranous colitis (PMC) is a severe form of the disease resulting in an endoscopic appearance of the bowel resembling thin membranes overlying the bowel wall. Due to protein loss, oedema may be detected. Extremely severe disease has been known to cause colonic perforation.

Diagnosis

Immunoassays to detect toxins A or B are the most commonly used diagnostic tests. They can be performed in less than two hours. Sensitivities and specificities are around 80–95% depending on the test used. Many test only for the presence of toxin A and so toxin A-negative, B-positive strains may go undetected. Culture of the organism is difficult (and hence its name) and is more expensive and takes longer (up to three days). Sigmoidoscopy may detect the pseudomembranes of PMC but the disease sometimes only affects more proximal large bowel. Therefore, a colonoscopy would be required to adequately exclude all such changes. Given the frailty of this population and the increased risk of colonic perforation in the presence of inflammation, this procedure can rarely be justified. A plain abdominal X-ray should be performed if megacolon is suspected.

Treatment

The causative antibiotic should be discontinued if possible. Oral metronidazole or vancomycin for 10 days are equally effective (as metronidazole is cheaper than vancomycin it is usually first-line therapy).[30] If unable to take oral medication, either intravenous (IV) metronidazole (not vancomycin) or oral medication via an NG tube may be tried. The role of probiotic agents (e.g. *Saccharomyces boulardii* and *Lactobacillus* species) is not well established.[30,31] They may have a benefit in reducing the chance of recurrent disease.[26] Agents that reduce bowel motility should be avoided. Supportive fluids and electrolytes are often necessary. Surgery is occasionally indicated for fulminant colitic forms of the disease. In this setting it is associated with high mortality rates; 48% in one case series.[29]

Relapse

Around 20% of patients will relapse several days after completion of their eradication therapy. This is most often due to reinfection by uncleared spores. A further 10-day course of antibiotics should be tried. Rarely, a colectomy is considered for unresponsive, progressive colonic disease. Recently, the technique of faecal transplantation has been tested.[32] Here donors' faeces were instilled into the rectum of patients with recurrent disease (via an NG tube) with apparent success.

Prevention

Antibiotic policies that reduce the exposure of susceptible individuals (e.g. the elderly) to the most common causative agents should be implemented. Antibiotics should only be prescribed when the clinical indication is well established and the shortest possible duration of treatment should be used. Hand washing between patients, isolation of cases and adequate ward cleaning to remove spores are all extremely important.

Faecal incontinence

Faecal incontinence (FI) is an embarrassing and debilitating problem that often goes undetected by healthcare professionals. It should be specifically asked about when other bowel symptoms are reported. It ranges in severity from occasional leakage of gas to regular loss of solid stools. The prevalence depends on the population studied and the definition employed. In community-dwelling people, when defined as losing control of 'bowels or gas' in the preceding year, a 2.2% prevalence has been detected.[33] When community-dwelling people over the age of 65 were studied, 3% reported difficulty controlling their bowels.[34] In a similar population, using a definition of stool leakage at least once a week or the requirement to wear a pad, a 7% prevalence was found.[35] When defined as losing control of the bowels within the past year sufficient to cause stained underwear or worse, it has been reported to have a prevalence of 12% in a community-based population with a mean age of 75 years.[36] The prevalence is increased in residential and nursing home settings, being 62% in one nursing home population.[37] Further, it represents a common reason for nursing home admission.

It is often associated with urinary incontinence (UI) in the elderly. When a population of 413 nursing home residents (mean age 84 years) was studied, there were prevalences for continence, UI and dual incontinence (DI) of 28%, 70% and 60%, respectively, with only 2% having FI alone.[37] The same study found that 90% of those with DI had cognitive impairment and 94% had transfer and mobility problems – values that were significantly higher than those in either the continent or UI-alone groups.

Faecal impaction or diarrhoea are both frequent precipitants within the nursing home population. In a community-based sample of people (aged 65–93 years) around 60% of those with FI had either an associated chronic diarrhoea or constipation.[35] Other risk factors include the presence of neurological disease, reduced mobility, cognitive decline, and advanced age.[38]

In the elderly it may be induced by diarrhoea or laxatives that cause stool liquefaction. Chronic diarrhoea has been found to be strongly correlated with FI.[36] It may occur with overflow diarrhoea secondary to faecal impaction (*see below*). Autonomic neuropathy in diabetes may induce diarrhoea and FI. It commonly develops in advanced dementia where, similar to urinary problems, there may be reduced mobility, decreased awareness of the need to defaecate or disinhibited behaviour. It frequently occurs in the early post-stroke period when both cognition and mobility may be affected. It may also be precipitated by neurological conditions affecting sphincter function. FI in older people is associated with a reduced anal resting pressure and reduced anal sensation.[39] It appears that internal anal sphincter dysfunction is an important factor. Rectal prolapse and subsequent disruption of the innervation can cause FI. It is more common in post-partum women, around half of whom will be incontinent of faeces.[40]

Faecal impaction

'Faecal impaction' is a term for a mass of hard faeces within the rectum that cannot be easily passed. The mechanism that provokes FI appears to be a reduced rectal sensation capacity secondary to the faecal mass rather than the faecal mass affecting internal anal sphincter function.[41] The causes are those of constipation (*see* Figure 7.1) but the frail elderly are particularly susceptible. It should be suspected when such a patient has an unexplained clinical deterioration, especially when bowel habit alters.[42] Specific presenting symptoms include nausea, vomiting, abdominal pain, paradoxical diarrhoea and subsequent FI, but non-specific presentations such as delirium are well recognised in the elderly. The faecal bulk may precipitate urinary retention or incontinence (*see* p 140). Rarely, pressure on the intestinal wall may provoke ulceration, bleeding or perforation. It is usually managed with a combination of laxatives and enemas. Infrequently, failed medical therapy necessitates manual evacuation. Recently a regimen of high-dose polyethylene glycol/electrolyte solution for up to three days has been shown to be effective in resolving impaction with minimal adverse effects.[43]

Assessment

History

The consistency and frequency of the stools should be established. A stool diary may help to quantify the problem. The patient may be aware of the need to pass stool but unable to reach the toilet in time (urgency) which may be compounded by mobility or environmental factors. Therefore, it is important to distinguish this from un-recognised, passive leakage of stools. When loose stools are reported, medical conditions or drugs that may be causative should be enquired about (*see* Table 7.2). Chronic diarrhoea has a prevalence of around 14% in the community-dwelling elderly.[35] When infrequent or difficult to pass stools precede the onset of FI, causes of constipation should be pursued (*see* Figure 7.1). The occurrence of rectal prolapse should be sought.

Table 7.2 Conditions and drugs that more commonly cause diarrhoea in the elderly

Conditions	*Drugs*
Irritable bowel syndrome (IBS)	Laxatives
Inflammatory bowel disease	Antibiotics (erythromycin)
Lactose intolerance	*C. difficile* (as a consequence of therapy)
Radiation enteritis	Proton pump inhibitors
	Donepezil

Examination

Rectal examination should be performed to exclude faecal impaction. A neuro-logical examination and cognitive assessment are often helpful.

Investigations

A stool sample should be obtained when diarrhoea is reported to exclude an infective cause. A change in bowel habit should raise concern that there is an underlying malignant lesion. Colonoscopy should be considered especially if there is associated weight loss or rectal bleeding. More detailed studies of anal structure and function, such as anal ultrasound and manometry or defecating proctograms, are usually unnecessary unless surgical intervention is being planned.

Treatment

A simple algorithm to guide the initial assessment and management of FI in the elderly is presented in Figure 7.3. When an underlying bowel condition has been identified, treatment should be undertaken to try and improve this. When FI is associated with faecal impaction, the use of laxatives and enemas to promote complete rectal emptying is associated with a reduction in the frequency of incontinent episodes.[44] Polyethylene glycol has been shown to be useful in the treatment of faecal impaction in a small, uncontrolled study ($n = 30$, age range 17–87 years).[45] If pharmacological disimpaction fails then manual evacuation (possibly under anaesthesia) may be required. When FI is associated with chronic diarrhoea, antimotility agents (e.g. loperamide or codeine) may be beneficial.

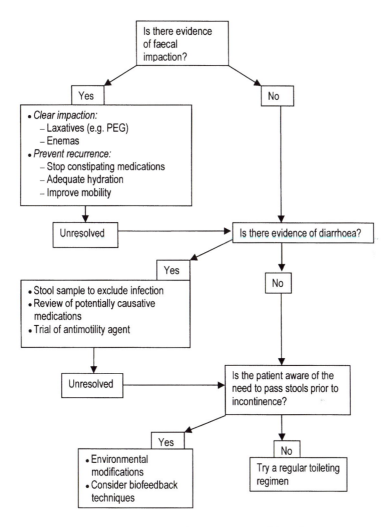

Figure 7.3 A simple scheme for the initial management of faecal incontinence (FI) in the elderly.

A regular toileting pattern can sometimes be produced by the alternating use of constipating drugs followed by enemas on a thrice-weekly basis. Alternatively regular toileting at times when the passage of stools is more likely (e.g. following meals) can sometimes establish an effective regimen.[46] When prompted-voiding (identical to that used for UI – see p 148) was tried in nursing home residents, no beneficial effect was demonstrated.[47] If the patient is aware of the need to pass stools but unable to access the toilet, simple environmental modifications should be tried, such as a bedside commode.

Occasionally, biofeedback or surgical intervention will be appropriate in older patients. These therapies are discussed below. Despite careful assessment and attempts at treatment, FI cannot always be improved. In this situation pads are often the most practical solution. Rarely, anal plugs are employed to prevent faecal leakage. These are often poorly tolerated by patients but may have a minor beneficial role in carefully selected people.[48]

Biofeedback training

Biofeedback techniques have been used to improve sphincter control in patients who are cognitively able to comply with such a programme. For a successful outcome there also needs to be some preserved rectal sensation and voluntary sphincter contraction. It aims to teach a method of increasing external anal sphincter closure in response to rectal filling. There have been reports of benefit in around 70% of well-selected groups of patients and no associated adverse effects have been noted.[46,49] However, a Cochrane review was unable to find sufficient high-quality evidence to endorse this approach.[50] Given the frequent association of dementia with FI in the elderly, it is unlikely to be a useful strategy in most older patients.

Surgical intervention

If there is an associated rectal prolapse with the FI, then this should be repaired. Around two-thirds of such patients will regain continence.[40] In cases where FI is due to sphincteric damage, for example after childbirth or a surgical procedure, an overlapping sphincter repair (sphincteroplasty) is often performed. There have been no randomised controlled trials of this therapy but data suggest that around two-thirds of such patients may benefit.[51] However, longer-term results may be less favourable as there is a tendency for this repair to break down.

An alternative technique is to transpose a muscle (usually the gracilis) so that it loops around the anus to form a new sphincter. This being a skeletal muscle, there are problems maintaining the prolonged contraction necessary to retain the bowel contents. Using an implantable stimulator can circumvent this problem. This combination is termed 'dynamic gracioplasty'. Unfortunately there is a high complication rate with this procedure, most commonly due to infection.[51]

Artificial anal sphincters have also been developed. These use an inflated balloon that can be deflated on demand by a switch positioned in the scrotum or labia. So far there are limited data available on outcomes with this technique, mainly coming from very small studies.[52] Sacral nerve stimulation, as used in UI, has also been used in FI.[53] The mechanism of action is unknown and, to date, there are only limited efficacy data. Injectable bulking agents, similar to those used in UI, have also been proposed but to date there are no randomised controlled trial data.[54]

If all else fails and it is deemed appropriate, colostomy has occasionally been performed for FI. The role of all of these surgical techniques in the management of FI in older people without anal sphincter traumatic injury is unclear. It seems likely that the vast majority of patients will not be suitable for such intervention.

Further reading

Riley TV. Nosocomial diarrhoea due to *Clostridium difficile. Curr Opin Inf Dis,* 2004; **17**(4): 323–327.

References

1   Schiller LR. Constipation and fecal incontinence in the elderly. *Gastroent Clin N Am,* 2001; **30**(2): 497–515.
2   Rao SSC. Constipation: evaluation and treatment. *Gastroent Clin N Am,* 2003; **32**: 659–683.
3   Whitehead WE, Drinkwater D, Cheskin LJ *et al.* Constipation in the elderly living at home: definition, prevalence, and relationship to lifestyle and health status. *JAGS,* 1989; **37**: 423–429.
4   Talley NJ, O'Keefe EA, Zinsmeister AR *et al.* Prevalence of gastrointestinal symptoms in the elderly: a population-based study. *Gastroenterology,* 1992; **102**: 895–901.
5   Heaton KW, Radvan J, Mountford RA *et al.* Defecation frequency and timing, and stool form in the general population: a prospective study. *Gut,* 1992; **33**: 818–824.
6   Wrenn K. Fecal impaction. *NEJM,* 1989; **321**(10): 658–662.
7   Monane M, Avorn J, Beers MH *et al.* Anticholinergic drug use and bowel function in nursing home patients. *Arch Int Med,* 1993; **153**: 633–638.
8   O'Donnell LJ, Virjee J and Heaton KW. Detection of pseudodiarrhoea by simple clinical assessment of intestinal transit rate. *BMJ,* 1990; **300**: 439–440.
9   Syn W, Tandon U and Ahmed MM. Colonoscopy in the very elderly is safe and worthwhile. *Age Ageing,* 2005; **34**: 510–513.
10 Cardin F, Barbato B and Terranova O. Outcomes of safe, simple colonoscopy in older adults. *Age Ageing,* 2005; **34**: 513–515.
11 Schiller LR. The therapy of constipation. *Aliment Pharmacol Ther,* 2001; **15**: 749–763.
12 Yuan C, Foss JF, O'Connor M *et al.* Methylnaltrexone for reversal of constipation due to chronic methadone use: a randomized controlled trial. *JAMA,* 2000; **283**(3): 367–372.
13 Ramkumar D and Rao SSC. Efficacy and safety of traditional medical therapies for chronic constipation: systematic review. *Am J Gastroent,* 2005; **100**(4): 936–971.
14 Petticrew M, Watt I and Brand M. What's the 'best buy' for treatment of constipation? Results from a systematic review of the efficacy and comparative efficacy of laxatives in the elderly. *Br J Gen Practice,* 1999; **49**: 387–393.
15 Tramonte SM, Brand MB, Mulrow CD *et al.* The treatment of chronic constipation in adults: a systematic review. *J Gen Int Med,* 1997; **12**: 15–24.
16 Xing JH and Soffer EE. Adverse effects of laxatives. *Dis Colon Rectum,* 2001; **44**(8): 1201–1209.
17 Elliot D and Glover GR. Large bowel perforation due to excessive bran ingestion. *Br J Clin Prac,* 1983; **37**: 32–33.
18 Lederle FA, Busch DL, Mattox KM *et al.* Cost-effective treatment of constipation in the elderly: a randomized double-blind comparison of sorbitol and lactulose. *Am J Med,* 1990; **89**: 597–601.
19 Passmore AP, Wilson-Davies K, Stoker C *et al.* Chronic constipation in long-stay elderly patients: a comparison of lactulose and a senna-fibre combination. *BMJ,* 1993; **307**: 769–771.
20 Corazziari E, Badiali D, Bazzocchi G *et al.* Long term efficacy, safety, and tolerability of low daily doses of isosmotic polyethylene glycol electrolyte balanced solution (PMF-100) in the treatment of functional chronic constipation. *Gut,* 2000; **46**: 522–526.
21 Attar A, Lemann M, Ferguson A *et al.* Comparison of a low dose polyethylene glycol electrolyte solution with lactulose for treatment of chronic constipation. *Gut,* 1999; **44**(2): 226–230.
22 Nusko G, Schneider B, Schneider I *et al.* Anthranoid laxative use is not a risk factor for colorectal neoplasia: results of a prospective case controlled study. *Gut,* 2000; **46**: 651–655.
23 McRorie JW, Daggy BP, Morel JG *et al.* Psyllium is superior to docusate sodium for treatment of chronic constipation. *Aliment Pharmacol Ther,* 1998; **12**(5): 491–497.
24 Hurdon V, Viola R and Schroder C. How useful is docusate in patients at risk for constipation? A systematic review of the evidence in the chronically ill. *J Pain Symptom Management,* 2000; **19**(2): 130–136.

25 Davies C. The use of phosphate enemas in the treatment of constipation. *Nursing Times*, 2004; **100**(18): 32–35.

26 Starr J. *Clostridium difficile* associated diarrhoea: diagnosis and treatment. *BMJ*, 2005; **334**: 498–501.

27 Dial S, Delaney JAC, Barkun AN *et al.* Use of gastric acid-suppressive agents and the risk of community-acquired *Clostridium difficile*-associated disease. *JAMA*, 2005; **294**(23): 2989–2995.

28 Cunningham R, Dale B, Undy B *et al.* Proton pump inhibitors as a risk factor for *Clostridium difficile* diarrhoea. *J Hosp Infect*, 2003; **54**: 243–245.

29 Longo WE, Mazuski JE, Virgo KS *et al.* Outcome after colectomy for *Clostridium difficile* colitis. *Dis Colon Rectum*, 2004; **47**(10): 1620–1626.

30 McFarland LV. Alternative treatments for *Clostridium difficile* disease: what really works? *J Med Micro*, 2005; **54**: 101–111.

31 Anonymous. Probiotics for gastrointestinal disorders. *Drugs and Therapeutics Bulletin*, 2004; **42**(11): 85–88.

32 Aas J, Gessert CE and Bakken JS. Recurrent *Clostridium difficile* colitis: case series involving 18 patients treated with donor stool administered via a nasogastric tube. *Clin Infect Dis*, 2003; **36**: 580–585.

33 Nelson R, Norton N, Cautley E *et al.* Community-based prevalence of anal incontinence. *JAMA*, 1995; **274**(7): 559–561.

34 Edwards NI and Jones D. The prevalence of faecal incontinence in older people living at home. *Age Ageing*, 2001; **30**: 503–507.

35 Talley NJ, O'Keefe EA, Zinsmeister AR *et al.* Prevalence of gastrointestinal symptoms in the elderly: a population-based study. *Gastroenterology*, 1992; **102**: 895–901.

36 Goode PS, Burgio KL, Halli AD *et al.* Prevalence and correlates of fecal incontinence in community-dwelling older adults. *JAGS*, 2005; **53**: 629–635.

37 Chiang L, Ouslander J, Schnelle J *et al.* Dually incontinent nursing home residents: clinical characteristics and treatment differences. *JAGS*, 2000; **48**(6): 673–676.

38 Chassagne P, Landrin I, Neveu C *et al.* Fecal incontinence in the institutionalized elderly: incidence risk factors, and prognosis. *Am J Med*, 1999; **106**: 185–190.

39 Barrett JA, Brocklehurst JC, Kiff ES *et al.* Anal function in geriatric patients with faecal incontinence. *Gut*, 1989; **30**: 1244–1251.

40 Madoff RD, Williams JG and Caushaj PF. Fecal incontinence. *NEJM*, 1992; **326**(15): 1002–1007.

41 Read NW and Abouzekry L. Why do patients with faecal impaction have faecal incontinence? *Gut*, 1986; **27**: 283–287.

42 Wrenn K. Fecal impaction. *NEJM*, 1989; **321**(10): 658–662.

43 Culbert P, Gillet H and Ferguson A. Highly effective new oral therapy for faecal impaction. *Br J Gen Pract*, 1998; **48**: 1599–1600.

44 Chassagne P, Jego A, Gloc P *et al.* Does treatment of constipation improve faecal incontinence in institutionalized elderly patients? *Age Ageing*, 2000; **29**: 159–164.

45 Culbert P, Gillett H and Ferguson A. Highly effective oral therapy (polyethylene glycol/electrolyte solution) for faecal impaction and severe constipation. *Clin Drug Invest*, 1998; **16**(5): 355–360.

46 Hinninghofen H and Enck P. Fecal incontinence: evaluation and treatment. *Gastroenterol Clin N Am*, 2003; **32**: 685–706.

47 Ouslander JG, Simmons S, Schnelle J *et al.* Effects of prompted voiding on fecal incontinence among nursing home residents. *JAGS*, 1996; **44**(4): 424–428.

48 Deutekom M and Dobben A. Plugs for containing faecal incontinence. Cochrane Database Syst Rev 2005, Issue 3. Art. No.: CD005086. DOI: 10.1002/14651858.CD005086.pub2.

49 Schiller L. Constipation and fecal incontinence in the elderly. *Gastroenterol Clin North Am*, 2001; **30**(2): 497–515.

50 Norton C, Hosker G and Brazzelli M. Biofeedback and/or sphincter exercises for the treatment of faecal incontinence in adults. Cochrane Database Syst Rev 2000, Issue 2. Art. No.: CD002111. DOI: 10.1002/14651858.CD002111.

51 Madoff RD. Surgical treatment options for fecal incontinence. *Gastroent*, 2004; **126**(1 Suppl.): S48–54.

52 O'Brien PE, Dixon JB, Skinner S *et al.* A prospective, randomized, controlled clinical trial of placement of the artificial bowel sphincter (Acticon Neosphincter) for the control of fecal incontinence. *Dis Colon Rectum*, 2004; **47**(11): 1852–1860.

53 Ganio E, Luc AR, Clerico G *et al.* Sacral nerve stimulation for treatment of fecal incontinence. *Dis Colon Rectum*, 2001; **44**(5): 619–631.

54 Vaizey CJ and Kamm MA. Injectable bulking agents for treatment of faecal incontinence. *Br J Surg*, 2005; **92**: 521–527.

Falls and related topics

Introduction

The first part of this section concerns dizziness (divided into lightheadedness and vertigo), falls, drop attacks and syncope. In this the following definitions will be used.

- *Fall*: unintentionally coming to rest on the ground or a lower level without apparent loss of consciousness.
- *Drop attack*: suddenly falling without warning, apparent cause or loss of consciousness.
- *Syncope*: an episode of loss of consciousness due to a transient global reduction in cerebral blood flow.
- *Lightheadedness*: an imbalance or pre-syncopal sensation often described by patients as feeling 'swimmy', 'woozy', 'giddy' or 'as though I was drunk'.
- *Vertigo*: a sensation of movement, usually the room spinning.

In elderly people a large overlap between lightheadedness, falls, drop attacks and syncope has been demonstrated.[1] Given this overlap, many components of assessment are common for all of these conditions. Single pathologies, such as carotid sinus syndrome, have been shown to be able to produce all of these presentations. Older people appear to be prone to such symptoms after minor insults (e.g. mild reductions in cerebral blood flow), which are insufficient to cause problems in younger individuals.[2] Their distinction is made more difficult due to a 30% occurrence of amnesia for unconsciousness in people experiencing syncope.[3] An assessment scheme that considers all of these diagnoses is shown later on (Figure 10.6).

The latter part of this section covers osteoporosis. As falls are the most common cause of fractures in the elderly, these subjects are clearly related. The National Institute for Clinical Excellence (NICE) guidelines recommend that the assessment and treatment of osteoporosis be incorporated into a comprehensive falls service.[4]

References

1 Shaw FE and Kenny RA. The overlap between syncope and falls in the elderly. *Postgrad Med J*, 1997; **73**: 635–639.
2 Kenny RA, Richardson DA, Steen N *et al.* Carotid sinus syndrome: a modifiable risk factor for nonaccidental falls in older adults (SAFE PACE). *J Am Coll Cardiol*, 2001; **38**(5): 1491–1496.
3 Kenny RA and Traynor G. Carotid sinus syndrome – clinical characteristics in elderly patients. *Age Ageing*, 1991; **20**: 449–454.
4 NICE guideline. Falls: the assessment and prevention of falls in older people. (Available at: www.nice.org.uk/CG021NICEguideline)

Chapter 8

Dizziness

Dizziness appears to have a very high prevalence among the elderly. In response to a postal questionnaire, a study found that 30% of people aged over 65 reported having experienced dizziness.[1] 'Dizziness' is a very vague term that is used to describe the symptoms of a wide range of conditions. For simplicity, here it will be divided into 'vertigo' and 'lightheadedness', as these can usually be distinguished by a careful history. Vertigo is a clear sensation of movement, usually the room spinning. Lightheadedness is a sensation of imbalance or pre-syncope that is often described as a giddiness, wooziness or drunkenness sensation. Both syndromes may coexist within a patient and both may be caused by some conditions, for example brainstem vascular disease.

The incidence of the various pathologies causing dizziness varies according to the subgroup studied. For example, a peripheral vestibular disorder is most likely to be diagnosed in older patients presenting to an ENT service.[2] In a study recruiting unselected dizzy older patients, lightheadedness or unsteadiness was reported in around two-thirds of patients with only one-third describing vertigo.[1] Also, when patients describing dizziness were subjected to both ENT and neurocardiovascular assessment, 28% were diagnosed with a cardiovascular condition compared to 18% receiving a diagnosis of a peripheral vestibular disorder.[3] In contrast, a study looking at a wide range of ages found the most common diagnoses made were vestibular and psychiatric disorders,[4] suggesting that these are more important causes of dizziness in younger people.

Vertigo

Vertigo can be caused by lesions affecting the inner ear, eighth nerve or vestibular nuclei in the brainstem. A simplified version of the vestibular system and its main connections is shown in Figure 8.1. More common potential causes are discussed below.

Specific conditions

Benign paroxysmal positional vertigo

The labyrinthine structures form a key part of the peripheral vestibular system. They include three semi-circular canals that contain sensory structures and fluid (*see* Figure 8.2). They are able to detect rotational movement. Benign paroxysmal positional vertigo (BPPV) is caused by free-floating debris within these semi-circular canals that causes inappropriate activation of the sensory structures. It presents as acute episodes of short-lived vertigo often induced by specific movements such as rolling over in bed or looking up to hang out washing. There may be

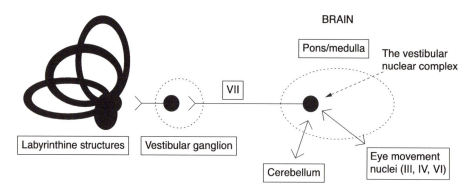

Figure 8.1 A simplified version of the vestibular system and its main connections.

associated nausea and vomiting. It may be diagnosed by the Hallpike test – *see* Figure 8.3. It is best treated by the Epley manoeuvre[5] – a series of movements that transfer the debris within the semi-circular canal into the utricle, where it no longer causes any symptoms.

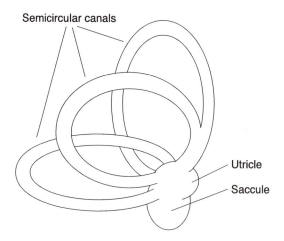

Figure 8.2 The peripheral vestibular system.

Vestibular neuronitis

Vestibular neuronitis is a poorly understood condition causing acute vertigo sometimes associated with nausea, vomiting and ataxia. It spontaneously resolves over several days. It is thought to be due to a viral infection of the vestibular pathway.

Ménière's disease

Ménière's disease is a condition that causes intermittent attacks of vertigo with associated tinnitus (usually unilateral at onset) and hearing deficit. The exact cause is unknown and treatment is often ineffective. The vertigo remits after several years in the majority of patients but the hearing deficit usually persists.

Brainstem vascular disease

Lesions affecting the central vestibular nuclei can cause vertigo, for example lateral medullary syndrome (*see* p 105). There will be associated neurological signs depending on the vascular territory involved, for example dysarthria, diplopia, hemianopia and sensory/motor signs. Vertigo in isolation is extremely unlikely to be due to a stroke.

Drug-induced

Ototoxic agents may cause vertigo. Some of the more common causative agents are listed below:

- furosemide
- gentamicin
- non-steroidal anti-inflammatory drugs (NSAIDs)
- quinine.

Cerebellopontine angle tumour

Cerebellopontine angle tumours (e.g. acoustic neuroma) usually present with unilateral sensorineural hearing loss due to compression of the eighth nerve. The trigeminal nerve may also be affected causing facial numbness and loss of the corneal reflex. When vertigo occurs it is usually a late feature.

Assessment

Clinical

History and examination will reveal clinical features leading to a diagnosis in most cases. Nystagmus is a physical sign often associated with vertigo. It is described by the direction of the fast (corrective) phase rather than the slow (pathological) phase. When it is caused by labyrinthine lesions it is usually horizontal in nature and the fast phase is in a direction away from the affected side. It is characteristically diminished on visual fixation of an object. In contrast, nystagmus associated with a cerebellar lesion usually has vertical and rotatory components and tends to be unaffected by visual fixation. The fast phase of the horizontal component is in a direction towards the affected side. There may also be other cerebellar signs. The Hallpike test is useful in the diagnosis of BPPV (*see* Figure 8.3).

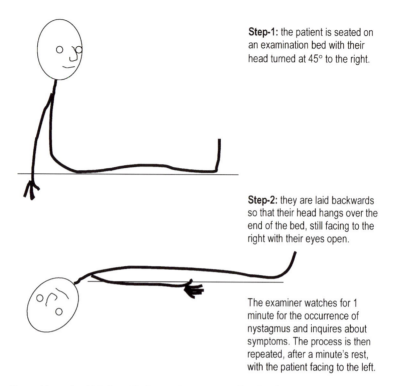

Step-1: the patient is seated on an examination bed with their head turned at 45° to the right.

Step-2: they are laid backwards so that their head hangs over the end of the bed, still facing to the right with their eyes open.

The examiner watches for 1 minute for the occurrence of nystagmus and inquires about symptoms. The process is then repeated, after a minute's rest, with the patient facing to the left.

A positive rest is one in which the patient's symptoms are reproduced and nystagmus is provoked.

Figure 8.3 The Hallpike test for benign paroxysmal positional vertigo (BPPV).

Investigations

Specialised vestibular testing including electronystagmography and detailed brain imaging with magnetic resonance imaging (MRI) have not proved to be good discriminators of the causes of vertigo within an elderly population.[6] Brain imaging is required when clinical features are suggestive of a cerebellopontine angle tumour or a brainstem stroke.

Treatment

If possible any underlying cause should be treated, for example discontinuation of causative medications or performing the Epley manoeuvre for BPPV.

Drugs

A wide range of medications has been tried in the management of vertigo with varying success.[7] The most commonly used are histamine receptor antagonists (e.g. cyclizine (H_1) and betahistine (H_3)). They may have a role in the short-term management of vertigo but prolonged use should be avoided as they may paradoxically worsen symptoms. Some of these drugs also have anticholinergic effects.

Reported side effects include sedation, confusion and dizziness. Newer antihistamine agents that are used in the management of allergies, such as loratadine, have fewer anticholinergic effects but do not cross the blood–brain barrier and so are not useful in the management of vertigo.

Vestibular rehabilitation

Vestibular rehabilitation is a form of exercise programme involving movements that induce the vertigo. These movements are taught by a nurse but then self-administered at home, the theory being that this invokes neurological adaptation that lessens the symptom impact. In a study looking at patients with chronic movement-provoked symptoms believed to be of inner ear origin, 67% of participants reported an improvement compared to 38% in the control group after three months.[8] However, there was no sham treatment in the control group and participants included had a number of different diagnoses and symptoms as well as many undiagnosed patients (71/170).

Lightheadedness

In the elderly, lightheadedness appears to be a more common reason for complaining of dizziness than vertigo.[1] The most common cause of this symptom is transient cerebral hypoperfusion in relation to neurocardiovascular disorders (e.g. orthostatic hypotension, vasovagal syndrome and carotid sinus hypersensitivity). The presence of posterior cerebral circulation atheromatous disease may make this symptom more likely to occur. Lightheadedness unrelated to postural change may be caused by brainstem cerebrovascular disease, drugs or, occasionally, by paroxysmal cardiac arrhythmias or psychological disorders. An overall scheme for the assessment of lightheadedness is shown later in Chapter 10 (Figure 10.6).

Specific conditions

Neurocardiovascular disorders

Neurocardiovascular disorders are discussed in Chapter 10. Orthostatic hypotension typically causes lightheadedness on standing from sitting or lying. Vasovagal syndrome typically causes symptoms following prolonged standing. Carotid sinus hypersensitivity classically presents following head turning but often no particular movement is noted prior to events. A reduction in blood pressure following meals (post-prandial hypotension)[9] has been noted in elderly subjects and this may be a factor in the aetiology of symptoms.

Brainstem vascular disease

Bilateral vertebrobasilar atherosclerotic disease frequently causes multiple similar transient ischaemic attack (TIA) episodes.[10] These may be triggered by any event further reducing blood flow, such as orthostatic hypotension on standing. They may also be provoked at rest by posterior circulation emboli or by cardiac dysrhythmias. The most common complaints caused are lightheadedness, blurred vision, and ataxia which is usually short-lived.[11] Patients presenting with these symptoms who have risk factors for vascular disease should be considered for secondary prevention measures, that is, antiplatelet and statin therapy (*see* Chapter 5). A number of patients who have sustained a brainstem stroke develop a chronic sensation of lightheadedness that is unaffected by postural change (sometimes termed 'central dizziness'). No effective treatment exists for this condition.

Subclavian steal syndrome is a potential, although rare, cause of similar symptoms. In some cases it may result in syncope.[12] It is caused by an occlusion of the proximal subclavian artery which results in retrograde blood flow in the ipsilateral vertebral artery ('steal' of the blood flow to the brainstem). In the vast majority of cases this is secondary to atheromatous disease. Characteristically, symptoms are provoked by vigorous exercise of the affected arm. Physical signs include absent pulses, a difference in blood pressure of >20 mmHg between the arms and a supraclavicular bruit. Diagnosis is made by demonstrating retrograde flow in the vertebral artery with Doppler studies and then proceeding to angiography. Treatment involves addressing vascular risk factors and considering revascularisation procedures such as percutaneous angioplasty.

Drugs

Many drugs are potentially causative. Some of the more common agents are listed below.

- *Antihypertensives* and *antidepressants*: as a cause of orthostatic hypotension (*see* p 201).
- *Antiarrhythmics* and *anticonvulsants*: causing paradoxical arrhythmias.

Cardiac arrhythmias

An arrhythmia fast or slow enough to cause reduced cerebral perfusion may provoke lightheadedness. Bradyarrhythmias may occur secondary to a neuro-cardiovascular mechanism. When 24-hour electrocardiograph (ECG) monitoring was used in the assessment of dizzy patients, two of 50 patients had a tachy-arrhythmia coinciding with symptoms (one fast atrial fibrillation (AF), one ventricular tachycardia (VT)).[3] A primary cardiac cause is more likely when the symptoms are intermittent and unrelated to postural change. Also, there is a greater chance with a previous history of cardiac disease, and pallor is often noted during these attacks.

Psychological disorders

Anxiety and depression are often cited as causes of dizziness. It is hard to know whether these are a cause or effect of the symptom. A lightheadedness that is constant in nature and unchanged by movement is most often reported. It would seem reasonable to screen such patients presenting with an unexplained lightheadedness for a psychiatric disorder and trying a course of therapy where indicated.

Assessment

Taking a careful history is vital. The events surrounding the symptoms give a clue to the diagnosis. A witness report is very useful when available. Lightheadedness caused by neurocardiovascular or cardiac mechanisms may be associated with facial pallor during the episodes. Investigation should be targeted at diagnosing or excluding potential causes (*see* Figure 10.6).

Treatment

Treatment is dependent on the underlying cause. The management of neuro-cardiovascular disorders is discussed in Chapter 10. Cardiac arrhythmias may be controlled with rate limiting medications ± cardiac pacemakers. Electrophysiology studies and implantable defibrillators may be indicated in cases of VT. If brainstem ischaemia is suspected, secondary stroke prevention measures should be instituted (*see* Chapter 5). Causative medications should be re-assessed for clinical need and alternative agents considered. If anxiety or depression is thought to be playing a significant role a trial of therapy should be considered (*see* Chapter 3).

References

1   Colledge NR, Wilson JA, MacIntyre CCA *et al.* The prevalence and characteristics of dizziness in an elderly community. *Age Ageing*, 1994; **23**: 117–120.
2   Katsarkas A. Dizziness in aging: a retrospective study of 1194 cases. *Otolaryn Head Neck Surg*, 1994; **110**(3): 296–301.
3   Lawson J, Fitzgerald J, Birchall J *et al.* Diagnosis of geriatric patients with severe dizziness. *JAGS*, 1999; **47**: 12–17.
4   Kroenke K, Lucas CA, Rosenberg ML *et al.* Causes of persistent dizziness: a prospective study of 100 patients in ambulatory care. *Ann Int Med*, 1992; **117**(11): 898–904.
5   Epley JM. The canalith repositioning procedure: for treatment of benign paroxysmal positional vertigo. *Otolaryn Head Neck Surg*, 1992; **107**(3): 399–404.
6   Colledge NR, Barr-Hamilton RM, Lewis SJ *et al.* Evaluation of investigations to diagnose the cause of dizziness in elderly people: a community based controlled study. *BMJ*, 1996; **313**: 788–792.
7   Darlington CL and Smith PF. Drug treatment for vertigo and dizziness. *NZ Med J*, 1998; **111**: 332–334.
8   Yardley L, Donovan-Hall M, Smith HE *et al.* Effectiveness of primary care-based vestibular rehabilitation for chronic dizziness. *Ann Int Med*, 2004; **141**(8): 598–605.
9   Lipsitz LA, Nyquist RP, Wei JY *et al.* Postprandial reduction in blood pressure in the elderly. *NEJM*, 1983; **309**(2): 81–83.
10 Shin H, Yoo K, Chang HM *et al.* Bilateral intracranial vertebral artery disease in the New England Medical Center Posterior Circulation Registry. *Arch Neurol*, 1999; **56**: 1353–1358.
11 Caplan LR, Wityk RJ, Glass TA *et al.* New England Medical Center Posterior Circulation Registry. *Ann Neurol*, 2004; **56**: 389–398.
12 Chan-Tack KM. Subclavian steal syndrome: a rare but important cause of syncope. *Southern Med J*, 2001; **94**(4): 445–447.

Chapter 9

Falls

Background

It has been shown that around 30% of people over the age of 65 will fall in any given year and that this figure increases to 40% of those aged over 80 years.[1,2] People in nursing homes seem at particular risk, an estimate has been made of 1.5 falls per bed per year.[3] Also, those recently discharged from hospital appear to have a higher chance of falling.[4] Even in the absence of injury, 47% of people over the age of 72 will be unable to get up after a fall at home.[5] Falls have been found to account for 39% of emergency department attendances in those over the age of 50 years.[6] A large proportion of falls in the elderly result in hospital admission and on discharge a significant number will be placed in residential facilities.[7]

The process of remaining upright depends on the interaction of multiple systems, including balance (visual, proprioceptive, vestibular and cerebellar components), co-ordination and limb power. There are also external factors that make falls more likely to occur, such as obstacles and uneven flooring. On top of this there are specific medical conditions that make falls more likely to occur, for example orthostatic hypotension (OH). Therefore, it is unsurprising that many falls are multi-factorial in nature and almost any acute illness can increase their likelihood. A comprehensive assessment tries to identify all of the factors that increase their probability. This is best performed by a multi-disciplinary team involving medical, nursing, physiotherapy and occupational therapy components.

A wide range of risk factors for falling has been identified. These include gait and balance disorders, visual impairment, arthritis, depression, cognitive impairment and old age itself.

Older people more often sustain injuries after a fall than younger people. This difference is partly attributed to blunted reaction times for protective reflexes, and a higher prevalence of osteoporosis. Serious complications of falling include hip fracture. Following a fall there is also a high incidence of 'fear of falling' that can lead to reduced mobility and social isolation. A negative spiral can develop where older people mobilise less due to this fear, and thereby become deconditioned. Then, on the occasions that they do walk, they are less steady on their feet and more likely to fall, further worsening the fear.

Assessment

History

The number of falls in the past year gives an idea of the scale of the problem.

- Onset of the symptoms – do any other factors coincide, for example medication changes or illnesses?

Try to get as much information about each fall as possible.

- *Activity at the time of falling*: syncope is occasionally provoked by actions such as coughing or micturition (situational syncope). Occurrence following prolonged standing suggests vasovagal syncope. Sudden head turning may trigger carotid sinus hypersensitivity (CSH). OH usually occurs after postural change (lying or sitting to standing). A drop in blood pressure can occur following a meal (post-prandial hypotension). Proximal myopathy or foot drop may cause tripping on going up stairs or whilst stepping over kerbstones. Falls at times when vision is reduced (e.g. whilst washing hair in the shower or under poor lighting at night) may suggest a proprioceptive problem.
- *Pattern of the falls*: is there a particular time of the day associated with falling? Visual and proprioceptive problems become worse in dim lighting, OH is characteristically worse in the mornings.
- *Preceding symptoms*: such as lightheadedness (suggestive of OH or syncope).
- *Loss of consciousness*: this may or may not be recalled. Ask the patient if they remember the act of falling. If available, a witness account is extremely useful; ask about colour change (neurocardiovascular causes often result in pallor, generalised seizures may cause cyanosis), the presence of seizure activity, duration of unconsciousness and the time taken to return to the normal self following arousal.
- *Consequence of the falls*: were any injuries sustained? Was the patient able to get up by him or herself? Have they resulted in a loss of confidence and subsequent social withdrawal?
- *Associated depression*: either as a contributory factor or a result of falling (*see* Chapter 3).

A full list of medications is particularly important, as many substances are likely to cause falls, in particular all psychotropic drugs[8] and all hypertension treatments (especially vasodilators and diuretics). Despite this, psychotropic agents are commonly prescribed in the elderly. A study of nursing home residents found that 36% were on an antidepressant, 24% on sedatives/hypnotics and 17% on antipsychotics.[9] There is no apparent benefit of atypical compared to typical neuroleptic agents in terms of fall risk. Fall hazard ratios (HR) have been found to be increased for typical antipsychotic agents (HR 1.35, 95% CI 0.87–2.09), risperidone (HR 1.32, 95% CI 0.57–3.06) and olanzapine (HR 1.74, 95% CI 1.04–2.90).[10] Tricyclic antidepressants (TCAs) and selective serotonin reuptake inhibitors (SSRIs) have been associated with similarly increased risks of hip fracture.[11] A systemic enquiry should look for factors associated with falls, such as urinary frequency or incontinence, cognitive decline and visual impairment. A past medical history may identify potentially causative illnesses.

A detailed social and functional history will help guide further assessments such as a home visit by an occupational therapist. In a study looking at community-dwelling people over the age of 70, 39% were found to have five or more safety hazards within their home with the bathroom being most often implicated.[12] Alcohol excess may also be a factor. Where syncope is suspected, establish if the patient is a current driver.

Examination

The following elements should be emphasised.

- *Cardiovascular*: pulse rate and rhythm, presence of murmurs (particularly that of aortic stenosis), blood pressure (lying and standing ideally done as part of an active stand test – *see* below), peripheral oedema and carotid bruits (if carotid sinus massage is being considered).
- *Neurological*: cerebellar signs, joint position sense, proximal or focal weakness, foot drop, spatial neglect and Parkinsonism.
- *Locomotor system*: reduced range of motion, pain/tenderness and deformity of joints.
- *Gait and balance*: observe the patient walking, note stride width, length, height, path deviation, arm swing and smoothness/steadiness of turning. A 'timed get up and go' test is a useful screening tool for gait abnormality[13] – see Figure 9.1. A normal, elderly individual would perform this in less than 20 seconds. It may also be used to measure response to interventions.
- *Vision*: using a Snellen chart, with and without glasses (where applicable). Visual impairment is associated with approximately a two-fold increase in falls risk.[14] Bifocal glasses may cause particular problems when negotiating stairs – they may need to be changed to a more appropriate type.

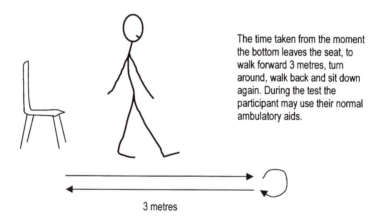

The time taken from the moment the bottom leaves the seat, to walk forward 3 metres, turn around, walk back and sit down again. During the test the participant may use their normal ambulatory aids.

3 metres

Figure 9.1 The 'timed get up and go' test.

Investigations

Baseline investigations should include the following.

- *Blood tests*: to exclude common contributory conditions such as anaemia, dehydration, hypoglycaemia, hypothyroidism and vitamin B_{12} deficiency.
- *Electrocardiogram* (ECG): to ensure sinus rhythm and a normal QT interval. An ECG suggesting previous cardiac disease may raise the suspicion of a cardiogenic aetiology.
- *Active stand*: the patient is connected to a beat-to-beat blood pressure monitor (digital plethysmography) and rested flat on a bed for at least five minutes. They

are then asked to stand up and remain standing for at least three minutes. The blood pressure is recorded when resting, on initial standing and then at 30-second intervals. The lowest recording is also noted (the nadir). Any symptoms experienced by the patient are recorded. Genuine OH is identified as a drop in blood pressure of more than 20 mmHg systolic and 10 mmHg diastolic that develops shortly after standing, remains present after a minute and is associated with symptoms such as lightheadedness. Very transient drops without associated symptoms are of doubtful clinical significance.

Further investigations should be guided by the findings from assessment so far. If loss of consciousness is detected or suspected then neurocardiovascular (head-up tilt (HUT) and carotid sinus massage (CSM)) or cardiological investigation (ambulatory ECG monitoring and electrophysiological studies (EPS)) may be performed. These are discussed in Chapter 10.

Treatment

The treatment of falls is primarily aimed at identifying and, where possible, improving all possible contributory mechanisms. Given the relationship between falls and syncope in the elderly, neurocardiovascular assessment is also often necessary. An algorithm integrating these approaches is shown in Figure 10.6.

Multi-factorial intervention programmes

Given the multifactorial nature of falls in the elderly, it is not surprising that a multi-factorial treatment strategy has been found to be most effective in meta-analyses.[15,16] An effect size of around a 33% reduction in the incidence of falls is characteristically seen. Most of these data come from community-based studies, which employed a number of different interventions tested together. Frequent components of these schemes include withdrawal of psychotropic medications, exercise ± gait and balance training, home environment adaptation, visual acuity assessment and information given to both patients and carers.

Further, a guideline has been devised by the National Institute for Clinical Excellence (NICE).[17] It is recommended that the following components be included in an intervention strategy: strength and balance training; home hazard assessment and modification; visual assessment and correction; and medication review and withdrawal, where appropriate. Also, information should be available in both written and oral forms for patients, their carers and healthcare staff. Topics covered should include strategies to avoid falls and ways to cope if a fall occurs. It is also recommended that an assessment of osteoporosis be incorporated into a falls programme. Osteoporosis is discussed in Chapter 11.

A study recruiting 981 nursing home residents with a mean age of 85 investigated the use of a multi-factorial intervention.[18] The intervention consisted of educational sessions for residents and staff, a review of environmental hazards, an exercise programme and the use of hip protectors (to which there was only a 28% adherence). They found a significant reduction in falls in the treatment arm (RR 0.55 (95% CI 0.41–0.73)). Therefore, it seems logical that such multi-factorial schemes should be implemented for both community-dwelling individuals and those in residential care.

A multi-component intervention has also been tested in a group of visually impaired people (acuity 6/24 or worse) aged 75 or over (mean age 84 years).[19] A combination of a home safety assessment and/or home exercise programme plus vitamin D supplementation or social visits only was implemented. The home safety element was effective at reducing falls (incidence rate ratio 0.59, 95% CI 0.42–0.83), but the other components were not.

It appears that multi-factorial intervention programmes, at present, are effective in reducing the incidence of falls by about a third. However, they are probably not effective for all people. In two community-based studies that included cognitively impaired patients, multi-factorial intervention programmes were not found to be effective (definitions of cognitive impairment were MMSE scores of less than 19 and 24, respectively).[20,21] This probably reflects the difficulty of this subgroup complying with interventions such as gait and balance training. So the selection of patients who are most likely to benefit is important. Some of the frequently incorporated components are discussed in more detail below.

Medication review

A wide range of medications can potentially contribute to falls. It is important to assess the risks versus benefits of all agents in a particular individual. For example, blood pressure-reducing medication may reduce the risk of a stroke but may also increase the risk of a fractured neck of femur, both of which may be fatal. Sedating medications such as benzodiazepines and neuroleptics are particularly harmful and their dose should be reduced and then discontinued whenever possible. A trial of 93 elderly patients (mean age 75 years) compared psychotropic drug withdrawal by gradual substitution with a placebo to a control group of usual care.[22] After a 44-week follow-up period a significant reduction in falls was demonstrated (relative hazard 0.34 (95% CI 0.16–0.74)).

Visual intervention

Some 70–79% of visual problems in the elderly are said to be correctable.[14] These are usually caused by cataracts and inadequate glasses. The other common causes are age-related macular degeneration, glaucoma and diabetic retinopathy. Treatment of these conditions is aimed at preventing deterioration in vision. There are no randomised controlled trials demonstrating efficacy of treatment in reducing falls but logic suggests that referral to an ophthalmologist is appropriate.

Strength and balance training

Strength and balance training regimens are common components of effective intervention programmes. The exact nature of the most effective format is unknown. One study failed to show a benefit of specific balance training over standard physiotherapy sessions in 198 individuals with a mean age of 83 years.[23] It could be that any form of neuromuscular improvement is beneficial. There is evidence that a once-weekly exercise regimen may be sufficient to provide this.[24] Physiotherapy input should also include guidance on how to get up after a fall.

Home environment assessment

A home visit performed by an occupational therapist may identify and subsequently improve environmental hazards. The types of simple interventions that have been found to be effective include removing rugs or poorly fitted carpets, installing bilateral stair rails and providing a raised toilet seat, a rubber shower mat, an emergency call alarm and nightlights for the bedroom and bathroom. A recent study recruited 360 community-dwelling people with a mean age of 82 years and a high risk of falling, and randomised them to either home environmental modifications or to a control group.[25] It demonstrated a significant reduction in fall incidence in the intervention arm (RR 0.69 (95% CI 0.51–0.97)).

Vitamin D

Deficiency in vitamin D is common among the elderly (*see* p 215). It has been associated with both proximal myopathy and falls.[26] A trial that compared vitamin D supplementation to placebo (both groups received calcium) in people in residential care (mean age 83 years) over a two-year period, found a reduction in falls in the treatment arm.[27] The participants recruited all had vitamin D levels in the low normal range (25–90 nmol/l). However, this was not associated with a significant reduction in fracture rates.

Preventing falls in hospitals

Whilst there is a large body of evidence supporting the efficacy of community-based fall-prevention schemes, there is far less knowledge about practice within the hospital setting.

A systematic review from the year 2000 identified two randomised controlled trials, one prospective study with a parallel control group and a further seven prospective studies with historical controls.[28] The randomised controlled trials investigated the single interventions of bed alarms and identification bracelets.[29,30] Neither demonstrated a significant reduction in falls. The remainder of the studies used a multi-faceted strategy including some or all of education programmes, environmental and equipment adjustment, high-risk identification signs/wrist bands, physical restraints and individualised care plans. The meta-analysis of all trials suggested a pooled effect rate ratio of 0.79 (95% CI 0.69–0.89). However, the majority of the positive studies used historical control groups for comparison. On further analysis, none of the interventions showed significant benefit when looked at in isolation. A later randomised controlled trial investigated the use of additional exercise training and an altered type of flooring without significant benefit.[31]

A more recent randomised controlled trial demonstrated a trend to reduction in number of falls (RR 0.78 (95% CI 0.56–1.06)) with a combination of a risk-alert card, information for patients, education sessions for staff, an exercise programme and hip protectors.[32] The difference between the groups was not apparent until after six weeks of intervention. There was no difference in fracture rates between groups, although the overall rate was low.

A further trial tested the introduction of a care plan consisting of a risk factor screening tool and appropriate interventions on alternate geriatric wards within a district general hospital with the other geriatric wards acting as a control group.[33] The mean age of patients was 81 years, the mean length of stay was 18 days on the control group wards and 21 days for the intervention group. Patients with a history of falls or those deemed to have either fallen or had a 'near miss' during their admission were targeted. The assessments included an eyesight screen, a review of medications, a lying and standing blood pressure measurement, a urine dip test, a mobility screen, an environment check (including bed rails, bed height and position on ward) and a footwear assessment. Appropriate interventions were then triggered according to the care plan. Comparing a preceding six-month evaluation period to a six-month period of intervention or control on both of the groups of wards, a significant reduction in the incidence of falls was seen in the intervention arm (RR 0.71 (95% CI 0.55–0.90) $p = 0.006$).

Risk assessment

Although broader policies, such as ward environment and prescribing practice adjustments, may affect all inpatients, it seems likely that specific interventions will only succeed if targeted at the highest risk patients. A review of fall risk-assessment tools found the following factors to be the best predictors of falls: lower limb weakness; gait instability; agitated confusion; urinary incontinence, increased frequency or the need for assisted toileting; a history of previous falls; and the use of sedative medications.[34] This, of course, does not confirm that the risk factors are also the causes of falls. The 'STRATIFY' assessment tool (*see* Table 9.1) has been validated with sensitivities and specificities of 92–93% and 68–88%, respectively, for a cut-off score of >2,[35] although it does not appear to be a good predictor of falls among patients who have sustained a stroke.[36]

Table 9.1   The STRATIFY risk assessment tool

Question	*Yes*	*No*
1. Did the patient present to the hospital with falls or has he or she fallen since admission?	1	0
2. Do you think the patient is agitated?	1	0
3. Do you think the patient is visually impaired to the extent that everyday function is affected?	1	0
4. Do you think the patient is in need of frequent toileting?	1	0
5. Does the patient have a transfer and mobility score* of 3 or 4?	1	0

*The transfer and mobility score is derived from the relevant sections of the Barthel index. The scores are added together to give a value between 0 and 6. Transfer score: 0 = unable, 1 = major help needed (one or two people, physical aids), 2 = minor help (verbal or physical), 3 = independent. Mobility score: 0 = immobile, 1 = independent with aid of wheelchair, 2 = walks with help of one person, 3 = independent.

Bed rails

The use of bed rails (also called 'cot sides') is commonplace within hospitals. One UK survey found that overall they were deployed on 32% of hospital beds, a figure that rose to 76% in acute geriatric wards.[37] Despite this, there is no randomised controlled trial evidence of efficacy in reducing falls and non-randomised studies have failed to demonstrate a benefit.[38] Where a policy of reducing their use has been implemented, there has been no apparent increase in fall or injury rates.[39] Also, they are not without the potential to cause harm, which may be that of falling from a greater height to the floor after scaling the rail, but also a number of fatal complications have been reported.[40] Given the absence of evidence of benefit and the fact that they represent a form of patient restraint, their use may be construed as unethical.[41]

In patients with a high risk of falling out of bed, an alternative strategy such as placing the mattress directly on the floor or the use of beds that can be lowered to ground level would appear more appropriate.

Restraints

Physical restraints, such as tying a patient down, have not been shown to reduce the incidence of falls,[42,43] act as a barrier to rehabilitation and are unethical. Their use should be strongly discouraged.

Prevention strategies

The following may be beneficial in reducing the incidence of falls in hospitalised patients.

- A screening proforma utilised to identify higher risk patients at the time of admission. The STRATIFY tool is simple and validated. Alternatively, the following information is likely to be a useful guide: falls history, a delirium screening test, urinary incontinence/frequency, gait assessment (e.g. timed get up and go) and potential culprit medication checklist.
- Patients in the high-risk group should then undergo the following interventions:
  - a risk identifier worn on their wrist or above their bed (a symbol rather than written information to try to help preserve patient confidentiality)
  - education in oral and written form on falls risk
  - preferential placement nearer the nursing station
  - a review of medications likely to increase falls risk, and a visual acuity assessment.
- Delirium and incontinence should be accurately diagnosed and treated (*see* Chapter 2 and Chapter 6).
- Education sessions for staff.
- Periodic review with ward team members of falls that have occurred.
- Exercise and balance training as deemed appropriate by the physiotherapist involved.
- Consideration of the falls risk when planning discharge, for example home assessment visits.

Drop attacks

The term 'drop attack' refers to events whereby the patient suddenly collapses to the ground without any preceding warning symptoms, and without apparent loss of consciousness. Unless an injury is sustained with the fall, there are no lasting effects and the patient is quickly back to normal. Such episodes probably account for around 20% of elderly patients presenting to a falls service.[44,45]

A wide range of conditions has been proposed as causative for these events, including otological disorders and forms of epilepsy.[46,47] It is likely that, along with other falls, they are often multi-factorial in nature. When older individuals with drop attacks have been systematically evaluated for neurocardiovascular disorders, 40% have been found to suffer from carotid sinus syndrome (CSS) and smaller numbers found to have OH and vasovagal syncope (VVS).[48] Therefore, in the elderly, drop attacks further blur the distinction between falls and syncope. Their assessment should be a combination of measures used in falls and syncopal events (*see* Figure 10.6). Treatment should be directed toward the underlying causative factors that are identified. Despite intensive investigation, around a third will go undiagnosed (sometimes termed 'cryptogenic drop attacks'), suggesting that we do not fully understand the aetiology of all such events.

References

1   Prudham D and Grimley Evans J. Factors associated with falls in the elderly: a community study. *Age Ageing*, 1981; **10**: 141–146.
2   Campbell AJ, Reinken J, Allan BC *et al*. Falls in old age: a study of frequency and related clinical factors. *Age Ageing*, 1981; **10**: 264–270.
3   Rubenstein LZ, Josephson KR and Robbins AS. Falls in the nursing home. *Ann Intern Med*, 1994; **121**: 442–451.
4   Mahoney J, Sager M, Dunham NC *et al*. Risk of falls after hospital discharge. *JAGS*, 1994; **42**: 269–274.
5   Tinetti ME, Liu W and Claus EB. Predictors and prognosis of inability to get up after falls among elderly persons. *JAMA*, 1993; **269**(1): 65–70.
6   Richardson DA, Bexton RS, Shaw FE *et al*. Prevalence of cardioinhibitory carotid sinus hypersensitivity in patients 50 years or over presenting to the accident and emergency department with 'unexplained' or 'recurrent' falls. *Pace*, 1997; **20** (Part II): 820–823.
7   Sattin RW, Lambert Huber DA, DeVito CA *et al*. The incidence of fall injury events among the elderly in a defined population. *Am J Epidem*, 1990; **131**(6): 1028–1037.
8   Leipzig RM, Cummings RG and Tinetti ME. Drugs and falls in older people: a systematic review and meta-analysis: I. Psychotropic drugs. *JAGS*, 1999; **47**(1): 30–39.
9   Gurwitz JH, Field TS, Avorn J *et al*. Incidence and preventability of adverse drug events in nursing homes. *Am J Med*, 2000; **109**: 87–94.
10 Hien LTT, Cummings RG, Cameron ID *et al*. Atypical antipsychotic medications and risk of falls in residents of aged care facilities. *JAGS*, 2005; **53**(8): 1290–1295.
11 Liu B, Anderson G, Mittmann N *et al*. Use of selective serotonin-reuptake inhibitors or tricyclic antidepressants and risk of hip fractures in elderly people. *Lancet*, 1998; **351**: 1303–1307.
12 Carter SE, Campbell EM, Sanson-Fisher RW *et al*. Environmental hazards in the homes of older people. *Age Ageing*, 1997; **26**: 195–202.
13 Podsiadlo D and Richardson S. The timed 'up and go': a test of basic functional mobility for frail elderly persons. *JAGS*, 1991; **39**(2): 142–148.
14 Harwood RH. Visual problems and falls. *Age Ageing*, 2001; **30** (Suppl. 4): 13–18.
15 Gillespie LD, Gillespie WJ, Robertson MC *et al*. Interventions for preventing falls in elderly people. Cochrane Database of Systematic Reviews 2003; issue 4.
16 Chang JT, Morton SC, Rubenstein LZ *et al*. Interventions for the prevention of falls in older adults: systematic review and meta-analysis of randomised clinical trials. *BMJ*, 2004; **328**: 680–683.
17 NICE guideline. Falls: the assessment and prevention of falls in older people. (Available at: www.nice.org.uk/CG021NICEguideline)
18 Becker C, Kron M, Lindemann U *et al*. Effectiveness of a multifaceted intervention on falls in nursing home residents. *JAGS*, 2003; **51**: 306–313.

19 Campbell AJ, Robertson MC, La Grow SJ *et al*. Randomised controlled trial of prevention of falls in people aged > 75 with severe visual impairment: the VIP trial. *BMJ,* 2005; **331**: 817–820.

20 Jensen J, Nyberg L, Gustafson Y *et al*. Fall and injury prevention in residential care – effects in residents with higher and lower levels of cognition. *JAGS,* 2003; **51**: 627–635.

21 Shaw FE, Bond J, Richardson DA *et al*. Multifactorial intervention after a fall in older people with cognitive impairment and dementia presenting to the accident and emergency department: randomised controlled trial. *BMJ,* 2003; **326**: 73–75.

22 Campbell AJ, Robertson MC, Gardner MM *et al*. Psychotropic medication withdrawal and a home-based exercise program to prevent falls: a randomized, controlled trial. *JAGS,* 1999; **47**(7): 850–853.

23 Steadman J, Donaldson N and Kalra L. A randomized controlled trial of an enhanced balance training program to improve mobility and reduce falls in elderly patients. *JAGS,* 2003; **51**: 847–852.

24 Taaffe DR, Duret C, Wheeler S *et al*. Once-weekly exercise improves muscle strength and neuromuscular performance in older adults. *JAGS,* 1999; **47**(10): 1208–1214.

25 Nikolaus T and Bach M. Preventing falls in community-dwelling frail older people using a home intervention team (HIT): results from the randomized falls-HIT trial. *JAGS,* 2003; **51**: 300–305.

26 Venning G. Recent developments in vitamin D deficiency and muscle weakness among elderly people. *BMJ,* 2005; **330**: 524–526.

27 Flicker L, MacInnis RJ, Stein MS *et al*. Should older people in residential care receive vitamin D to prevent falls? Results of a randomized trial. *JAGS,* 2005; **53**: 1881–1888.

28 Oliver D, Hooper A and Seed P. Do hospital fall prevention programs work? A systematic review. *JAGS,* 2000; **48**: 1679–1689.

29 Tideiksaar R, Feiner CF and Maby J. Falls prevention: the efficacy of a bed alarm system in an acute care setting. *Mt Sinai J Med,* 1993; **60**: 522–527.

30 Mayo NE, Gloutney L and Levy AR. A randomised trial of identification bracelets to prevent falls among patients in a rehabilitation hospital. *Arch Phys Med Rehab,* 1994; **75**: 1302–1308.

31 Donald I and Shuttleworth H. Preventing falls on an elderly care rehabilitation ward. *Clin Rehab,* 2000; **14**: 178–185.

32 Haines TP, Bennell KL, Osborne RH *et al*. Effectiveness of targeted falls prevention programme in subacute hospital setting: randomised controlled trial. *BMJ,* 2004; **328**: 676–679.

33 Healey F, Monro A, Cockram A *et al*. Using targeted risk factor reduction to prevent falls in older in-patients: a randomised controlled trial. *Age Ageing,* 2004; **33**: 390–395.

34 Oliver D, Daly F, Martin FC *et al*. Risk factors and risk assessment tools for falls in hospital in-patients: a systematic review. *Age Ageing,* 2004; **33**: 122–130.

35 Oliver D, Britton M, Seed P *et al*. Development and evaluation of evidence based risk assessment tool (STRATIFY) to predict which elderly inpatients will fall: case control and cohort studies. *BMJ,* 1997; **315**: 1049–1053.

36 Smith J, Forster A and Young J. Use of the 'STRATIFY' falls risk assessment in patients recovering from acute stroke. *Age Ageing,* 2006; **35**(2): 138–143.

37 Mildner R, Snell A, Arora A *et al*. The prevalence of bedrail use in British hospitals. *Age Ageing,* 2002; **31**: 555–556.

38 Capezuti E, Maislin G, Strumpf N *et al*. Side rail use and bed-related fall outcomes among nursing home residents. *JAGS,* 2002; **50**(1): 90–96.

39 Hanger HC, Ball MC and Wood LA. An analysis of falls in the hospital: can we do without bedrails? *JAGS,* 1999; **47**(5): 529–531.

40 Parker K and Miles SH. Deaths caused by bedrails. *JAGS,* 1997; **45**: 797–802.

41 Oliver D. Bed falls and bedrails – what should we do? *Age Ageing,* 2002; **31**: 415–418.

42 Tinetti ME, Liu W and Ginter SF. Mechanical restraint use and fall-related injuries among residents of skilled nursing facilities. *Ann Intern Med,* 1992; **116**: 369–374.

43 Ejaz FK, Jones JA and Rose MS. Falls among nursing home residents: an examination of incident reports before and after restraint reduction programs. *JAGS,* 1994; **42**: 960–964.

44 Sheldon JH. On the natural history of falls in old age. *BMJ,* 1960; **2**: 1685–1690.

45 O'Mahony D and Foote C. Prospective evaluation of unexplained syncope, dizziness, and falls among community-dwelling elderly adults. *J Gerontology: Med Sci,* 1998; **53A**(6): M435–440.

46 Ishiyama G, Ishiyama A, Jacobson K *et al.* Drop attacks in older patients secondary to an otologic cause. *Neurology,* 2001; **57**: 1103–1106.

47 Gambardella A, Reutens DC, Andermann F *et al.* Late-onset drop attacks in temporal lobe epilepsy: a re-evaluation of the concept of temporal lobe syncope. *Neurology,* 1994; **44**: 1074–1078.

48 Parry SW and Kenny RA. Drop attacks in older adults: systematic assessment has a high diagnostic yield. *JAGS,* 2005; **53**: 74–78.

Chapter 10

Syncope

Syncope is defined as an episode of loss of consciousness due to a transient global reduction in cerebral blood flow. In elderly, institutionalised individuals (mean age 87 years) it has been found to occur in around 6% of people per year.[1] Its community prevalence is hard to establish because of the frequent amnesia for unconsciousness in people who present with simple falls.

One of the differential diagnoses is epilepsy. The distinction can be made more difficult by the presence of associated seizure-like movements with the onset of syncope (usually myoclonic jerks). In situations where the hypoxia is prolonged, for example if the subject is propped up rather than being laid flat following the onset, seizure activity is more likely. Clinical features that are more suggestive of syncope than epilepsy include preceding symptoms of nausea or lightheadedness, a pallid appearance, a brief ictal phase without rhythmic clonic movements, and a rapid recovery phase without significant confusion or disorientation. Epileptic seizures may be associated with a preceding aura (e.g. a peculiar smell), a cyanotic appearance and tongue biting. When patients with a questionable diagnosis of epilepsy (due to poor response to treatment or atypical clinical features) were evaluated for syncopal conditions, around 40% were assigned an alternative diagnosis.[2] A suggested assessment algorithm is shown in Figure 10.6.

Subclavian steal syndrome is a rare cause of syncope (*see* p 182). Occasionally, metabolic disorders such as hypoglycaemia can present as syncope. Clinical features and baseline investigations should exclude such conditions. Rarely, psychiatric conditions present with similar symptoms to syncope. This group of patients tends to be younger. Conditions implicated include conversion reactions and somatisation disorders related to anxiety and depression.[3] Despite extensive investigation, a number of patients presenting with syncope will remain undiagnosed.

Syncope can impair an individual's ability to drive safely. Guidelines on what is approved within the UK are available at the DVLA website (www.dvla.gov.uk/at_a_glance/ch1_neurological.htm). Essentially, the guidance reflects the risk of recurrence whilst seated behind the wheel of a vehicle. Patients who drive should be made aware of the guidelines that apply to them. Web resources for driving regulations in countries outside the UK are shown in Box 1.2.

Assessment

The assessment of patients with suspected syncope begins with a clinical evaluation the same as for those presenting with falls (*see* Chapter 9). Additional investigations that are useful in determining the cause of suspected syncope are discussed below.

Head-up tilt

The head-up tilt (HUT) test is used to diagnose vasovagal syncope. After a 5-minute period of lying flat, the patient is placed at an angle of 70° from the horizontal on a special table (Figure 10.1). The blood pressure (BP) and heart rate (HR) are carefully monitored. This position is maintained for around 40 minutes.[4] Provocation substances such as glycerol trinitrate (GTN) spray or isoprenaline infusions may be used to increase the sensitivity (a 'provoked HUT'). However, these may reduce the specificity of the test – it is critical that the reproduction of symptoms, rather than haemodynamic consequences alone, is sought. A positive test shows a gradually declining BP, with or without a change in heart rate, which ultimately produces unconsciousness with the reproduction of the same symptoms previously experienced by the patient. These changes have been found to occur at a mean time of 24 minutes into the investigation.[5] On production of a positive result, the bed is rapidly lowered and the patient's legs are raised until the symptoms pass (Figure 10.2). A variant of this test in which the patient receives GTN provocation after 20 minutes of unprovoked tilting has also been described.[6]

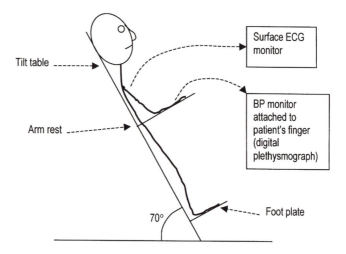

Figure 10.1 The set-up for a head-up tilt (HUT) test.

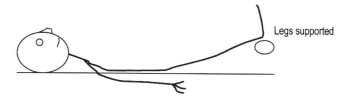

Figure 10.2 Recovery position after a positive head-up tilt (HUT) test.

Carotid sinus massage

Carotid sinus massage (CSM) is a test used to diagnose carotid sinus syndrome (CSS). It is recommended that it should not be performed in people who have sustained a stroke, transient ischaemic attack (TIA) or myocardial infarction (MI) within the past three months or in people with a history of ventricular dysrhythmias.[4] There is a reported 1% risk of inducing transient neurological symptoms with a 0.1% risk of stroke, which the patient needs to be made aware of during the consent process.[7] For this reason the neck is auscultated for carotid bruits and if present a carotid Doppler scan is recommended prior to proceeding in order to assess patient risk and advise on safety (in the absence of definitive evidence this is considered best practice).[4] The patient's neck is then palpated to identify the point of maximal carotid pulsation. This approximates to the location of the carotid sinus and is usually at the level of the cricoid cartilage, medial to the sternocleidomastoid muscle (Figure 10.3). Whilst continuously monitoring the BP and HR, the point of maximal pulsation is rubbed (firm, longitudinal pressure is recommended) for five seconds on the right side, with the patient lying flat on a bed. The right side is assessed first as this has been found to be more sensitive than the left.[8] If a positive result is not produced, the process is repeated at an interval of more than one minute on the left, and subsequently on the right and then left whilst tilted at 70° on a special table. A 31% additional benefit of detecting CSS by performing the test at 70° has been demonstrated.[9] A positive result is a pause in HR of more than three seconds or a drop in systolic BP of more than 50 mmHg. If a positive result occurs, then steps as for the HUT should be commenced. Atropine and equipment for external cardiac pacing should be available for the unlikely event of a prolonged cardiac pause.

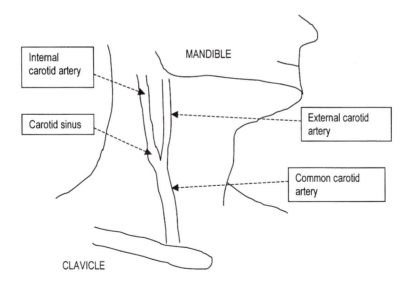

Figure 10.3   The position of the carotid sinus.

Ambulatory ECG

Ambulatory electrocardiograph (ECG) recording may be useful if a paroxysmal cardiac arrhythmia is suspected. The standard 24-hour ECG will only be reliable if symptoms occur on a daily basis. The less frequent the symptoms, the less likely that the abnormal rhythm will be captured. An alternative method, also using adhesive surface electrodes, is an event recorder. The patient wears this device for periods of up to several weeks. On the occurrence of a symptomatic episode, the patient activates the device and the heart beat over the preceding 10 minutes is stored in its memory for later analysis.

Implantable loop recorder

An implantable loop recorder is useful when symptoms are infrequent, and a longer recording period is necessary. This device is placed under the skin much like a pacemaker. Similar to surface event recorders, it can be activated following a symptomatic episode, the advantage of the device being that it can be used reliably for periods of up to two years. The obvious disadvantages are the requirement for a minor surgical procedure and the financial cost involved.

Electrophysiological studies

Electrophysiological studies (EPS) are techniques for identifying abnormal cardiac rhythms (e.g. ventricular tachycardia) that have not been detected by less invasive methods. They involve the percutaneous placement of a catheter that is fed through the femoral vein to the right atrium and ventricle. Electric stimulation or intravenous medications can then be used to try to stimulate abnormal heart rhythms. A positive test is one causing the reproduction of symptoms at the same time as a significant arrhythmia. Yield is highest in patients with either a history of cardiac disease or an abnormal baseline ECG.[10]

Ambulatory blood pressure recording

Ambulatory BP recording is unlikely to help with the diagnosis of the aetiology of falls or syncope. Its main use is to guide BP treatment in cases of orthostatic hypotension. It is discussed in more detail on p 201.

Neurocardiovascular syncope

There is a great deal of overlap amongst the neurocardiovascular disorders, suggesting similarities in causative mechanisms. In a group of patients with CSS, a 27% prevalence of orthostatic hypotension (OH) and a 20% prevalence of vasovagal syndrome (VVS) were also detected.[11] These conditions also appear to be more common in people with neurodegenerative dementias, possibly suggesting a common neurotransmitter deficit in their aetiology.[12] This association may explain the feature of loss of consciousness in patients with dementia with Lewy bodies (DLB) (*see* p 76).

Vasovagal syncope

VVS is produced by an autonomic reflex that leads to hypotension and bradycardia, resulting in a temporary reduction in cerebral perfusion. The precise mechanism is incompletely understood. When normal individuals are standing, there is a gradual gravity-driven accumulation of interstitial fluid in the legs. This is usually compensated for by peripheral vasoconstriction. This is mainly driven by baroreceptor activation and increased vagally mediated parasympathetic actions (*see* Figure 10.4). In susceptible individuals, this corrective reflex malfunctions, leading to VVS.

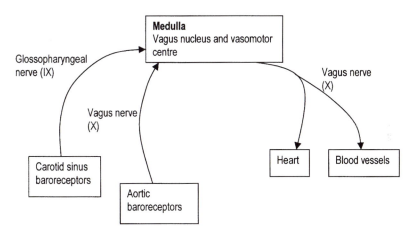

Figure 10.4   Vagally mediated blood pressure homeostasis.

VVS is classically triggered by periods of prolonged standing. There are several variants of this condition. It is proposed that young individuals may have a *hyper*-sensitive autonomic reflex which, when triggered, causes a rapid drop in BP. This pattern is associated with a history of fainting since childhood. Older individuals who develop symptoms may have a *hypo*-sensitive reflex that causes a gradual reduction in BP on prolonged standing.[3] Alternative triggers may be situations that cause increased abdominal pressure (*see* p 202) and painful or anxiety-causing stimuli (e.g. cannulation or the sight of blood). It is commonly associated with preceding symptoms of sweating and nausea and a pallid facial appearance.

The diagnostic test is the HUT. If a standard HUT is negative then provocation substances such as GTN may be used to try and reproduce symptoms. The test has not been associated with significant complications apart from rare reports of arrhythmias on provocation with isoprenaline. The reproducibility of the HUT test is significantly less than 100%.

Differential diagnoses that have been identified during head-up tilt, attributed to an absence of associated BP change, include psychogenic and hyperventilation syncope.[10,13] The latter appears to be mediated by cerebral vasoconstriction in response to a reduced pCO_2. Both of these conditions are more common in younger age groups.

Treatment

The first stage of management is education and reassurance. A number of lifestyle adjustments have been found to reduce the occurrence of symptoms. They are discussed, along with other treatment options, on p 203.

Carotid sinus syndrome

The carotid sinus is an area of dilatation of the internal carotid artery just distal to the carotid bifurcation (Figure 10.3). It contains a number of nerve receptors that sense change in pressure within the vessel wall (baroreceptors). Signals from these travel in a branch of the glossopharyngeal nerve (IX) to the medulla. From here a vagally mediated response can be triggered (Figure 10.4). As a response to increased pressure within the vessel wall the resultant effect is peripheral vasodilatation and a reduction in HR, leading to a drop in BP. In normal individuals this important mechanism maintains homeostasis of BP during changing physical activities.

CSS (also known as 'carotid sinus hypersensitivity') is a condition of abnormal activation of this structure which causes symptoms due to changes in HR and BP that lead to cerebral hypoperfusion. It appears to be increasingly common with advancing years, probably due to a combination of increased baroreceptor sensitivity and reduced cerebral autoregulatory mechanisms. The resultant presentations include lightheadedness, falls, drop attacks and syncope. A study that systematically evaluated elderly patients (mean age 78, range 67–89 years) with these complaints, found that around 25% had CSS.[8] When patients presenting to an emergency department with unexplained or recurrent falls were evaluated, 23% were found to have the cardio-inhibitory (*see below*) variant of CSS.[14] It appears to have significant consequences, with one study demonstrating a prevalence of 36% in patients hospitalised following a fractured neck of femur.[15]

It is subdivided into three categories:

- *Cardio-inhibitory CSS* (CICSS): the primary result of CSM is a pause in HR of >3 seconds.
- *Vasodepressor CSS* (VDCSS): the primary result is a drop in systolic BP of 50 mmHg or more.
- *Mixed CSS*: a simultaneous combination of both.

In a study of 64 elderly patients (mean age 81 years) with CSS, 37% had VDCSS, 29% CICSS and 34% had a mixed picture.[11] The same study found that the most common precipitants of CSS were head movements and prolonged standing, and that 25% of patients with CSS had had a previous associated fracture. Amnesia for witnessed syncope is well recognised in this population.[8,11]

CSS seems to be able to result in a range of presentations, namely syncope, falls, drop attacks and lightheadedness.[8] In a study systematically applying CSM to a group of elderly patients with any of these symptoms (mean age 79 years), a positive result was detected in 18% of subjects.[16] The yield was higher in the syncope and falls groups than in those with dizziness alone.

Treatment

Pacemakers

A group of 60 patients (mean age 70) with syncope attributed to either CICSS or mixed type CSS were randomly assigned to either pacemaker insertion or a control group.[17] After three years of follow-up there was a 57% recurrence of syncope in the control subjects compared to only 9% in the paced group ($p = 0.0002$).

The role of cardiac pacing in CICSS appears not to be limited to those with syncope. A study compared dual-chamber pacemaker insertion to standard care in a series of 175 patients (mean age 73 years) presenting to the emergency department with an unexplained fall and who were subsequently tested and found to have CICSS.[18] It was found that over the following one-year period there was a significant reduction in the likelihood of falling within the treatment group (OR 0.42, 95% CI 0.23–0.75). The authors speculated that this improvement in falls rather than syncope may be due, in part, to amnesia for actual syncope or may be because older people are more likely to fall with smaller reductions in cerebral perfusion that are insufficient to cause syncope in younger individuals.

Vasodepressor subtype

Treatment for VDCSS is less well established. Education and reassurance about the condition are important. Simple lifestyle adjustments, as outlined in Table 10.1, should be tried. Any culprit medications (e.g. antihypertensives) should be reduced or discontinued if possible. If these measures fail, a trial of medical therapy as used in orthostatic hypotension may be warranted for frequent events or patients at a high risk of injury.

Orthostatic hypotension

OH is a condition of low BP occurring on postural change that results in reduced cerebral perfusion and associated symptoms. When defined as a drop in BP of >20 mmHg, with or without symptoms, it appears to have a prevalence of 33% in geriatric inpatients.[19]

It is believed that approximately 500–700 ml of blood is pooled in the capacitance blood vessel in the legs and the splanchnic and pulmonary circulations whilst sitting or lying down.[20] On standing this causes a reduced venous return to the heart and, therefore, a lower cardiac output. In normal individuals, baroreceptors in the walls of the major blood vessels detect this change and initiate a reflex by increasing sympathetic nervous activity. The resultant constriction of peripheral blood vessels and increase in HR prevents a drop in BP. This process can be disturbed in a number of clinical situations (Figure 10.5).

Autonomic neuropathy impairs the ability to increase sympathetic nervous responses. This deficiency is associated with Parkinson's disease and diabetes. Also, a number of medications can affect this system, in particular anticholinergic (e.g. TCAs) and dopaminergic (e.g. levodopa) agents.

Chronic hypertension decreases the sensitivity of baroreceptors to change in intravascular pressure and also causes reduced vessel wall and vascular compliance.[20] For these reasons OH and hypertension often occur together. Also, cerebral blood flow autoregulation appears to be affected by prolonged hypertension,

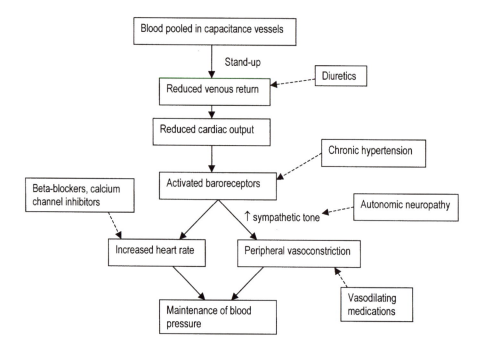

Figure 10.5 The causative mechanisms of orthostatic hypotension (OH). Solid arrows represent the normal physiological steps and dashed arrows represent unhelpful factors.

resulting in small changes in BP dramatically affecting cerebral blood flow.[21] Further, all BP-lowering medications are likely to worsen this problem. Particular culprits are vasodilators and diuretics (by reducing intravascular volume), and agents with peak and trough levels due to having short half-lives.[22] This combination of OH and hypertension is particularly difficult to treat (*see* p 244).

Post-prandial hypotension

A post-prandial reduction in BP in elderly subjects (mean age 87 years) has been noted.[23] This appears to occur between 30 and 60 minutes after a meal, with a mean maximum decrease in systolic BP of 25 mmHg. It was found in symptomatic and asymptomatic subjects but not in a young control group (mean age 27). There was no associated increase in HR, suggesting that this may be related to an impaired autonomic mechanism. In some individuals this reduction is sufficient to cause syncope.

Situational syncope

A range of stimuli can trigger a vasovagal-type reaction resulting in VVS. These are usually attributed to a rise in intra-abdominal pressure secondary to coughing, micturating or defaecating. They are sometimes referred to accordingly, for example 'cough syncope'. Treatment should be to reduce the precipitant, for example treating chest disorders, constipation and prostatism. Other treatment as for VVS should then be considered for ongoing symptoms.

Postural orthostatic tachycardia syndrome

Postural orthostatic tachycardia syndrome (POTS) is a condition that has been described in younger individuals (mean age 30, range 14–56 years).[24] It appears to cause symptoms of weakness and lightheadedness with associated tachycardia (a rise of 30 beats per minute or more within 10 minutes) but only minor changes in BP on postural change. It is believed to be autonomically mediated and is diagnosed by the HUT. Treatments that may be helpful include fludrocortisone and beta-blockers.

Treatment of OH, VDCSS and VVS

OH, VDCSS and VVS have similar causative mechanisms and so their treatment is similar. The first step is education and reassurance of the patient. A list of things to avoid or to try is given in Table 10.1. The second step is to reduce or discontinue any potentially causative medications (all anticholinergics, dopaminergics and antihypertensive agents, in particular vasodilators, diuretics and drugs with short half-lives). Compression hosiery (preferably full-length stockings) may be tried to reduce the effects of fluid pooling in the legs. In the case of OH, if the above steps do not improve symptoms, a trial of fludrocortisone or midodrine may be warranted. Paroxetine has been proposed as a treatment of VVS (*see below*).

Table 10.1 Lifestyle measures to help with the symptoms of episodic low blood pressure

Things to avoid to prevent hypotensive episodes:
  fluid depletion
  prolonged standing
  large meals
  hot rooms
  alcohol
  rapid postural change

Things to try to improve symptoms:
  small, frequent meals
  increased salt intake (not if history of heart failure)[25]
  raising the head of the bed (provides gravitational exposure during sleep)[26]
  lying flat and elevating legs at the onset of symptoms

Fludrocortisone

Fludrocortisone is a synthetic mineralocorticoid, and its main mechanism of action is by promoting renal sodium retention (in exchange for potassium). Its dose is usually started at 100 µg and titrated up to 400 µg if required. Main side effects are provocation of congestive cardiac failure (CCF) and hypertension (due to fluid retention) and hypokalaemia.

Midodrine

Midodrine is an alpha-adrenergic agonist that causes an increase in BP via vasoconstriction of arterioles and venous capacitance vessels. It is absorbed from the gastrointestinal tract and metabolised into its active metabolite (desglymidodrine) in the liver. Its onset of action is about 40 minutes after ingestion and its effects last for four to six hours. Therefore it is taken two to three times a day.[27] The dose is titrated upwards from 2.5 mg tds to 10 mg tds if required and supine BP permits. It does not cross the blood–brain barrier and so has no central side effects.[28]

In studies, a 10 mg dose of midodrine caused a mean increase in systolic BP of 28–34 mmHg one hour after ingestion.[28,29] This was associated with symptomatic improvement in small cohorts with OH.[28–30]

The most problematic side effect is supine hypertension; others include a scalp tingling sensation, pruritis, urinary urgency and a goose bumps sensation due to a piloerection. Midodrine does not have a licence for use in the UK, therefore it can only be prescribed by falls specialists on a named-patient basis.

Paroxetine

A single, small study ($n = 68$, mean age 45 years) has demonstrated a benefit of the selective serotonin reuptake inhibitor (SSRI) paroxetine in VVS.[31] Given the potential adverse effects of this medication in the elderly, a larger study confirming this finding in older individuals is required before this treatment can become recommended practice.

Cardiogenic syncope

Cardiogenic syncope generally carries a worse prognosis than other causes of syncope.[21] There are two broad diagnostic groups of causative conditions. These are structural lesions causing reduced left ventricular outflow, and arrhythmias. The most likely structural lesion in the elderly is aortic stenosis. Likely causative dysrhythmias in the elderly include complete heart block, sick sinus syndrome and ventricular tachycardia. In younger people conditions such as long QT syndrome and Brugada syndrome[32] (a cause of sudden death, associated with a characteristic ECG pattern) are more likely to be causative. A number of medications may worsen the situation, for example drugs that prolong the QT interval predispose individuals to torsade de pointes.

Cardiogenic syncope is more likely when there is a history of cardiac disease or a family history of sudden death or in the presence of an abnormal ECG.[33] Symptoms suggestive of a cardiac cause include onset during exertion. Exercise results in peripheral vasodilatation and outflow tract impairment can prevent an appropriate increase in cardiac output resulting in syncope. Alternatively ischaemia-related ventricular tachycardia may be triggered. Cardiogenic syncope, unlike most neuro-cardiovascular syncope, is characteristically unrelated to either postural change or head movements and so should be suspected in individuals with symptom onset whilst sitting or lying still. A sensation of palpitations may be associated.

Specific assessments should begin with auscultation of the heart and a standard ECG. When structural disease is suspected, an echocardiogram should be performed. With exercise-induced symptoms an exercise test should be considered. If an arrhythmia is suspected and symptoms are occurring at least every 24 hours, a standard ambulatory ECG should be performed. If symptoms are less frequent a longer period of ambulatory monitoring or an implantable loop recorder can be tried. Some devices are triggered by the patient following a syncopal event and are able to retrospectively record the last 10 or so minutes. An alternative is EPS to try and induce the arrhythmia. If underlying cardiac ischaemia is thought to be triggering an arrhythmia, than an angiogram may be performed.

Treatment should be directed to the underlying cause (Figure 10.6). Potentially worsening medications should be withdrawn if possible. Recurrent VT may be treated with an implantable defibrillator. Ischaemia-related arrhythmias may require revascularisation. Bradyarrhythmias may be appropriate for pacemaker insertion. Surgical options should be explored for structural lesions. For inoperable aortic stenosis, symptoms may be improved by discontinuing any vasodilatory medications.

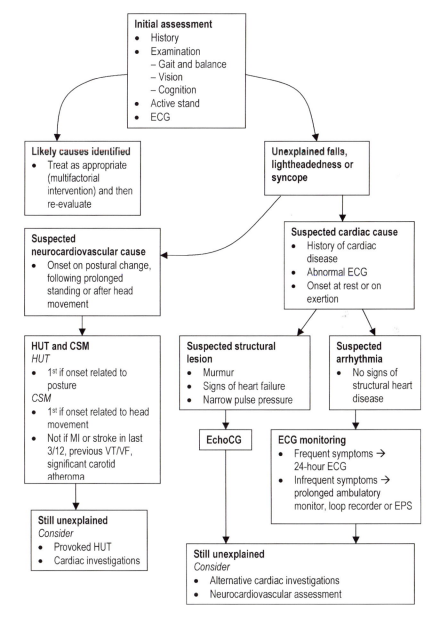

Figure 10.6 Suggested procedure for the assessment of elderly patients with falls, lightheadedness or syncope.

References

1 Lipsitz LA, Wei JY and Rowe JW. Syncope in an elderly, institutionalised population: prevalence, incidence, and associated risk. *Q J Med*, 1985; **55**: 45–54.

2 Zaidi A, Clough P, Cooper P *et al.* Misdiagnosis of epilepsy: many seizure-like attacks have a cardiovascular cause. *J Am Coll Cardiol*, 2000; **36**(1): 181–184.

3 Brignole M, Alboni P, Benditt D *et al.* Guidelines on management (diagnosis and treatment) of syncope. *Eur Heart J*, 2001; **22**(15): 1256–1306.

4 Kenny RA, O'Shea D and Parry SW. The Newcastle protocols for head-up tilt table testing in the diagnosis of vasovagal syncope, carotid sinus hypersensitivity, and related disorders. *Heart*, 2000; **83**: 564–569.

5 Fitzpatrick AP, Theodorakis G, Vardas P *et al.* Methodology of head-up tilt testing in patients with unexplained syncope. *J Am Coll Cardiol*, 1991; **17**(1): 125–130.

6 Del Rosso A, Bartoli P, Bartoletti A *et al.* Shortened head-up tilt testing potentiated with sublingual nitroglycerin in patients with unexplained syncope. *Am Heart J*, 1998; **135**: 564–570.

7 Richardson DA, Bexton R, Shaw FE *et al.* Complications of carotid sinus massage – a prospective series of older patients. *Age Ageing*, 2000; **29**: 413–417.

8 Kenny RA and Traynor G. Carotid sinus syndrome – clinical characteristics in elderly patients. *Age Ageing*, 1991; **20**: 449–454.

9 Parry SW, Richardson DA, O'Shea D *et al.* Diagnosis of carotid sinus hypersensitivity in older adults: carotid sinus massage in the upright position is essential. *Heart*, 2000; **83**: 22–23.

10 Petersen MEV, Williams TR and Sutton R. Psychogenic syncope diagnosed by prolonged head-up tilt testing. *Q J Med*, 1995; **88**: 209–213.

11 McIntosh SJ, Lawson J and Kenny RA. Clinical characteristics of vasodepressor, cardioinhibitory, and mixed carotid sinus syndrome in the elderly. *Am J Med*, 1993; **95**: 203–208.

12 Ballard C, Shaw F, McKeith I *et al.* High prevalence of neurovascular instability in neurodegenerative dementias. *Neurology*, 1998; **51**: 1760–1762.

13 Naschitz JE, Gaitini L, Mazov I *et al.* The capnography-tilt test for the diagnosis of hyperventilation syncope. *Q J Med*, 1997; **90**: 139–145.

14 Richardson DA, Bexton RS, Shaw FE *et al.* Prevalence of cardioinhibitory carotid sinus hypersensitivity in patients 50 years or over presenting to the accident and emergency department with 'unexplained' or 'recurrent' falls. *Pace*, 1997; **20** (Part II): 820–823.

15 Ward CR, McIntosh S and Kenny RA. Carotid sinus hypersensitivity – a modifiable risk factor for fractured neck of femur. *Age Ageing*, 1999; **28**: 127–133.

16 Kumar NP, Thomas A, Mudd P *et al.* The usefulness of carotid sinus massage in different patient groups. *Age Ageing*, 2003; **32**(6): 666–669.

17 Brignole M, Menozzi C, Lolli G *et al.* Long-term outcome of paced and nonpaced patients with severe carotid sinus syndrome. *Am J Cardiol*, 1992; **69**: 1039–1043.

18 Kenny RA, Richardson DA, Steen N *et al.* Carotid sinus syndrome: a modifiable risk factor for nonaccidental falls in older adults (SAFE PACE). *J Am Coll Cardiol*, 2001; **38**(5): 1491–1496.

19 Palmer KT. Studies into postural hypotension in elderly patients. *NZ Med J*, 1983; **96**: 43–45.

20 Lipsitz LA. Orthostatic hypotension in the elderly. *NEJM*, 1989; **321**: 952–957.

21 Kapoor WN. Syncope in older persons. *JAGS*, 1994; **42**: 426–436.

22 MacFadyen RJ, Lees KR and Reid JL. Differences in first dose response to angiotensin converting enzyme inhibition in congestive heart failure: a placebo controlled study. *Br Heart J*, 1991; **66**: 206–211.

23 Lipsitz LA, Nyquist RP, Wei JY *et al.* Postprandial reduction in blood pressure in the elderly. *NEJM*, 1983; **309**(2): 81–83.

24 Grubb BP, Kosinski DJ, Boehm K *et al.* The postural orthostatic tachycardia syndrome: a neurocardiogenic variant identified during head-up tilt table testing. *Pacing Clin Electrophysiol*, 1997; **20**(1): 2205–2212.

25 El-Sayed H and Hainsworth R. Salt supplementation increases plasma volume and orthostatic tolerance in patients with unexplained syncope. *Heart*, 1996; **75**: 134–140.

26 Ten Harkel ADJ, Van Lieshoult JJ and Weiling W. Treatment of orthostatic hypotension with sleeping in the head-up tilt position, alone and in combination with fludrocortisone. *J Int Med*, 1992; **232**: 139–145.

27 Benditt DG, Fahy GJ, Lurie KG *et al.* Pharmacotherapy of neurally mediated syncope. *Circulation*, 1999; **100**(11): 1242–1248.

28 Wright RA, Kaufmann HC, Perera R *et al.* A double-blind, dose-response study of midodrine in neurogenic orthostatic hypotension. *Neurology*, 1998; **51**(1): 120–124.

29 Jankovic J, Gilden JL, Hiner BC *et al.* Neurogenic orthostatic hypotension: a double-blind, placebo controlled study with midodrine. *Am J Med*, 1993; **95**: 38–48.

30 Low PA, Gilden JL, Freeman R *et al.* Efficacy of midodrine vs placebo in neurogenic orthostatic hypotension: a randomized, double-blind multicenter study. *JAMA*, 1997; **277**(13): 1046–1051.

31 Di Girolamo E, Di Iorio C and Sabatini P. Effects of paroxetine hydrochloride, a selective serotonin reuptake inhibitor, on refractory vasovagal syncope: a randomized, double-blind, placebo-controlled study. *J Am Coll Cardiol*, 1999; **33**(5): 1227–1230.

32 Antzelevitch C, Brugada P, Brugada J *et al.* Brugada syndrome: 1992–2002. *J Am Coll Cardiol*, 2003; **41**(10): 1665–1671.

33 Sagrista-Sauleda J, Romero-Ferrer B, Moya A *et al.* Variations in diagnostic yield of head-up tilt test and electrophysiology in groups of patients with syncope of unknown origin. *Eur Heart J*, 2001; **22**(10): 857–865.

Chapter 11

Osteoporosis

Osteoporosis is a condition of reduced bone density that is associated with micro-architectural changes that reduce bone quality. The process of bone loss begins after attaining peak bone mass around the age of 25–30 years. A gradual decline then occurs in all people as they age, mediated by a relative excess of bone resorption compared to bone formation (Figure 11.1). The definition of when this is a pathological condition is based on bone mineral density (BMD) measurements. A BMD of less than 2.5 standard deviations (SD) below the normal value for a person of the same sex aged 25 is defined as osteoporosis, and between 1 SD and 2.5 SD below the norm is termed 'osteopaenia'. Using this definition, around 30% of post-menopausal women are classified as having osteoporosis.[1] These data are derived from studies looking at Caucasian women and their applicability to other groups is uncertain. The major significance of osteoporosis is the increased risk of fractures as bone density declines. People who fulfil this definition may have either failed to reach a normal peak bone mass, have a condition that has accelerated bone loss or have simply lived long enough for their bone density to have declined below this arbitrary level.

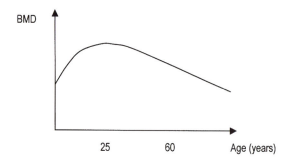

Figure 11.1 Changes in bone mineral density (BMD) over time in normal individuals.

The causes of osteoporosis has been subdivided into primary and secondary. The primary causes have been further divided into type I (post-menopausal) and type II (related to ageing). Important secondary causes or contributory factors in elderly people with osteoporosis are shown in Table 11.1. There are also genetic factors – a family history of osteoporosis increases an individual's risk. The majority of osteoporosis occurs in women due to the accelerated bone loss that occurs after the menopause.

Fragility fractures are those that occur following minimal trauma, which is conventionally acknowledged as falling from one's own height or less. The occurrence of such a fracture in an elderly person is highly suggestive of osteoporosis.

Severe osteoporosis is defined as a BMD <2.5 SD below the normal reference plus one or more fragility fractures.

Table 11.1 Important secondary causes of osteoporosis

Causative factor	Comments
Steroids	Usually following exogenous oral steroids for >3 months in a year; occasionally secondary to inhaled formulations; plus the other causes of Cushing syndrome
Osteomalacia	Reduced sunlight exposure, dietary deficiency, malabsorption (e.g. coeliac disease), phenytoin
Hyperparathyroidism	Primary or secondary (e.g. chronic renal disease); paraneoplastic (parathyroid hormone (PTH)-related peptide)
Hyperthryroidism	Over-replacement is also possible
Hypogonadism	For example, pan-hypopituitarism
Multiple myeloma	
Smoking	A meta-analysis has suggested that smokers have an additional 0.2% BMD ↓ per year compared to non-smokers;[2] this may be due to an associated poor diet[3]
Excessive alcohol	Alcohol probably has a direct effect causing the suppression of bone formation when taken in large quantities; alcoholism is also associated with vitamin D deficiency
Immobility	
Low body weight	The risk of hip fracture is elevated in thin women[4]
Heparin	
Low calcium intake	Probably less important than vitamin D deficiency

Osteoporosis in men

Osteoporotic fractures are less common in men than women. The key to this difference is the absence of a post-menopausal acceleration of bone loss in men. Other factors include a higher peak bone mass and a lower incidence of falls.[5] However, the precise incidence of osteoporosis in men is not known. The standard definition of osteoporosis is based on comparing BMD measurements to those of young women. This criterion may result in an underestimation of the incidence as men have a higher peak bone mass. If a comparison is made to the BMD of young men, then an age-adjusted prevalence of 6% is estimated for male osteoporosis.[6] The lifetime fracture risk for men is estimated at 13–25% compared to nearly 50% for women.[6] However, it should be noted that many of these fractures will occur in younger people without osteoporosis and that fractures occurring at a younger age are more common in men than women. The lifetime risk of hip fracture in the UK is 5% in men compared to 12% in women.[5] Given the infrequent measurement of BMD in older men, it is not surprising to find that asymptomatic osteoporosis is rarely detected and it usually presents with symptoms associated with a fracture.

The secondary causes of osteoporosis are similar to those of women but are more common in men with osteoporosis. Alcohol excess, glucocorticoids and hypogonadism are reported to cause 40–50% of cases.[6]

In relation to hypogonadism, testosterone levels appear to decline from about the fourth decade at a rate that has been estimated to be between 0.5% and 1.6% per year.[7] This is also coupled with a rise in sex hormone binding globulin (SHBG) that has a combined effect in reducing free testosterone levels by 2–3% per year. Plus, there is evidence that testosterone levels transiently reduce at times of intercurrent illness. Other factors, including obesity and diabetes, may also affect levels of free testosterone. The actual number of older men defined as having testosterone deficiency is dependent on the value that is considered as normal. It is estimated that 80-year-old men have a mean testosterone level that is half that of 20-year-olds.[8] Men have been found to suffer progressive BMD reductions after castration.[9] Testosterone replacement has been show to increase bone mass in deficient males.[8]

It has also been suggested that a relative deficiency in oestrogens is an important factor in osteoporosis in men. Bioavailable oestradiol levels decline in men with advancing age, similar to testosterone.[10] Osteoporosis has been described in young men who have had either inherited oestrogen deficiencies (through lacking the aromatase enzyme) or resistance syndromes.[6] A study comparing the levels of testosterone and oestradiol in younger and older men relative to changes in BMD found that serum oestradiol levels better correlated to bone loss than serum testosterone levels.[11]

The metabolic pathway of testosterone is shown in Figure 11.2. Testosterone is produced by the Leydig cells of the testes under the influence of luteinising hormone (LH). It may then directly interact with androgen receptors or may be converted to dihydrotestosterone (DHT) by the enzyme 5-alpha reductase, which acts on a subset of androgen receptors. DHT appears to have actions on the prostate and for this reason 5-alpha reductase inhibitors (e.g. finasteride) are used in the treatment of benign prostatic hyperplasia. Some testosterone is converted to oestradiol by the enzyme aromatase. Testosterone replacement has been shown to produce a rise in oestradiol levels. It may be this increase that mediates the rise in BMD that has been observed.

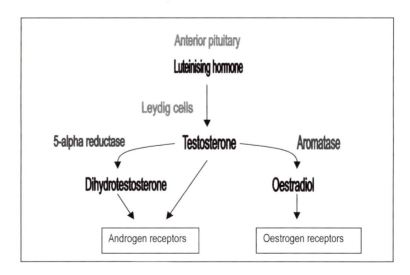

Figure 11.2 The metabolic pathway of testosterone.

Physiology

The key components of bone are proteins (especially collagen), cells and calcium salts. Osteoblasts are the cells that form new bone and osteoclasts are the cells that resorb it. They work in balance and in normal bone this produces a constant remodelling process. Their action is co-ordinated by a number of growth factors, cytokines and hormones. There are two distinct types of bone, termed 'cortical' and 'cancellous' (or 'trabecular'). Long bones are mainly composed of cortical bone and bones of other shapes are mainly composed of cancellous bone (e.g. the pelvis and vertebrae).

The metabolism of bone is influenced by a number of external factors. Bone acts as a reservoir of calcium. Vitamin D and parathyroid hormone (PTH) influence its turnover in order to regulate serum calcium levels. The relationship between vitamin D and PTH is shown in Figure 11.3. They are discussed further, along with calcitonin, below.

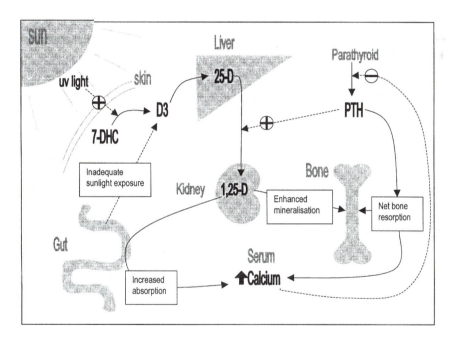

Figure 11.3 Simplied schematic of the interactions between vitamin D and parathyroid hormone (PTH) in calcium metabolism. D3 = cholecalciferol; 25-D = 25-hydroxy-cholecalciferol; 1,25-D = 1,25-dihydroxycholecalciferol; 7-DHC = 7-dehydroxycholesterol; + = an enhancing effect; – = an inhibitory effect.

Vitamin D

Vitamin D is not a true vitamin as most of it is created within the skin in normal adults by the action of ultraviolet (UV) light from the sun on 7-dehydroxy-cholesterol to form cholecalciferol (D_3). The remainder comes from dietary intake. If sunlight exposure is inadequate then this intestinal source becomes more important. This precursor is then converted to 25-hydroxycholecalciferol in the liver. This is further hydroxylated in the kidney to form 1,25-dihydroxycholecalciferol (also know as 'calcitriol'), which is the active form of vitamin D. The main actions of vitamin D are on the bowel and on bone. In the bowel it causes an increase in both calcium and phosphate absorption by inducing an increase in binding proteins in the intestinal epithelial cells. Its actions on bone are complex but appear to result in enhanced bone mineralisation. Vitamin D receptors have also been found on striated muscle cells. Their role is unclear but vitamin D deficiency is associated with proximal myopathy and an increased risk of falls (*see* p 189).[12]

Parathyroid hormone

PTH is secreted from the parathyroid glands. It also has complex actions on bone but the net result is increased bone resorption. This causes the release of calcium and phosphate into the circulation. PTH also has a mild inhibitory effect on renal calcium excretion but conversely increases renal phosphate loss. The overall effect is to increase serum calcium and reduce serum phosphate levels. PTH also has a major role in controlling the metabolism of vitamin D as it stimulates the conversion of 25-hydroxy to 1,25-dihydroxycholecalciferol in the kidney. PTH secretion is controlled by negative feedback on the parathyroid glands by serum calcium. Therefore, its secretion is reduced when serum calcium levels are elevated.

Calcitonin

Calcitonin is a poorly understood hormonal agent that is excreted by the C cells of the thyroid gland. Its effect is essentially the opposite of PTH – it causes a reduction in bone resorption by inhibiting osteoclasts and its release is stimulated by rising serum calcium levels. However, its precise physiological role in humans is, as yet, undefined and people who have undergone a thyroidectomy appear to be able to survive without any.

Clinical features

The three most common osteoporosis-associated fractures in order of frequency are vertebral, hip and distal radius (Colle's fracture), respectively.

Vertebral fractures

Vertebral fractures most commonly occur in the low thoracic to upper lumbar region. They may be asymptomatic, being detected only on X-rays, or present as progressive spinal curvature with height loss, chronic back pain, or acute back pain following minor trauma. Occasionally spinal cord compression can occur. Patterns of vertebral changes are shown in Figure 11.4. As a consequence of multiple fractures, a spinal kyphosis can cause further complications, for example reduced lung capacity provoking respiratory problems or reduced abdominal wall muscle efficacy leading to constipation. Treatment is usually with analgesia alone. Nasal salmon calcitonin may have a role as an analgesic agent in this situation (*see* p 219).

Normal

Biconcave deformity

Wedge deformity

Crush deformity

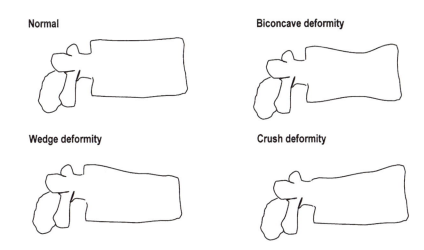

Figure 11.4   Patterns of vertebral deformity seen with osteoporosis.

A technique of percutaneous correction or 'vertebroplasty' is being increasingly employed. This involves the injection of cement into the damaged vertebral body in order to stabilise it and reduce associated pain. Small, non-randomised studies have shown promising results.[13,14] The technique appears to be well tolerated in the elderly. Potential complications include cement pulmonary emboli and nerve root or spinal cord compression due to cement leakage around the vertebra.

Hip fractures

Hip fractures usually occur after falling from the patient's own height or less (a fragility fracture). Overall mortality is between 10% and 20%, being highest in those most frail and those with comorbidities. In those who survive, there is significant associated functional impairment. In a cohort of 536 patients who had sustained a hip fracture (mean age 79.8 years, mean length of hospital stay 18 days) only 54% were independently mobile at one year, compared to 87% pre-admission.[15] Often these patients present with a classical leg shortening and external rotation but an undisplaced or impacted fracture may only cause pain on attempted weight-bearing. Treatment is by surgical fixation – either joining the broken bones back together with a dynamic hip screw or replacing the broken section of bone with a hemi-arthroplasty.

Hip protectors

Hip protectors are devices that consist of an underwear-like garment with protective pads overlying the hips on either side. They have been proposed to reduce the likelihood of sustaining a hip fracture following a fall. The evidence here remains inconclusive. When subjected to a Cochrane review, it appeared that a benefit was seen in cluster-randomised trials within institutional care homes with a high background incidence of hip fractures but this was not seen in trials with individual patient randomisation or with community-dwelling individuals.[16] The most recent data are less favourable for their use than earlier studies.[17] A major problem with this kind of device is patient concordance due to discomfort when wearing them and difficulty getting them on and off. This latter problem may be a particular issue in patients with an overactive bladder. It seems hard to justify the costs in terms of patient comfort as well as economics on the basis of available evidence.

Distal radius fractures

Distal radius fractures occur when there is an attempt to lessen the impact of a fall by using an outstretched arm. The treatment of this type of fracture is usually by placing the limb in a cast. Occasionally open or closed reduction is necessary for proper alignment. It does not usually necessitate hospital admission. However, in the elderly living alone, normal functioning may be impaired.

Assessment

Blood and urine tests

Blood and urine tests should be used to try to exclude secondary causes of osteoporosis. Thyroid stimulating hormone (TSH), calcium, phosphate, alkaline phosphatase (ALP), vitamin D, PTH, serum electrophoresis and urinary Bence–Jones protein are appropriate. A short synacthen test should be performed if Cushing syndrome is suspected.

Dual-energy X-ray absorptiometry scans

Dual-energy X-ray absorptiometry (DEXA) scan measurements taken from the hips of young Caucasian women form the basis of the standard definition of osteoporosis. This technique evaluates the amount of radiation that passes through the tested bone. The calculated density is inversely proportional to this value. Ideally this is done at at least two different sites (e.g. spine and hip). This measurement may give inaccurately high readings in the presence of structural abnormalities, such as vertebral compression fractures. By comparing the data obtained with reference tables, T and Z scores are derived. T scores are based on comparison with the mean value for young people; Z scores are based on age-matched mean values. Readings at particular sites best predict fracture risk at that site; that is, a low femoral neck BMD is a better predictor of hip fracture than a low vertebral BMD. A 2.6 times increased risk of fractured neck of femur is estimated for each SD drop in femoral neck BMD.[18]

Smaller, more portable units are available to scan peripheral sites such as the radius. These are quicker to use and expose the patient to less radiation. The disadvantage is that they may be less accurate and do not allow comparison of the data to the standard reference tables for hip values.

Whilst DEXA scanning has a clear role in the diagnosis of osteoporosis, it is less clear what its usefulness is in monitoring response to treatment. Random variations in BMD results obtained may make it a poor guide to the real effects of treatment.[19] Also, there is growing evidence that the relationship between fracture risk and

BMD is not a linear one.[20] Treatments may improve bone strength through micro-architectural changes with only small increases in BMD scores.

Quantitative CT

Quantitative computerised tomography (CT) measurements are usually taken at the spine. It allows accurate bone density assessment (expressed as g/cm^3) but is associated with increased costs and radiation exposure.

Quantitative US

Quantitative ultrasound (US) measurements are taken at peripheral sites, such as the calcaneum. It is a simple, quick and radiation-free technique but its accuracy has not been fully proven.

Bone biopsy

A bone biopsy may be considered when there is diagnostic uncertainty. This can exclude certain conditions, including malignancy, but is rarely performed.

Biochemical markers of bone turnover

Biochemical markers of bone turnover have been detected in serum and urine samples. They may have the advantage of reflecting responses to treatment faster, before BMD changes are detectable on DEXA. They include bone-specific ALP and various breakdown products of collagen. They are often utilised in the setting of clinical trials but are infrequently used in routine practice.

Treatment options

Ideally, osteoporosis or osteopaenia is detected by screening BMD measurements in at-risk groups and treatment is preventative. However, often the first presentation is following a fracture. Non-pharmacological measures include increasing activity levels, stopping smoking and reducing alcohol consumption. If a secondary cause of osteoporosis is identified, this should also be targeted. The pharmacological agents in current use are discussed below. They can be broadly divided into three categories. These are supplementation (calcium and vitamin D), anti-resorptive (e.g. bisphos-phonates) and bone-formation stimulation (e.g. PTH).

Calcium and vitamin D

A diet deficient in calcium is associated with bone demineralisation. This is more likely to occur in older adults. Vitamin D is mainly derived from the action of sunlight on the skin. In elderly people who may have reduced mobility and subsequent reduced sunlight exposure, possibly coupled with a diet low in vitamin D, deficiency is a genuine problem. The number of people who are defined as deficient in vitamin D depends on what numerical value is used. For a value of <25 nmol/l in people over the age of 65 years living in the UK, 10–15% who live in private residences and around 30% of those residing in residential care are deficient.[3] However, there is evidence that at levels <50 nmol/l there are increased PTH levels and bone resorption.[21] Using this value, around 55% and 80% of those aged over 65 in private homes or residential care, respectively, are deficient.[3] Trials that have looked at calcium or vitamin D alone have been inconclusive.[21–23] Two of the larger trials using a combination of therapy are discussed below.

The daily supplementation with calcium (1.2 g) and vitamin D (800 IU) of 3270 ambulatory women, with a mean age of 84 years, who lived in nursing homes or apartment houses for the elderly in France has been studied.[24] At baseline, all the subjects had a low calcium intake (less than 800 mg/day) and 44% had low serum 25-hydroxycholecalciferol levels. After 18 months, a 43% lower incidence of hip fractures ($p = 0.043$) and 32% lower total non-vertebral fracture incidence ($p = 0.015$) was seen in the treatment arm. This was associated with a 2.7% increase in femoral BMD compared to a 4.6% reduction in the placebo arm ($p<0.001$). The PTH levels significantly reduced in the treatment group and increased in the placebo group over this time period. This would be compatible with a rise in PTH being induced by a low intake of calcium with resultant bone resorption to maintain serum calcium levels (i.e. secondary hyperparathyroidism).

A study that recruited 3314 women over the age of 70, with at least one risk factor for hip fracture, gave either daily calcium (1 g) and vitamin D_3 (800 IU) supplementation or placebo.[25] Exclusions were the presence of cognitive impairment or a life expectancy of less than six months. After a median follow-up of 25 months, there were no significant differences in the incidence rates of overall fractures, hip fractures or falls.

Recently, a meta-analysis of trials of vitamin D supplementation with or without calcium found evidence for a benefit with 700–800 IU per day, but not 400 IU per day.[26] The size of the effect was a recurrence risk reduction of 26% for hip fractures. The variation in doses used within trials may partially explain the mixed results. A component of the Women's Health Initiative study randomised 36 282 healthy women aged between 50 and 79 (mean age 62 years) to receive either calcium (1 g) and vitamin D_3 (400 IU) or placebo over a follow-up period of seven years.[27] It was found that there was a small but statistically significant rise in BMD, but not a significant reduction in fracture rates. There was also a rise in the rate of renal stones in the treatment arm.

So, there have been conflicting results in trials of calcium and vitamin D. Their supplementation may only benefit certain subgroups, such as those with deficiencies at baseline and those who are housebound or in residential care. However, the majority of trials looking at osteoporosis interventions other than calcium or vitamin D also used supplementation with these agents. Therefore, to practise evidence-based medicine, calcium and vitamin D should be added to treatment regimens. The cost is low and side effects are infrequent with the doses commonly used. The role of vitamin D in the prevention of falls is discussed on p 189.

Bisphosphonates

Bisphosphonate molecules bind to hydroxyapatite crystals and act by reducing osteoclast activity (probably by inducing apoptosis) and thereby reduce bone resorption. They have a poor oral absorption and are best taken on an empty stomach without other medication to maximise their bioavailability. The current most commonly used agents are alendronate and risedronate. Both of these are available in once-weekly preparations, which appear to have similar efficacy to the daily versions. The main advantage of these preparations is to reduce the inconvenience for the patient.

Risedronate 2.5 mg and 5 mg daily doses were compared to placebo in 2458 ambulant post-menopausal women (mean age 69 years), with either two or more vertebral fractures on X-ray or a BMD T score of ≤ 2 plus one vertebral fracture, over a three-year period.[28] All participants also received calcium and vitamin D if baseline levels were low. The 2.5 mg dose arm was discontinued after one year. The 5 mg group had a lower vertebral fracture incidence (11.3%) compared to the placebo group (16.3%), which was significant (RR 0.59; 95% CI 0.42–0.82; $p = 0.03$) and a lower non-vertebral fracture rate (5.2%) compared to placebo (8.4%), which was also significant (RR 0.61; 95% CI 0.39–0.94; $p = 0.02$). BMD was also significantly increased compared to placebo at the lumbar spine (5.4% vs 1.1%) and femoral neck (1.6% vs −1.4%). There did not appear to be any difference in adverse-event rates between the treatment and placebo groups.

Risedronate was also compared to placebo in two groups of elderly women at a high risk of hip fracture over a three-year period (the Hip Intervention Program Study Group).[29] Some 5445 women aged between 70 and 79 years (mean age 74) with marked osteoporosis (a T score ≤ 4 or ≤ 3 plus a non-skeletal risk factor for hip fracture) and 3886 women over the age of 80 (mean age 83) with either a non-skeletal risk factor for hip fracture or marked osteoporosis (a T score of at least ≤ 3) were recruited. All participants also received calcium and vitamin D if baseline levels were low. Overall there was a reduction in hip fracture incidence from 3.9% in the placebo arm to 2.8% in the treatment arm (RR 0.7; 95% CI 0.6–0.9; $p = 0.02$). However, there was no benefit in the subgroup of patients without a low BMD score.

Alendronate has been compared to placebo in 2027 women (mean age 71 years, range 55–81 years) with a T score of ≤ 2.1 on BMD and X-ray evidence of previous vertebral fracture over a three-year period (the Fracture Intervention Trial).[30] Women with a history of peptic ulcer disease or dyspepsia were excluded. Participants deemed to have a low calcium intake (82% of the cohort) were given calcium and vitamin D supplements. The incidence of new vertebral fractures was 8.0% in the alendronate group and 15.0% in the placebo group (RR 0.53; 95% CI 0.41–0.68; $p<0.001$). The incidence of hip fracture was also reduced (RR 0.49; 95% CI 0.23–0.99; $p = 0.047$). There did not appear to be any difference in adverse-event rates (including gastrointestinal events) between the treatment and placebo groups.

Another arm of the above study looked at the effect of alendronate compared to placebo in 4432 women with low BMD scores but no evidence of prior vertebral fracture over a four-year period.[31] There was an associated significant increase in BMD scores, but only the subgroup of people with a T score of ≤ 2.5 had a significant reduction in clinical fracture incidence. This suggests that treating osteopaenic women with bisphosphonates may not be cost-effective – a point upheld by a recent economic evaluation.[32]

Side effects

Erosive oesophagitis and ulceration have been reported with alendronate.[33] Risk factors for this complication appear to be inadequate water intake with the tablet, lying down after ingestion and a history of oesophageal disorders. For this reason patients with gastric or oesophageal problems were excluded from many of the studies and they should not be prescribed alendronate. It is advised that patients consume at least 200 ml of water after ingestion and do not lie down for at least 30 minutes. The medication should be discontinued if oesophageal symptoms develop. This association has not been found with risedronate but similar precautions should be observed whilst taking this medication.

There have been no head-to-head comparison studies between these two agents but meta-analyses do not suggest a significant difference in treatment effects between them.[20] They both appear to significantly reduce vertebral and non-vertebral fracture incidence in osteoporotic women.

Oestrogen

Osteoblasts and osteoclasts have been found to have oestrogen receptors. Oestrogen has been shown to inhibit osteoclast activity and this mechanism is thought to be important in post-menopausal osteoporosis. It is, therefore, not surprising to find that oestrogen replacement therapy has been shown to be beneficial in increasing BMD in older women. In order to reduce the risk of endometrial carcinoma, women who have not had a hysterectomy also take cyclical progestins.

A meta-analysis of trials found a mean increase in BMD compared to control groups of 6.8% at the spine and 4.1% at the femoral neck.[34] There were non-significant trends towards reduced vertebral (RR 0.66; 95% CI 0.41–1.07) and non-vertebral (RR 0.87; 95% CI 0.71–1.08) fracture rates.

The problem with oestrogen therapy is the associated effects on other organ systems. Previously it was thought that oestrogens may increase the risk of breast cancer but were thought to be cardioprotective. A recent large randomised controlled study of women between the ages of 50 and 79 years showed a significant increase in cardiovascular morbidity (coronary heart disease, stroke and pulmonary embolism) as well as breast cancer.[35,36] These were partially offset by significant reductions in hip fractures and colorectal cancer. In those who had not had a hysterectomy, after a mean follow-up of 5.2 years, the hazard ratios were 1.22 (95% CI 1.09–1.36) for total cardiovascular disease, 1.03 (95% CI 0.90–1.17) for total cancer, 0.76 (95% CI 0.69–0.85) for combined fractures and 0.98 (95% CI 0.82–1.18) for mortality.[35] Although overall mortality is not significantly increased, the absolute number of adverse cardiovascular events appears to outweigh the bone protection benefit. They are also associated with an increase in urinary incontinence incidence and severity (*see* Box 6.1). Therefore, it no longer seems reasonable to use these agents routinely in the management of osteoporosis.

Selective oestrogen receptor modulators

Selective oestrogen receptor modulators include tamoxifen, which is used in the management of breast cancer, as well as raloxifene, which is used in the management of post-menopausal osteoporosis. Raloxifene is thought to be a useful agent as it has similar actions to oestrogen on bone but an inhibitory effect at the different oestrogen receptor subtype found on breast and endometrial tissue.

The Multiple Outcomes of Raloxifene Evaluation (MORE) trial recruited 7705 women (mean age 67, range 31–80 years) with osteoporosis (defined by BMD scores or radiographic evidence of vertebral fractures) to compare raloxifene (60 mg or 120 mg) to placebo over a three-year period.[37] The participants also received calcium and vitamin D supplements. They found a significant reduction in vertebral fracture incidence (RR for the 60 mg raloxifene group 0.7; 95% CI 0.5–0.8). There was an associated increase in BMD at the femoral neck and spine by around 2.5%. However, there was no significant benefit in terms of non-vertebral fracture reduction (RR 0.9; 95% CI 0.8–1.1). A continuation of the trial to four years did not show a significant change to the above data in either vertebral or non-vertebral fracture incidence.[38]

The most serious side effect encountered was a significant increased risk of venous thrombo-embolism (RR 3.1; 95% CI 1.5–6.2). Other side effects occurring more commonly in the raloxifene group included hot flashes, leg cramps and peripheral oedema. There was a lower incidence of breast cancer in the treatment group (RR 0.3; 95% CI 0.2–0.6). No association with either endometrial hyperplasia or carcinoma was detected.

The role of raloxifene in the management of post-menopausal osteoporosis is unclear. The actual size of the increase in bone density seen appears to be less than that seen with bisphosphonates.[39] This may suggest that it is useful only when bisphosphonates are not tolerated. Combination therapy has not been assessed in clinical trials. The increase in venous thrombo-embolism is certainly a concern, especially in high-risk groups such as hospitalised elderly patients.

Calcitonin

Calcitonin has been proposed as a useful agent in the management of osteoporosis as it has an inhibitory effect on osteoclast activity. It is usually given as salmon calcitonin as this has a 40–50 times greater potency than the human version. It cannot be given by the oral route and is usually taken as a nasal spray or as a subcutaneous injection. It is expensive and long-term use may be associated with the development of antibodies that could negate its efficacy.

The largest study looking at the role of calcitonin in post-menopausal osteo-porosis was the PROOF trial.[40] Some 1255 women (mean age 68 years) with osteoporosis were given salmon calcitonin nasal spray at a dose of 100, 200 or 400 IU per day or placebo over a five-year period. All participants also received calcium and vitamin D supplements. Results for the 100 IU and 400 IU doses were not signifi-cantly different from the placebo group. Strangely, the 200 IU daily group had a reduction in vertebral fracture incidence compared with placebo (RR 0.67; 95% CI 0.47–0.97; $p = 0.03$). There was an associated increase in BMD. Rhinitis was the only adverse effect reported. However, it should be noted that there was a 59% drop-out rate in this trial. A meta-analysis of trials found a large heterogeneity in results, raising the concern of publication bias.[41]

There is some evidence for a role in the management of pain associated with acute vertebral crush fractures. A study recruiting 100 men and women (mean age 73 years) who had sustained an osteoporotic vertebral fracture within the past five days gave either nasal salmon calcitonin (200 IU daily) or placebo over a 28-day period.[42] It found a significant reduction in pain and an increase in early mobilisation in the calcitonin group. During the trial the patients were only allowed to take paracetamol as an additional analgesic. No significant adverse effects were reported.

Parathyroid hormone

PTH appears to have both bone creation and bone resorption effects. When bone is exposed to high levels of PTH for long time periods the net effect is bone loss. However, when bone is exposed to intermittently raised levels of PTH it results in osteoblast expression of growth factors and the promotion of new bone formation. It is this finding that underlies the theory for the use of PTH in osteoporosis. It is the only treatment option currently available that acts exclusively by stimulating new bone formation rather than inhibiting resorption. A form of the PTH molecule that includes only the first 34 amino acids (PTH (1–34)) has been developed. It has been produced by recombinant DNA technology and is also known as 'teriparatide'. It is believed that this part of the molecule causes most of its biological effects. It is given parenterally, usually by subcutaneous injections. Long-term safety has not yet been established and its administration to rats at supra-physiological levels was associated with an increase in osteosarcoma development.

It has previously been shown to have beneficial effects on BMD in younger women treated with gonadotrophin-releasing hormone (GnRH) analogues for endometriosis.[43] A more recent study (the Fracture Prevention Trial) recruited 1637 post-menopausal women (mean age 69 years) and gave either PTH (1–34) at a dose of 20 or 40 µg/day or placebo.[44] Participants were also given calcium and vitamin D supplements. After a mean duration of 18 months' treatment the subset receiving 20 µg/day of PTH had a significant reduction in vertebral and non-vertebral fracture incidence compared to placebo (RR 0.35; 95% CI 0.22–0.55 and RR 0.47; 95% CI 0.25–0.88, respectively). There was no significant additional benefit at the higher dose of PTH and it had the cost of increased side effects. The study was stopped early because of concerns about the elevated osteosarcoma incidence in animal models. There were no cases of osteosarcoma within this study. Side effects occurring more commonly in the treatment group than in the placebo group included: nausea, headaches, dizziness and leg cramps. The benefit of this treatment appears to last to some degree up to at least 18 months beyond its discontinuation.[45] When PTH is discontinued, there is evidence that commencing anti-resorptive therapy with a bisphosphonate prevents subsequent reduction in BMD.[46]

So, the role of PTH has not yet been established, in part due to safety concerns. Currently it may be a beneficial treatment for osteoporosis over short periods of administration. Drawbacks to its use include high cost and the need for daily subcutaneous injections.

Strontium

Strontium was first used in the treatment of osteoporosis in the 1950s but fell out of favour due to concerns that it caused bone mineralisation defects and inhibited the synthesis of calcitriol.[47] The development of a new compound, strontium ranelate, has led to the re-emergence of this therapeutic agent. It is believed to promote bone formation whilst also inhibiting bone resorption. Tissues undergoing osteogenesis actively absorb it. The precise mechanism of action is unknown but may involve, in part, interaction with the calcium-sensing receptor and the suppression of PTH secretion.

Due to the heavy atomic weight of strontium, the X-rays utilised in DEXA scanning are more readily absorbed. This leads to artificially elevated BMD estimations. This problem is tackled by using a formula to adjust the readings to more comparative values.

A study involving 1649 post-menopausal women (mean age 69 years) with osteoporosis (defined by BMD) and at least one vertebral fracture gave either 2 g/day of strontium or placebo over a three-year period.[48] Participants were also given calcium and vitamin D supplements. It found a significant reduction in new vertebral fractures (RR 0.59; 95% CI 0.48–0.73) with an associated increase in adjusted BMD of 8.1% at the lumbar spine.

The recent treatment of peripheral osteoporosis study (TROPOS) recruited 5091 women (mean age 77) with osteoporosis (defined by BMD) who were given either 2 g/day of strontium ranelate or placebo over a three-year period.[49] Participants were also given calcium and vitamin D supplements. It found an overall 16% relative risk (RR) reduction in non-vertebral fractures ($p = 0.04$), with a RR reduction for hip fractures of 36% ($p = 0.046$). Side effects observed more frequently in the treatment group included nausea, diarrhoea, headache, dermatitis and eczema.

Therefore, it appears that strontium is a promising therapy for post-menopausal osteoporosis, with benefits in reducing both vertebral and non-vertebral fractures, but data on the long-term safety and efficacy are not yet available.

Statins

Statins (HMG CoA reductase inhibitors) have been linked to increased BMD, possibly by interference with the mevalonate pathway. Two analyses of epidemiological data have suggested that older individuals on current statin therapy have a reduced risk of fractures.[50,51] However, a secondary analysis of the LIPID study did not demonstrate a difference in fracture rate.[52] Randomised controlled trials are required to investigate this association.

Treatment of male osteoporosis

There is very little trial evidence for the treatment of male osteoporosis. Similarly to women, the role of calcium and vitamin D alone is unclear but they have been used in conjunction with other treatments in most trials and so should be considered a standard component of therapy.

Bisphosphonates

A trial has been conducted using alendronate versus placebo in 241 osteoporotic men (mean age 63, range 31–87 years) over a two-year period.[53] All participants were also given calcium and vitamin D supplements. Men with a history of peptic ulcer or oesophageal disease within the past year were excluded. They found mean increases in BMD at the lumbar spine and femoral neck of 7.1% and 2.5% in the alendronate group compared to 1.8% and –0.1% in the placebo group, respectively ($p<0.001$ for both sites). Further, there was a reduction in vertebral fracture incidence from 7.1% in the placebo group to 0.8% in the alendronate group ($p = 0.02$). There was no significant difference in side-effect rates between the two groups.

Parathyroid hormone

Although there are no available data to show a benefit in terms of fracture reduction in men, the effects on bone density appear to be more favourable than those seen with alendronate.[54] After 24 months of treatment of osteoporotic men (mean age 58, range 46–85) an increase in BMD at the femoral neck of 9.7% was seen with PTH compared to 3.2% with alendronate ($p<0.001$). The same trial failed to show an additional benefit of combining these two treatments. All participants received vitamin D supplements and additional calcium supplementation if their dietary intake was thought to be inadequate (less than 1 g per day).

Testosterone

An age-related reduction in testosterone has been described earlier in the chapter (*see* p 209). A number of problems have been attributed to this reduction, including reduced libido, erectile dysfunction, anaemia, and reduced muscle mass and bone density. It has been proposed that testosterone replacement may benefit all of these. However, the effects of replacement of this decline may be quite different to the replacement of testosterone in other deficiency states, such as pan-hypopituitarism. Testosterone is available in oral, transdermal and injectable preparations.[55]

- *Injections*: need to be given regularly and cause fluctuations in serum levels that may increase the risk of some adverse effects, for example erythrocytosis.
- *Transdermal*: easy to administer and results in consistent serum levels. May cause skin irritation beneath patches, this is less severe with a gel form of the drug.
- *Oral*: associated with hepatotoxicity and neoplasia and for this reason is seldom used.

A study of 108 healthy men over the age of 65 years (mean age 73) looked at the effect of a testosterone patch on BMD.[8] It was found that overall BMD was not increased but there was a positive effect in those individuals who had a low baseline testosterone level. A study using two-weekly intramuscular testosterone injections in hypogonadal men with a mean age of 71 over a three-year period found a significant increase in BMD compared to placebo.[56] There were mean increases of 10.2% and 2.7% at the spine and total hip in the testosterone group compared to 1.3% and –0.2%, respectively, in the placebo group ($p<0.001$ and $p = 0.02$). During this study there were significant rises in both haematocrit (mean 42.5% to 48.6%) and PSA levels (mean 1.0 to 1.4) in the testosterone group compared to baseline. Thirty per cent of subjects in the testosterone group required a dose reduction due to a haematocrit level above 52%. There are no studies demonstrating a reduced fracture incidence in osteoporotic men treated with testosterone.

Adverse effects

To date there is no clear evidence that testosterone levels correlate with either cardiovascular disease risk or serum lipid levels. But, given the problems associated with female hormone replacement therapy (*see* p 218) it would seem prudent to use caution with male replacement until long-term safety data are available. Also, there is little evidence that it induces prostatic hyperplasia and subsequent urinary voiding problems. Some of the problems it does cause are listed below.

- *Polycythaemia*: testosterone appears to have an action on bone marrow and higher levels have been found to induce erythropoiesis. The higher peak levels seen with injected doses confer a higher risk. The clinical significance of this is unclear but it is recommended that the haematocrit be monitored during therapy.
- *Prostate cancer*: the efficacy of anti-testosterone treatments in the management of prostate cancer has lead to concerns that elevating testosterone levels may induce such cancers. To date the available evidence does not support this; however, data from large studies and over long time periods are not yet available. It is recommended that prostate-specific antigen (PSA) level monitoring be performed during therapy.
- *Hepatotoxicity and neoplasia*: appear to be related to oral preparations only.
- *Sleep apnoea*: testosterone use has been associated with the development or worsening of sleep apnoea in at-risk individuals. This may be mediated by a central mechanism.
- *Fluid retention*: caution may be needed in the presence of cardiac or renal failure.

Monitoring is recommended at three- to six-month intervals. This should include questioning about the above side effects and measurement of the haematocrit and PSA levels.

B_{12} and folate

A study of Japanese stroke survivors over the age of 65 years has found a reduction in fracture risk with the use of folate and B_{12} supplementation.[57] The theory behind this finding is that low levels of these agents are associated with raised levels of homocysteine, which is associated with osteoporosis. These findings will need to be validated in other cohorts before this becomes standard practice.

Combinations of therapy

The majority of trials investigating therapeutic agents for osteoporosis have used calcium and vitamin D supplements concurrently. Therefore, the combination of any anti-resorptive agent or PTH with calcium and vitamin D is standard practice. Trials that have looked at a combination of PTH and alendronate have failed to show a benefit of the two agents together.[54,58] This is probably due to alendronate blocking the PTH-induced stimulation of bone formation. The combination of other agents has not been adequately assessed.

Treatment recommendations

If a secondary or contributory cause for osteoporosis is identified then correcting or improving this should also be attempted. A treatment strategy is suggested below and in Figure 11.5. In the subgroup of patients with osteopaenia detected on DEXA scanning, optimal treatment is unproven. Given the questionable cost benefits of anti-resorptive therapy,[32] an alternative strategy may be non-pharmacological measures and the commencement of calcium and vitamin D with repeat BMD measurement in two years' time.

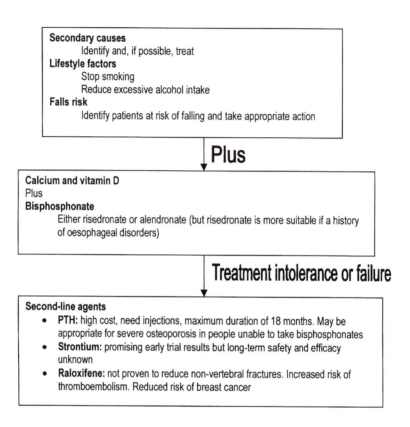

Figure 11.5   Suggested strategy to manage osteoporosis in the elderly.

Pharmacological

Currently, the best evidence for efficacy and long-term safety is with the combination of calcium, vitamin D and a bisphosphonate. Appropriate bisphosphonates are risedronate and alendronate. There appears to be little to choose between the two agents but alendronate should be avoided in people with a history of oesophageal disease. If a bisphosphonate is not tolerated then the choice of second-line agents includes PTH and strontium. Trials studying the efficacy of raloxifene have not demonstrated a clear benefit in reducing non-vertebral fractures. The reason for this may be partly due to the younger age (mean 67 years) of women in the MORE study.[20] However, it must be considered that an older population may also have a significant increase in adverse events, especially venous thrombo-embolism. Raloxifene may be best suited to people who are at an increased risk of breast cancer and a lower risk of thrombo-embolism. Available data do not support the combination of agents other than calcium and vitamin D with other osteoporosis treatments. Oestrogens, testosterone, calcitonin and statins do not have a major role in the management of osteoporosis at the present time.

Non-pharmacological

Lifestyle measures include stopping smoking and reducing excessive alcohol intake. Exercise in earlier life may confer a BMD gain. Increasing activity once osteoporosis has developed is less likely to be beneficial. However, exercise programmes may have a role in the prevention of falls. Those at risk of falls should undergo appropriate risk assessment and intervention (*see* Chapter 9). The role of hip protectors remains controversial.

Prognosis

In the year following a vertebral fracture, osteoporotic women appear to have a 19% risk of sustaining a further vertebral fracture.[59] This risk is increased in women with lower BMD scores and a history of previous fractures. Five-year survival rates are significantly reduced after either hip or vertebral fractures but appear to be unaffected following distal radius fractures.[60]

References

1 Cranney A, Tugwell P, Wells G *et al.* Systematic reviews of randomized trials in osteoporosis: introduction and methodology. *Endocrine Reviews,* 2002; **23**(4): 497–507.
2 Law MR and Hackshaw AK. A meta-analysis of cigarette smoking, bone mineral density and risk of hip fracture: recognition of a major effect. *BMJ,* 1997; **315**: 841–846.
3 Hirani V and Primatesta P. Vitamin D concentrations among people aged 65 years and over living in private households and institutions in England: population survey. *Age Ageing,* 2005; **34**: 485–491.
4 Williams AR, Weiss NS, Ure CL *et al.* Effect of weight, smoking, and estrogen use on the risk of hip and forearm fractures in postmenopausal women. *Obst Gynae,* 1982; **60**(6): 695–699.
5 Seeman E. Osteoporosis in men: epidemiology, pathophysiology, and treatment possibilities. *Am J Med,* 1993; **95** (Suppl. 5A): 22S–28S.
6 Bilezikian JP. Osteoporosis in men. *J Clin Endocr Met,* 1999; **84**(10): 3431–3434.
7 Allan CA and McLachlan RI. Age-related changes in testosterone and the role of replacement therapy in older men. *Clin Endocr,* 2004; **60**(6): 653–670.
8 Snyder PJ, Peachey H, Hannoush P *et al.* Effect of testosterone treatment on bone mineral density in men over 65 years of age. *J Clin Endocr Met,* 1999; **84**(6): 1966–1972.
9 Stepan JJ, Lachman M, Zverina J *et al.* Castrated men exhibit bone loss: effect of calcitonin treatment on biochemical indices of bone remodelling. *J Clin Endocr Met,* 1989; **69**(3): 523–527.
10 Ferrini RL and Barrett-Connor E. Sex hormones and age: a cross-sectional study of testosterone and estradiol and their bioavailable fractions in community-dwelling men. *Am J Epidem,* 1998; **147**(8): 750–754.
11 Khosla S, Melton LJ, Atkinson EJ *et al.* Relationship of serum sex steroid levels to longitudinal changes in bone density in young versus elderly men. *J Clin Endocr Met,* 2001; **86**(8): 3555–3561.
12 Venning G. Recent developments in vitamin D deficiency and muscle weakness among elderly people. *BMJ,* 2005; **330**: 524–526.
13 Grados F, Depriester C, Cayrolle G *et al.* Long-term observations of vertebral osteoporotic fractures treated by percutaneous vertebroplasty. *Rheumatology,* 2000; **38**: 1410–1414.

14 Diamond TH, Champion B and Clark WA. Management of acute osteoporotic vertebral fractures: a nonrandomized trial comparing percutaneous vertebroplasty with conservative therapy. *Am J Med*, 2003; **114**: 257–265.

15 Magaziner J, Simonsick EM, Kashner TM *et al.* Predictors of functional recovery one year following hospital discharge for hip fracture: a prospective study. *J Gerontol*, 1990; **45**(3): M101–107.

16 Parker MJ, Gillespie WJ and Gillespie LD. Hip protectors for preventing hip fractures in older people. The Cochrane Database of Systematic Reviews 2005, Issue 3. Art. No.: CD001255. DOI: 10.1002/14651858.CD001255.pub3.

17 Parker MJ, Gillespie WJ and Gillespie LD. Effectiveness of hip protectors for preventing hip fractures in elderly people: systematic review. *BMJ*, 2006; **332**: 571–573.

18 Cummings SR, Black DM and Nevitt MC. Bone density at various sites for prediction of hip fractures. *Lancet*, 1993; **341**(9): 72–75.

19 Cummings SR, Palmero L, Browner W *et al.* Monitoring osteoporosis therapy with bone densitometry: misleading changes and regression to the mean. *JAMA*, 2000; **283**(10): 1318–1321.

20 Boonen S, Body J, Boutsen Y *et al.* Evidence-based guidelines for the treatment of postmenopausal osteoporosis: a consensus document of the Belgian Bone Club. *Osteopor Int*, 2005; **16**: 239–254.

21 Anderson F. Vitamin D for older people: how much, for whom and – above all – why? *Age Ageing*, 2005; **34**: 425–426.

22 Shea B, Wells G, Cranney A *et al.* Meta-analysis of calcium supplementation for the prevention of postmenopausal osteoporosis. *Endocr Rev*, 2002; **23**(4): 552–559.

23 Papadimitropoulos E, Wells G, Shea B *et al.* Meta-analysis of the efficacy of vitamin D in preventing osteoporosis in postmenopausal women. *Endocr Rev*, 2002; **23**(4): 560–569.

24 Cahpuy MC, Arlot ME, Duboeuf F *et al.* Vitamin D3 and calcium to prevent hip fractures in elderly women. *NEJM*, 1992; **327**(23): 1637–1642.

25 Porthouse J, Cockayne S, King C *et al.* Randomised controlled trial of supplementation with calcium and cholecalciferol (vitamin D3) for prevention of fractures in primary care. *BMJ*, 2005; **330**: 1003–1006.

26 Bischoff-Ferrari HA, Willet WC, Wong JB *et al.* Fracture prevention with vitamin D supplementation: a meta-analysis of randomized controlled trials. *JAMA*, 2005; **293**(18): 2257–2264.

27 Jackson RD, LaCroix AZ, Gass M *et al.* Calcium plus vitamin D supplementation and the risk of fractures. *NEJM*, 2006; **354**(7): 669–683.

28 Harris ST, Watts NB, Genant HK *et al.* Effects of risedronate treatment on vertebral and nonvertebral fractures in women with non-vertebral osteoporosis: a randomized controlled trial. *JAMA*, 1999; **282**(14): 1344–1352.

29 McClung MR, Geusens P, Miller PD *et al.* Effect of risedronate on the risk of hip fracture in elderly women. *NEJM*, 2001; **344**(5): 333–340.

30 Black DM, Cummings SR, Karpf DB *et al.* Randomised trial of effect of alendronate on risk of fracture in women with existing vertebral fractures. *Lancet*, 1996; **348**: 1535–1541.

31 Cummings SR, Black DM, Thompson DE *et al.* Effect of alendronate on risk of fracture in women with low bone density but without osteoporosis: results from the fracture intervention trial. *JAMA*, 1998; **280**(24): 2077–2082.

32 Schousboe JT, Nyman JA, Kane RL *et al.* Cost-effectiveness of alendronate therapy for osteopenic postmenopausal women. *Ann Intern Med*, 2005; **142**(9): 734–741.

33 de Groen PC, Lubbe DF, Hirsch LJ *et al.* Esophagitis associated with the use of alendronate. *NEJM*, 1996; **335**: 1016–1021.

34 Wells G, Tugwell P, Shea B *et al.* Meta-analysis of the efficacy of hormone replacement therapy in treating and preventing osteoporosis in postmenopausal women. *Endocr Rev*, 2002; **23**(4): 529–539.

35 Writing Group for the Women's Health Initiative Investigators. Risks and benefits of estrogen plus progestin in healthy postmenopausal women: principal results from the Women's Health Initiative randomized controlled trial. *JAMA*, 2002; **288**(3): 321–333.

36 Women's Health Initiative Steering Committee. Effects of conjugated equine estrogen in postmenopausal women with hysterectomy: the Women's Health Initiative randomized controlled trial. *JAMA*, 2004; **291**(14): 1701–1712.

37 Ettinger B, Black DM, Mitlak BH *et al*. Reduction of vertebral fracture risk in postmenopausal women with osteoporosis treated with raloxifene: results from a 3-year randomized clinical trial. *JAMA*, 1999; **282**(7): 637–645.

38 Delmas PD, Ensrud KE, Adachi JD *et al*. Efficacy of raloxifene on vertebral fracture risk reduction in postmenopausal women with osteoporosis: four-year results from a randomized clinical trial. *J Clin Endocr Met*, 2002; **87**(8): 3609–3617.

39 Cranney A, Tugwell P, Zytaruk N *et al*. Meta-analysis of raloxifene for the prevention and treatment of postmenopausal osteoporosis. *Endocr Rev*, 2002; **23**(4): 524–528.

40 Chesnut CH, Silverman S, Andriano K *et al*. A randomized trial of nasal spray salmon calcitonin in postmenopausal women with established osteoporosis: the prevent recurrence of osteoporotic fractures study. *Am J Med*, 2000; **109**: 267–276.

41 Cranney A, Tugwell P, Zytaruk N *et al*. Meta-analysis of calcitonin for the treatment of postmenopausal osteoporosis. *Endocr Rev*, 2002; **23**(4): 540–551.

42 Lyritis GP, Paspati I, Karachalios T *et al*. Pain relief from nasal salmon calcitonin in osteoporotic vertebral crush fractures. *Acta Orthop Scand*, 1997; **68** (Suppl. 275): 112–114.

43 Finkelstein JS, Klibanski A, Arnold AL *et al*. Prevention of estrogen deficiency-related bone loss with human parathyroid hormone – (1–34): a randomized controlled trial. *JAMA*, 1998; **280**(12): 1067–1073.

44 Neer RM, Arnaud CD, Zanchetta JR *et al*. Effect of parathyroid hormone (1–34) on fractures and bone mineral density in postmenopausal women with osteoporosis. *NEJM*, 2001; **344**(19): 1434–1441.

45 Lindsay R, Scheele WH, Neer R *et al*. Sustained vertebral fracture risk reduction after withdrawal of teriparatide in postmenopausal women with osteoporosis. *Arch Intern Med*, 2004; **164**: 2024–2030.

46 Black DM, Bilezikian JP, Ensrud KE, *et al*. One year of alendronate after one year of parathyroid hormone (1–34) for osteoporosis. *NEJM*, 2005; **353**(6): 555–565.

47 Fuleihan GE. Strontium ranelate – a novel therapy for osteoporosis or a permutation of the same? *NEJM*, 2004; **350**(5): 504–506.

48 Meunier PJ, Roux C, Seeman E *et al*. The effects of strontium ranelate on the risk of vertebral fracture in women with postmenopausal osteoporosis. *NEJM*, 2004; **350**(5): 459–468.

49 Reginster JY, Seeman E, De Vernejoul MC *et al*. Strontium ranelate reduces the risk of nonvertebral fractures in postmenopausal women with osteoporosis: treatment of peripheral osteoporosis (TROPOS) study. *J Clin Endocr Metab*, 2005; **90**(5): 2816–2822.

50 Meier CR, Schlienger RC, Kraenzlin ME *et al*. HMG-CoA reductase inhibitors and the risk of fractures. *JAMA*, 2000; **283**(24): 3205–3210.

51 Wang PS, Solomon DH, Mogun H *et al*. HMG-CoA reductase inhibitors and the risk of hip fractures in elderly patients. *JAMA*, 2000; **283**(24): 3211–3216.

52 Reid IR, Hague W, Emberson J *et al*. Effect of pravastatin on frequency of fracture in the LIPID study: secondary analysis of a RCT. *Lancet*, 2001; **357**: 509–512.

53 Orwoll E, Ettinger M, Weiss S *et al*. Alendronate for the treatment of osteoporosis in men. *NEJM*, 2000; **343**(9): 604–610.

54 Finkelstein JS, Hayes A, Hunzelman JL *et al*. The effects of parathyroid hormone, alendronate, or both in men with osteoporosis. *NEJM*, 2003; **349**(13): 1216–1226.

55 Rhoden EL and Morgentaler A. Risks of testosterone-replacement therapy and recommendations for monitoring. *NEJM*, 2004; **350**(5): 482–492.

56 Amory JK, Watts NB, Easley KA *et al*. Exogenous testosterone or testosterone with finasteride increases bone mineral density in older men with low serum testosterone. *J Clin Endocr Met*, 2004; **89**(2): 503–510.

57 Sato Y, Honda Y, Iwamoto J *et al*. Effect of folate and mecobalamin on hip fractures in patients with stroke: a randomized controlled trial. *JAMA*, 2005; **293**(9): 1082–1088.

58 Black DM, Greenspan SL, Ensrud KE *et al*. The effects of parathyroid hormone and alendronate alone or in combination in postmenopausal osteoporosis. *NEJM*, 2003; **349**(13): 1207–1215.

59 Lindsay R, Silverman SL, Cooper C *et al*. Risk of new vertebral fracture in the year following a fracture. *JAMA*, 2001; **285**(3): 320–323.

60 Cooper C, Atkinson EJ, Jacobsen SJ *et al*. Population-based study of survival after osteoporotic fractures. *Am J Epidemiol*, 1993; **137**: 1001–1005.

Part D

Cardiovascular

Chapter 12

Heart failure

Heart failure occurs when the heart is no longer able to pump blood at the rate required to meet the body's metabolic requirements. It has been estimated to have a prevalence of around 1% in adults in their 50s, and this rises to around 10% in those in their 80s.[1] This failure is attributed to a combination of age-related changes to the cardiovascular system and a higher prevalence of cardiovascular diseases. These changes include increased stiffness of the heart and blood vessels caused by reductions in the amount of elastin with increased collagen deposition. This results in impaired cardiac diastolic relaxation and subsequent inefficient filling. In normal individuals these changes do not affect the resting cardiac output but do reduce the ability to increase the output at times of increased demand (e.g. physical exertion).

Frequent cardiac causes of heart failure are ischaemic, hypertensive and valvular heart diseases. Atrial fibrillation (AF) is also more common in the elderly – usually in association with atrial enlargement secondary to elevated intracardiac pressures. The loss of co-ordinated atrial contraction may further reduce the efficacy of cardiac filling even if the ventricular rate is normal. Another factor increasing risk in the elderly may be the deterioration seen in renal function with advancing years.

Diastolic heart failure is a term used to describe the clinical features of heart failure in individuals with preserved ejection fractions (greater than 50%). It appears to account for 30–50% of those with heart failure.[2,3] It occurs more commonly in the elderly probably because of the increased vascular stiffness. In reality, both systolic and diastolic dysfunction probably co-exist to some degree in many older patients with heart failure. Other factors increasing risk include female sex and a history of hypertension, whereas it is less common in people with a history of ischaemic heart disease.[3]

Assessment

History

Classically, heart failure symptoms are breathlessness on exertion, ankle swelling and orthopnoea. Precipitating medications such as non-steroidal anti-inflammatory drugs (NSAIDs) (which impair renal salt handling and increase fluid overload) should be identified.

Examination

Signs include a raised jugular venous pressure (JVP), a third heart sound, pitting ankle oedema and basal chest crepitations. Their interpretation can be more difficult in the elderly. For example, leg oedema can be due to calcium channel blockers, a low albumin, or venous congestion, and basal chest crepitations can be a normal variant.

Investigations

An electrocardiograph (ECG) will usually be abnormal with signs of previous ischaemia or chamber enlargement (*see* Figure 12.1). A chest X-ray may show ventricular enlargement, oedema, effusions, Kerley lines or venous congestion. Thyroid disease and anaemia should be excluded by standard blood tests.

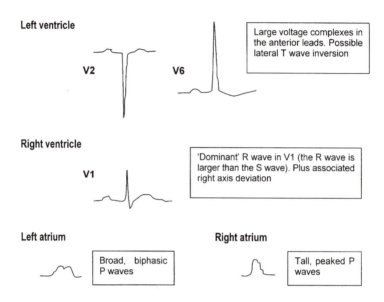

Figure 12.1 Electrocardiograph (ECG) signs of heart chamber enlargement.

The natriuretic peptides are a group of naturally occurring, structurally related hormones that include brain natriuretic peptide (BNP), atrial natriuretic peptide (ANP) and C-type natriuretic peptide (CNP) variants. They have a physiological role in the maintenance of fluid homeostasis. Despite its name, BNP comes mainly from the cardiac ventricles – released in response to cardiac wall stretching. It has been proposed as a marker of cardiac failure that can be measured from blood samples.[4] However, it is a non-specific test as levels may rise with other cardiac (e.g. ischaemia and arrhythmias)[5] and non-cardiac conditions (e.g. pulmonary emboli, or, to a lesser degree, with normal ageing), and so it is unclear whether this adds to the information gained form clinical, ECG and chest X-ray evaluation. Currently its role in clinical practice is not fully defined. It also exists in a recombinant form (nesiritide) that has been used as a treatment for acute heart failure. At present this has a high cost and large-sized randomised controlled trials demonstrating a long-term benefit are lacking.

Echocardiography should be performed in all patients with a new diagnosis of heart failure. Its functions include the ability to identify any valvular lesions and to distinguish between diastolic and systolic dysfunction. Standard techniques for estimating ejection fraction tend to overestimate its value in the presence of left ventricular enlargement (and associated change in shape).

Treatment

A management programme should include patient education, including how to identify the signs of worsening disease and the importance of medication adherence.

If any precipitating factors have been identified, then attempts should be made to improve them. These may include minor changes such as stopping unhelpful medications or major procedures such as valvular or revascularisation surgery. Secondary prevention of vascular disease with anti-platelets, statins and adequate blood pressure (BP) control may also be appropriate. Smokers should be advised to stop. Left ventricular impairment increases the risk of thrombo-embolism in the presence of AF. Therefore these patients should be carefully considered for warfarinisation (*see* p 251).

Medications

Most of the evidence for pharmacological management of heart failure is based on trials enrolling patients with systolic dysfunction. There is little direct evidence for the treatment of diastolic problems but it currently appears that similar strategies are probably appropriate.

Loop diuretics

Loop diuretics (e.g. furosemide or bumetanide) are highly effective at reducing the fluid overload of heart failure. Their site of action is shown in Figure 12.2. They are effective at treating the symptoms of heart failure and improve the quality of patients' lives. They are usually the first medications to be commenced. However, they do not alter the progress or outcome of the condition. Patients with co-existent renal impairment may require large doses for clinical effect.

Patients with bowel oedema due to right heart failure may not absorb furosemide well. In this situation either intravenous furosemide or oral bumetanide may be more effective.

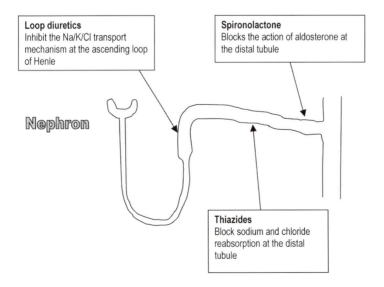

Figure 12.2   Sites of action of diuretic drugs.

Thiazide diuretics

Thiazide diuretics are more effective as BP-lowering agents than loop diuretics but are less effective at reducing fluid overload (*see* Figure 12.2). Therefore, they are not used as first-line therapy. However, in combination with loop diuretics they can be highly effective for patients with oedema that is difficult to control by loop diuretics alone. This is due to their different site of action leading to 'sequential nephron blockade'. Suitable agents include bendroflumethiazide or metolazone at low doses. Their use needs to be closely monitored as fluid loss may be profound and electrolyte disturbances (hyponatraemia and hypokalaemia) are common.

Angiotensin-converting enzyme inhibitors

Angiotensin-converting enzyme (ACE) inhibitors have been proven to be effective in the treatment of patients with heart failure. In a study of 2569 patients (mean age 61 years) with ejection fractions below 35% (mean 25%), treatment with enalapril compared to placebo resulted in significantly better mortality rates over a 41-month period (35% vs 40%).[6] A meta-analysis of data from over 12 000 patients with heart failure (mean age 61 years, mean ejection fraction 29%) demonstrated lower mortality rates with ACE inhibitors compared to placebo over an average follow-up period of 35 months (23% vs 27%).[7]

They have also been found to be beneficial in reducing myocardial infarction (MI), stroke or cardiovascular death in patients with vascular risk factors but not known to have left ventricular impairment.[8]

Side effects include a persistent dry cough due to an increase in bradykinin formation caused by raised levels of angiotensin I (*see* Figure 12.3). This may be severe enough to lead to discontinuation of the medication in up to 10% of patients. They may also cause deteriorating renal function in those with renal artery stenosis. This is due to high renin levels being important for maintaining renal perfusion in these patients. A further potential problem is hyperkalaemia – which may be worse in combination with aldosterone antagonists (e.g. spironolactone). Hypotension is common following initiation of therapy and patients should be warned to avoid rapid postural change. For this reason doses are started low and only gradually increased.

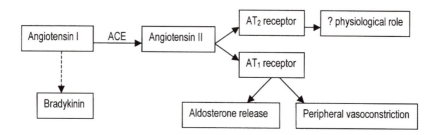

Figure 12.3 Normal physiological actions of angiotensin. ACE = angiotensin-converting enzyme; AT_1 = angiotensin II type I, AT_2 = angiotensin II type 2.

The commencement of these agents may result in a rise in serum creatinine level. It is generally considered insignificant with a rise of less than 30% from the baseline.

Angiotensin type II receptor blockers

Angiotensin type II receptor blockers (ARBs) act by directly inhibiting receptor activation (*see* Figure 12.4). As they do not prevent the breakdown of bradykinins, they are not associated with a dry cough.

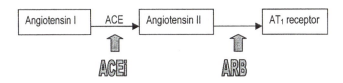

Figure 12.4 The sites of action of angiotensin-converting enzyme (ACE) inhibitors and angiotensin receptor blockers (ARB). AT_1 = angiotensin II type I.

In a trial that compared the addition of valsartan or placebo to standard therapy in 5010 people with advanced heart failure, a significant reduction in the combined endpoint of mortality and morbidity (but not mortality alone) was seen in the treatment arm (RR 0.87; 95% CI 0.77–0.97).[9] A similar study compared the addition of candesartan or placebo to the treatment of 7599 patients (mean age 66 years) with heart failure.[10] It also demonstrated a benefit with the ARB in cardiovascular death or non-fatal MI compared to placebo (HR 0.87; 95% CI 0.79–0.96). The benefit appeared to be seen even in those patients concurrently taking ACE inhibitors (41% of the participants at baseline).

A trial that recruited 3152 patients (mean age 71 years) with systolic heart failure compared the addition of losartan or captopril to standard medical management.[11] Over an 18-month period they found no difference in mortality rates but fewer patients discontinued therapy because of adverse events in the losartan group (9.7% vs 14.7%) – mainly due to a lower incidence of cough.

Therefore, it seems that ARBs are a reasonable choice of second-line agent for those already on or intolerant to ACE inhibitors.

Beta blockers

Reduced bodily tissue perfusion results in the activation of the sympathetic nervous system. This process is helpful when the reduction is due to profound blood loss but is counterproductive in the case of heart failure. It may actually reduce cardiac function, and increase the risk of ischaemia and arrhythmias. For these reasons beta-blockers have been tried in heart failure.

Carvedilol was compared to placebo in 1094 patients with chronic systolic heart failure in addition to standard medical therapy over a follow-up period of 6–12 months.[12] A significantly lower mortality rate was found in the carvedilol group (3.2% vs 7.8%).

The CIBIS-II trial randomised 2647 patients (mean age 61 years) with chronic systolic heart failure to receive either bisoprolol (slowly titrated up to 10 mg per day) or placebo in addition to standard therapy over a period of 1.3 years.[13] It found a lower mortality rate in the bisoprolol group compared to the placebo arm (11.8% vs 17.3%; HR 0.66; 95% CI 0.54–0.81).

The MERIT-HF study randomised 3991 patients (mean age 64 years) with chronic systolic heart failure to receive either metoprolol (slowly titrated up to 200 mg once daily) or placebo in addition to their usual medications over a one-year period.[14] It also found a lower mortality rate with the beta-blocker compared to placebo (7.2% vs 11.0%; RR 0.66; 95% CI 0.53–0.81).

The patients recruited in the above studies were relatively young. However, data derived from a number of randomised controlled trials suggest that these benefits are maintained amongst older patients.[15] Also, a more recent study randomised 2128 patients over the age of 70 (mean age 76 years) with heart failure to receive either nebivolol or placebo over a 21-month period.[16] This found a reduction in all-cause mortality and cardiovascular hospital admissions with beta-blocker therapy (HR 0.86; 95% CI 0.74–0.99).

Doses should be gradually increased at two-weekly intervals. Their use is contraindicated in patients with reversible airway disease, marked bradycardia, or second- or third-degree heart block.

Spironolactone

Spironolactone is a potassium-sparing diuretic that acts by inhibiting the action of aldosterone by blocking the binding with its receptor (*see* Figure 12.2).

A study has compared low-dose spironolactone (25 mg daily) to placebo in 1663 patients with systolic heart failure also on standard medical therapy over a two-year period.[17] The mortality rate was significantly lower in the spironolactone group (35% vs 46%; RR 0.70; 95% CI 0.60–0.82). Spironolactone use was associated with a 10% incidence of gynaecomastia and a 2% incidence of serious hyperkalaemia. The mechanism of the apparent beneficial effects of spironolactone is not fully understood. At the low dose used it has very little diuretic effect. It may have a cardioprotective role. The higher serum potassium levels seen with spironolactone compared to placebo may lead to a lower rate of cardiac arrhythmias induced by hypokalaemia.

Digoxin

Digoxin is proposed to have a mechanism that causes an increased intracellular calcium concentration leading to improved cardiac muscle contraction. Side effects include nausea and vomiting, diarrhoea and arrhythmias. The risk of toxicity is increased in association with hypokalaemia.

It (mean daily dose 0.25 mg) has been compared to placebo in 6800 patients with systolic heart failure on standard medical therapy over a three-year period.[18] It did not result in any improvement in mortality rates but was associated with a significantly lower rate of hospitalisation than placebo (RR 0.72; 95% CI 0.66–0.79).

Hydralazine and nitrates

In patients who are intolerant of ACE inhibitors, the combination of hydralazine and nitrates may, occasionally, be a suitable alternative. A study of 642 patients (mean age 58 years) who received either hydralazine (300 mg per day) and isosorbide dinitrate (160 mg per day), prazosin (20 mg per day) or placebo over a mean period of 2.3 years found a reduction in mortality with hydralazine-isosorbide (26%) compared to placebo (34%) or prazosin.[19] However, this combination is significantly less effective than ACE inhibitors.[20] The high doses used in the trials are unlikely to be tolerated by many older patients.

Cardiac resynchronisation

The use of biventricular pacemaker devices to restore a more physiological timing of ventricular contraction has been proposed for people with severe heart failure whose ECGs show sinus rhythm plus bundle branch block. This involves pacing the right ventricle in the normal way and also placing a lead through the coronary sinus to be able to pace the left ventricle,[21] the rationale being that improved timing of contractions will improve cardiac output.

In a trial of 813 patients (median age 67 years) in New York Heart Association class III or IV with ejection fractions below 35% and QRS durations of at least 120 ms (median 160 ms), individuals were randomised to receive medical therapy alone or in combination with cardiac resynchronisation over a mean period of 29 months.[22] The primary outcome of death or unplanned hospitalisation for a cardiovascular event occurred in 39% of the resynchronisation group compared to 55% of the controls (HR 0.63; 95% CI 0.51–0.77; $p<0.001$). This suggests that this treatment is beneficial in such patients, although cost-effectiveness is unclear. They may also be combined with implantable defibrillators to reduce the risk of sudden death due to arrhythmias (*see below*).

Implantable cardioverter-defibrillators

Sudden death caused by cardiac arrhythmias is common in patients with advanced heart failure. In the past some physicians have advocated regular oral amiodarone to prevent this complication. A recent study compared the use of amiodarone to implantable cardioverter-defibrillator (ICD) insertion or placebo in 2521 patients (median age 60 years) with advanced heart failure and ejection fractions at or below 35%.[23] After 46 months of follow-up, the amiodarone group fared no better than those given placebo (28 and 29% mortality, respectively), but the ICD group did significantly better (22% mortality).

Palliative care

It is a requirement of the National Service Framework for Coronary Heart Disease (*see* the website www.dh.gov.uk/assetRoot/04/05/75/23/04057523.pdf) that palliative care be incorporated into a patient's heart failure care. Patients who are reaching the palliative stage of their condition typically have had a number of admissions due to uncontrolled heart failure, no clear precipitant for deterioration, worsening renal function, and a poor response to optimal medical management.[24]

Prevention

The adequate control of hypertension has been associated with a reduction in the incidence of heart failure.[25]

Prognosis

The prognosis of heart failure is poor. One-year and five-year survival rates are around 60% and 30%, respectively, and older age is associated with a worse outcome.[26]

References

1 Kannel WB and Belanger AJ. Epidemiology of heart failure. *Am Heart J*, 1991; **121**(3): 951–957.

2 Aurigemma GP and Gaasch WH. Diastolic heart failure. *NEJM*, 2004; **351**(11): 1097–1105.

3 Hogg K, Swedberg K and McMurray J. Heart failure with preserved left ventricular systolic function. *J Am Coll Cardiol*, 2004; **43**(3): 317–327.

4 De Denus S, Pharand C and Williamson DR. Brain natriuretic peptide in the management of heart failure: the versatile neurohormone. *Chest*, 2004; **125**(2): 652–668.

5 McKie PM and Burnett JC. B-type natriuretic peptide as a biomarker beyond heart failure: speculations and opportunities. *Mayo Clin Proc*, 2005; **80**(8): 1029–1036.

6 The SOLVD Investigators. Effect of enalapril on survival in patients with reduced left ventricular ejection fractions and congestive heart failure. *NEJM*, 1991; **325**(5): 293–302.

7 Flather MD, Yusuf S, Kober L *et al.* Long-term ACE-inhibitor therapy in patients with heart failure or left-ventricular dysfunction: a systematic overview of data from individual patients. *Lancet*, 2000; **355**: 1575–1581.

8 The Heart Outcomes Prevention Evaluation Study Investigators. Effects of an angiotensin-converting-enzyme inhibitor, ramipril, on cardiovascular events in high-risk patients. *NEJM*, 2000; **342**(3): 145–153.

9 Cohn JN andTognoni G. A randomized trial of the angiotensin-receptor blocker valsartan in chronic heart failure. *NEJM*, 2001; **345**(23): 1667–1675.

10 Demers C, McMurray JJV, Swedberg K *et al.* Impact of candesartan on non-fatal myocardial infarction and cardiovascular death in patients with heart failure. *JAMA*, 2005; **294**(14): 1794–1798.

11 Pitt B, Poole-Wilson PA, Segal R *et al.* Effect of losartan compared with captopril in mortality in patients with symptomatic heart failure: randomised trial – the Losartan Heart Failure Survival Study ELITE II. *Lancet*, 2000; **355**: 1582–1587.

12 Packer M, Bristow MR, Cohn JN *et al.* The effect of carvedilol on morbidity and mortality in patients with chronic heart failure. *NEJM*, 1996; **334**(21): 1349–1355.

13 CIBIS-II Investigators and Committees. The Cardiac Insufficiency Bisoprolol Study II (CIBIS-II): a randomised trial. *Lancet*, 1999; **353**: 9–13.

14 MERIT-HF Study Group. Effect of metoprolol CR/XL in chronic heart failure: Metoprolol CR/XL Randomised Intervention Trial in Congestive Heart Failure (MERIT-FH). *Lancet*, 1999; **353**: 2001–2007.

15 Dulin BR, Haas SJ, Abraham WT *et al.* Do elderly systolic heart failure patients benefit from beta blockers to the same extent as the non-elderly? Meta-analysis of >12,000 patients in large-scale clinical trials. *Am J Cardiol*, 2005; **95**: 896–898.

16 Flather MD, Shibata MC, Coats AJS *et al.* Randomized trial to determine the effect of nebivolol on mortality and cardiovascular hospital admission in elderly patients with heart failure (SENIORS). *Eur Heart J*, 2005; **26**(3): 215–225.

17 Pitt B, Zannad F, Remme WJ *et al.* The effect of spironolactone on morbidity and mortality in patients with severe heart failure. *NEJM*, 1999; **341**(10): 709–717.

18 The Digitalis Investigation Group. The effect of digoxin on mortality and morbidity in patients with heart failure. *NEJM*, 1997; **336**(8): 525–533.

19 Cohn JN, Archibald DG, Ziesche S *et al.* Effect of vasodilator therapy on mortality in chronic congestive heart failure. *NEJM*, 1986; **314**(24): 1547–1552.

20 Cohn JN, Johnson G, Ziesche S *et al.* A comparison of enalapril with hydralazine-isosorbide dinitrate in the treatment of chronic congestive heart failure. *NEJM*, 1991; **325**(5): 303–310.

21 Chow AWC, Lane RE and Cowie MR. New pacing technologies for heart failure. *BMJ*, 2003; **326**: 1073–1077.

22 Cleland JGF, Daubert J, Erdmann E *et al.* The effect of cardiac resynchronization on morbidity and mortality in heart failure. *NEJM*, 2005; **352**(15): 1539–1549.

23 Bardy GH, Lee KL, Mark DB *et al.* Amiodarone or an implantable cardioverter-defibrillator for congestive heart failure. *NEJM*, 2005; **352**(3): 225–237.

24 Ellershaw J and Ward C. Care of the dying patient: the last hours or days of life. *BMJ*, 2003; **326**: 30–34.

25 Moser M and Herbert PR. Prevention of disease progression, left ventricular hypertrophy and congestive heart failure in hypertension treatment trials. *J Am Coll Cardiol*, 1996; **27**: 1214–1218.

26 Nieminen MS and Harjola V. Definition and epidemiology of acute heart failure syndromes. *Am J Cardiol*, 2005; **96** (Suppl.): 5G–10G.

Chapter 13

Hypertension

Epidemiology

Hypertension is a common problem, especially in the elderly, yet it is often under-recognised and undertreated. Data from the Framingham Heart Study found that it had a prevalence of 27% in those below age 60 years, rising to 63% of those aged 60–79, and 74% in those aged over 80.[1] Only 32% of hypertensive subjects were on adequate treatment to control their blood pressure (BP) below 140/90 mmHg. Even normotensive people aged 55–65 years have a 90% chance of developing hypertension at some stage in their lifetime.[2] Isolated systolic hypertension (ISH) is defined as having a systolic BP above 140 mmHg with a diastolic below 90 mmHg. It appears to be particularly common in the elderly, probably due to an increase in stiffness of large arteries.[3] This is mediated by a reduction in elastin and increase in collagen proteins within vessel walls.

Assessment

It is advised that BP estimates are based on an average of at least two readings whilst seated, on at least two different occasions.[3] Orthostatic hypotension (OH) is frequently associated with hypertension in the elderly (see p 201). Standing BP readings, especially in those with postural symptoms, may demonstrate it, but an active stand test would provide a more accurate evaluation (see p 186). 24-hour BP monitoring sometimes provides additional information and is discussed below.

A physical examination may detect signs of end-organ damage, such as hypertensive retinopathy (see Table 13.1), evidence of left ventricular enlargement or proteinuria on urinalysis. Electrocardiograph (ECG) or chest X-ray tests may provide further signs of left ventricular hypertrophy.

Table 13.1 The classification of hypertensive retinopathy

Grade	
I	Narrowing of retinal arterioles
II	Arteriovenous 'nipping'
III	Soft exudates or flame haemorrhages
IV	Papilloedema

24-hour blood pressure monitoring

Several BP recording devices are available for the patient to carry around with them over a period of, usually, 24 hours. They take measurements at regular intervals (usually set to hourly) and these data can be downloaded and analysed when the machine is returned to the hospital. The use of such devices has led to the discovery of different patterns of BP that have differing effects on cardiovascular risk. O'Brien *et al.* have provided a useful review of this topic.[4] The main variants are discussed below.

'Normal' blood pressure

BP usually varies throughout the day with lower values occurring during the night. Normal individuals are currently defined as having an average daytime BP that is at or below 135/85 mmHg and a night-time dip to 120/70 mmHg or less. However, a truly normal BP is hard to define (*see* p 244). (*See* Figure 13.1.)

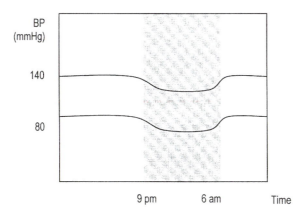

Figure 13.1   Representation of a 24-hour pattern of a 'normal' blood pressure (BP).

Hypertension

Hypertension is defined as an average daytime BP of greater than 140/90 mmHg (this value is adjusted for people who have vascular disease (such as a stroke) and those who have diabetes – *see below*). A diurnal variation is usually maintained. A mean nocturnal BP of over 125/75 mmHg is considered abnormal. (*See* Figure 13.2.)

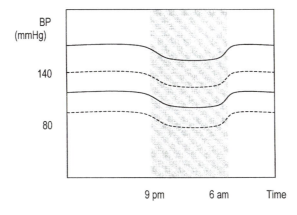

Figure 13.2   Representation of hypertension over 24 hours with preserved diurnal variation. Dashed lines represent upper limits of the normal range.

White coat hypertension

This is a term that is used to describe a pattern of hypertension with initial high readings in the presence of a healthcare professional (traditionally a doctor – hence 'white coat'). The BP will then normalise if repeated later. It is estimated to occur in 15–30% of the population but is more common in elderly people. Its significance is not fully understood but it does not appear to be associated with a major cardio-vascular risk. It is represented in Figure 13.3.

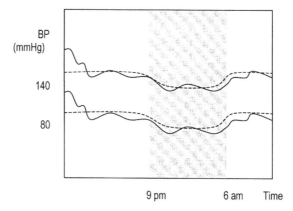

Figure 13.3 Representation of a 24-hour blood pressure (BP) recording in a person with 'white coat' hypertension.

Loss of diurnal variation

A number of people seem to have lost the normal pattern of BP variation. This pattern appears to be associated with an increased vascular and end organ damage risk,[5] including vascular dementia.[6] The term 'non-dippers' has been used for these people (compared to the normal 'dippers'). (*See* Figure 13.4.)

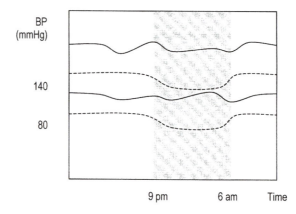

Figure 13.4 Representation of a 24-hour blood pressure (BP) recording in a person with hypertension associated with a loss of diurnal variation.

Nocturnal hypertension

Some people have higher night time BP readings than their daytime values. Similarly to those with a loss of diurnal variation, they appear to be at an increased risk of vascular events. (*See* Figure 13.5.)

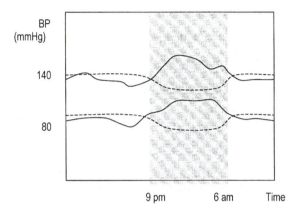

BP (mmHg)

140

80

9 pm   6 am   Time

Figure 13.5 Representation of a 24-hour blood pressure (BP) recording in a person with nocturnal hypertension.

Twenty-four hour BP monitoring probably has a number of roles in clinical practice. Among those are the enabling of identification of white coat and nocturnal hypertension, guiding the commencement of treatment in patients with borderline BP readings, and assessing the overall control of BP in people with mixed spine hypertension and OH.

The use of ambulatory BP values rather than conventional measurement has been compared.[7] Over a six-month period the ambulatory BP group was prescribed fewer anti-hypertensive medications with similar resultant blood pressures and no evidence of an increase in left ventricular size (assessed by ECG and echocardiography measurements). Another study found that 24-hour recordings offered additional information to predict cardiovascular risk to that derived from conventional measurements alone.[8] The night-time BP reading may be of particular predictive value due to its unfluctuating nature during normal sleep. So, it appears to be an appropriate alternative to conventional methods in selected patients.

Treatment

Reducing elevated BP has been shown to reduce the risk of vascular adverse events, in particular stroke (*see* p 105). Estimates of around a 40% reduction in stroke and 15% reduction in MI with adequate BP treatment have been made.[9] Such benefits appear to be maintained in elderly populations[10] and in those with ISH.[11] These patients have also been found to have a significantly lower rate of heart failure after

BP treatment compared to placebo over a 4.5-year period (RR 0.51; 95% CI 0.37–0.71).[12] Trial evidence regarding the treatment of those over the age of 80 years is limited, but a meta-analysis of data from people in this age group who were enrolled in antihypertensive randomised controlled trials suggests a maintained benefit.[13] Once hypertension has been identified it should be treated immediately, as delays are associated with an excess of cardiovascular adverse events.[14]

BP targets

There is no apparent 'normal' BP value below which there is no additional treatment benefit, that is, the lower the blood pressure the lower the vascular risk. A meta-analysis of studies suggests that lowering blood pressure down to at least 115/75 mmHg continues to reduce vascular risk.[15] Below this value there are few available data. Between the ages of 40 and 69 years there is a doubling of vascular death rates for every elevation of 20 mmHg systolic, or 10 mmHg diastolic BP.[15] After this age the relative risk reduction is less but the absolute risk is higher and so a significant benefit is still attained. Accepted target blood pressures are better than 140/85 mmHg in non-diabetics and better than 130/80 mmHg in those with diabetes.[9] Recently the lower target of 130/80 mmHg has also been recommended for patients with evidence of secondary organ damage (vascular disease, abnormal renal function, retinopathy, or evidence of left ventricular enlargement on ECG or echocardiogram).[16] The actual benefit of treatment is proportional to the baseline risk of cardiovascular disease. Indicators of elevated risk include signs of target organ damage (e.g. left ventricular hypertrophy, proteinuria or retinopathy) or associated comorbidities (e.g. diabetes, stroke or renal impairment). More than 50% of people over 65 years in most populations are defined as hypertensive by such targets.[9] Even if these targets cannot be safely achieved (e.g. because of associated OH (*see* Chapter 10)), there is still a benefit from smaller BP reductions and so, in some elderly people less stringent targets may be more appropriate.

Non-pharmacological intervention

Some lifestyle measures can reduce the impact of hypertension. These include weight reduction in the obese, avoiding excess alcohol intake, increasing physical activity, and dietary factors (fresh vegetables, low saturated fat and reduced salt).[9] Additional changes to reduce the chance of vascular disease, such as stopping smoking, are also clearly logical.

Pharmacological intervention

Despite the above measures, pharmacological therapy is almost always required. The question remains as to which agent or combination of agents is most effective. Analysis of the trials performed suggests that any method of BP reduction will have cardiovascular benefits, and the degree of reduction rather than the drugs used is the key factor.[17] Most patients will require more than one agent to achieve adequate control – especially if the starting BP is above 160/100 mmHg,[3] and 30% will need three or more agents.[9] Other vascular prevention strategies are also of proven benefit in many of these patients (e.g. antiplatelets[18] and statins[19]). This all adds to the burden of polypharmacy seen in elderly people (*see* p 277). Given the lack of obvious benefit to the individual patient, medication adherence is a particular problem with these drugs, and patient education is especially important. Two recent, large hypertension trials are discussed below.

ALLHAT

The ALLHAT trial randomised 33 357 people over the age of 55 (mean age 67 years) with hypertension and at least one other vascular risk factor to receive either a thiazide (chlorthalidone), angiotensin-converting enzyme (ACE) inhibitor (lisinopril) or a calcium channel-blocker (amlodipine) over a mean follow-up of 4.9 years.[20] After this time, there was no significant difference in the primary outcome (combined fatal coronary heart disease and non-fatal myocardial infarction (MI)) with any of the agents. Chlorthalidone resulted in a small but significantly significant greater reduction in systolic BP than either lisinopril (2 mmHg) or amlodipine (0.8 mmHg). The conclusion of this trial was that, due to their low cost and proven efficacy, thiazides should be considered as first-line agents for BP control.

ASCOT

The ASCOT trial randomised 19 257 people (mean age 63, range 40–79 years) with hypertension plus other vascular risk factors to receive either amlodipine with perindopril if required or atenolol plus bendroflumethiazide if required over a five-year period.[21] The mean initial BP was 164/95 mmHg and this was reduced to 136/77 mmHg in the amlodipine arm and 139/79 mm Hg in the atenolol arm. The primary endpoint of non-fatal MI and fatal coronary heart disease failed to reach significance in favour of the amlodipine regimen (8.1 vs 9.2 events per 1000 people-years; $p = 0.11$). However, there were significant reductions in total cardiovascular events and procedures (27.4 vs 32.8; $p<0.0001$), stroke (6.2 vs 8.1; $p = 0.0003$) and overall mortality (13.9 vs 15.5; $p = 0.025$). Only 53% of participants achieved their target BP, which was set at 140/90 mmHg for non-diabetics and 130/80 mmHg for diabetics (of whom only 32% achieved the target). On average 2.2 and 2.3 BP-lowering agents were used in the amlodipine and atenolol groups, respectively. Eight per cent of the subjects were on four or more agents at the end of the study. Twenty-five per cent of each group stopped a treatment because of side effects. Adverse events occurring more often in the amlodipine arm included cough (19% vs 8%) and oedema (23% vs 6%). Adverse events occurring more often in the atenolol arm included bradycardia (6% vs <1%), dizziness (16% vs 12%), dyspnoea (10% vs 6%), fatigue (16% vs 8%) and cold peripheries (6% vs 1%).

The mean difference in blood pressure of 2.7/1.9 mmHg between the groups would explain at least some of the difference in outcomes. Other metabolic features that differed between the groups included a higher mean glucose (raised by 0.2 mmol/l), body mass index (by 0.3 kg/m^2) and lower HDL cholesterol (by 0.1 mmol/l) in the atenolol group.

PROGRESS

This trial is of particular relevance to BP control post-stroke and is discussed on p 112.

Individual drugs

The mechanisms of action and main side effects of the most commonly used agents are discussed in Chapter 12.

Thiazide diuretics

Thiazide diuretics are considered a first-line agent for the management of hypertension in the elderly[9] – especially in those with ISH. They were used in the ALLHAT, ACSOT and PROGRESS trials as outlined earlier.

ACE inhibitors

ACE inhibitors were used in the ALLHAT, ACSOT and PROGRESS trials as outlined earlier.

Calcium channel-blockers

Dihydropyridines (e.g. amlodipine) are suitable for the management of hypertension, especially in the elderly.[9] Non-dihydropyridines (e.g. diltiazem) are probably less effective in this situation. In the ALLHAT study a calcium channel-blocker compared less favourably to a thiazide for the prevention of heart failure.

Beta-blockers

A recent meta-analysis of trials into the use of atenolol has brought into question the use of beta-blockers for the treatment of hypertension.[22] In randomised controlled trials comparing atenolol to placebo, despite improvements in BP, no significant reductions in cardiovascular events or mortality were detected. In comparison to alternative antihypertensive agents, there was a significantly higher mortality with atenolol (RR 1.13; 95% CI 1.02–1.25).

Less lipid-soluble agents (e.g. atenolol, bisoprolol and metoprolol) are less likely to cause neuropsychiatric side effects (sedation, sexual dysfunction and depression) than lipid-soluble alternatives (e.g. propranolol).[3]

Angiotensin receptor blockers (ARBs)

A trial recruiting 15 245 patients compared valsartan to amlodipine (plus other antihypertensive agents as required) in patients aged over 50 years (mean age 67) with hypertension and other vascular risk factors over a mean period of 4.2 years.[23] The amlodipine regimen proved to be more effective at lowering BP (by a mean of 1.5/1.3 mmHg) and was associated with a non-significant lower rate of attaining the combined end-point of cardiac mortality and morbidity (10.4% vs 10.6%).

Losartan has been compared to atenolol in 1326 patients (mean age 70, range 55–80 years) with ISH and evidence of left ventricular hypertrophy in the LIFE study.[24] Other agents (mainly thiazide diuretics) could be added if required for better BP control. Despite similar reductions in blood pressure (28/9 mmHg in both arms), after a mean period of 4.7 years, there was a non-significantly reduced incidence of the combined endpoint of cardiovascular death, stroke or MI in the losartan arm

(RR 0.75; 95% CI 0.59–1.01; p = 0.06). This suggests that ARBs may be useful BP-lowering agents, but given the emerging evidence that beta-blockers may be less effective than alternatives (*see above*), the more expensive and less well studied ARBs remain second-line agents. They may be effectively used in combination with ACE inhibitors.[25]

Recently there has been concern that ARBs may be associated with an increased risk of MI.[26] However, a meta-analysis of studies comparing the use of ARBs to either placebo or ACEis did not support such a link.[27]

Interpretation of pharmacological data

The benefits seen after BP-lowering are probably mostly due to the degree of pressure reduction rather than any factors related to the class of medications themselves. The above studies suggest that, either alone or (more commonly) in combination, any of thiazide diuretics, ACE inhibitors and dihydropyridine calcium channel-blockers (e.g. amlodipine) are suitable first-line agents for the management of hypertension in the elderly. The actual agents chosen may be dictated by the presence of comorbidities, for example ACE inhibitors may be of additional benefit in those with renal impairment, thiazides may be avoided in those with gout. Certain agents (e.g. vasodilators and diuretics) and those in shorter-acting formulations are particularly likely to cause OH (*see* p 202). This may influence the choice of drug in selected patients. An additional factor influencing prescribing should be cost – as cheaper agents are the more cost-effective.[9]

Beta-blockers should no longer be considered first-line agents unless there is another reason to justify their use – such as the prevention of angina or rate control in AF. ARBs are probably a reasonable choice of second-line agent, or for those intolerant of but with an indication for ACE inhibitors. Alpha-blockers (e.g. doxazosin) may also be appropriate in some patients but the evidence is less clear and an increased association with orthostatic hypotension may limit their use in the elderly. Other drugs, such as central alpha-agonists (e.g. methyldopa and clonidine) or vasodilators (e.g. hydralazine), will occasionally be appropriate but there is less randomised controlled trial evidence of efficacy and side effects are likely to be significant.

Current guidelines for the British Hypertension Society recommend either a calcium channel-blocker or thiazide diuretic as first-line therapy in the elderly (>55 years).[9] The second step would be to add an ACE inhibitor (or an ARB if ACE inhibitor-intolerant) or a beta-blocker. The third step is to add either a calcium channel-blocker or thiazide (whichever has not already been used), and the final step is to add an alpha-blocker or a non-thiazide diuretic.

References

1 Lloyd-Jones DM, Evans JC and Levy D. Hypertension in adults across the age spectrum: current outcomes and control in the community. *JAMA*, 2005; **294**(4): 466–472.

2 Vasan RS, Beiser A, Seshadri S *et al*. Residual lifetime risk of developing hypertension in middle-aged women and men: the Framingham Heart Study. *JAMA*, 2002; **287**(8): 1003–1010.

3 Dickerson LM and Gibson MV. Management of hypertension in older persons. *Am Family Phys*, 2005; **71**(3): 469–476.

4 O'Brien E, Coats A, Owens P *et al*. Use and interpretation of ambulatory blood pressure monitoring: recommendations of the British Hypertension Society. *BMJ*, 2000; **320**: 1128–1134.

5 Verdecchia P, Schillaci G, Guerrieri M *et al*. Circadian blood pressure changes and left ventricular hypertrophy in essential hypertension. *Circulation*, 1990; **81**: 528–536.

6 Yamamoto Y, Akiguchi I, Oiwa K *et al*. The relationship between 24-hour blood pressure readings, subcortical ischemic lesions and vascular dementia. *Cerebrovasc Dis*, 2005; **19**: 302–308.

7 Staesseu JA, Byttebier G, Buntinx F *et al*. Antihypertensive treatment based on conventional or ambulatory blood pressure measurement: a randomised controlled trial. *JAMA*, 1997; **278**(13): 1065–1072.

8 Staessen JA, Thijs L, Fagard R *et al*. Predicting cardiovascular risk using conventional vs ambulatory blood pressure in older patients with systolic hypertension. *JAMA*, 1999; **282**(6): 539–546.

9 Williams B, Poulter NR, Brown MJ *et al*. Guidelines for management of hypertension: report of the fourth working party of the British Hypertension Society, 2004-BHS IV. *J Human Hypertension*, 2004; **18**: 139–185.

10 Leeper SC. Aggressive hypertension management in patients of advancing and advanced age. *Southern Med J*, 2005; **98**(8): 805–808.

11 Perry HM, Davis BR, Price TR *et al*. Effect of treating isolated systolic hypertension on the risk of developing various types and subtypes of stroke: the Systolic Hypertension in the Elderly Program (SHEP). *JAMA*, 2000; **284**(4): 465–471.

12 Kostis JB, Davis BR, Cutler J *et al*. Prevention of heart failure by antihypertensive drug treatment in older persons with isolated systolic hypertension. *JAMA*, 1997; **278**(3): 212–216.

13 Gueyffier F, Bulpitt C, Boissel JP *et al*. Antihypertensive drugs in very old people: a subgroup meta-analysis of randomised controlled trials. *Lancet*, 1999; **353**: 793–796.

14 Staessen JA, Thijs L, Fagard R *et al*. Effects of immediate versus delayed antihypertensive therapy on outcome in the Systolic Hypertension in Europe Trial. *J Hypertension*, 2004; **22**: 847–857.

15 Prospective Studies Collaboration. Age-specific relevance of usual blood pressure to vascular mortality: a meta-analysis of individual data for one million adults in 61 prospective studies. *Lancet*, 2002; **360**: 1903–1913.

16 Joint British Societies' guidelines on prevention of cardiovascular disease in clinical practice. *Heart*, 2005; **91** (Suppl. V): v1–v52.

17 Blood Pressure Lowering Treatment Trialists' Collaboration. Effects of different blood-pressure-lowering regimens on major cardiovascular events: results of prospectively-designed overviews of randomised trials. *Lancet*, 2003; **362**: 1527–1535.

18 Hansson L, Zanchetti A, Carruthers SG *et al*. Effects of intensive blood-pressure lowering and low-dose aspirin in patients with hypertension: principal results of the Hypertension Optimal Treatment (HOT) randomised trial. *Lancet*, 1998; **351**: 1755–1762.

19 Sever PS, Dahlof B, Poulter NR *et al*. Prevention of coronary and stroke events with atorvastatin in hypertensive patients who have average or lower-than-average cholesterol concentrations, in the Anglo-Scandinavian Cardiac Outcomes Trial – Lipid Lowering Arm (ASCOT-LLA): a multicentre randomised controlled trial. *Lancet*, 2003; **361**: 1149–1158.

20 The ALLHAT Officers and Coordinators for the ALLHAT Collaborative Research Group. Major outcomes in high-risk hypertensive patients randomized to angiotensin-converting enzyme inhibitor or calcium channel blocker vs diuretic: the Antihypertensive and Lipid-Lowering Treatment to Prevent Heart Attack Trial (ALLHAT). *JAMA*, 2002; **288**(23): 2981–2997.

21 Dahlof B, Sever PS, Poulter NR *et al*. Prevention of cardiovascular events with an antihypertensive regimen of amlodipine adding perindopril as required versus atenolol adding bendroflumethiazide as required, in the Anglo-Scandinavian Cardiac Outcomes Trial – Blood Pressure Lowering Arm (ASCOT-BPLA): a multicentre randomised controlled trial. *Lancet*, 2005; **366**: 895–906.

22 Carlberg B, Samuelsson O and Lindholm LH. Atenolol in hypertension: is it a wise choice? *Lancet*, 2004; **364**: 1684–1689.

23 Julius S, Kjeldsen SE, Weber M *et al*. Outcomes in hypertensive patients at high cardiovascular risk treated with regimens based on valsartan or amlodipine: the VALUE randomised trial. *Lancet*, 2004; **363**: 2022–2031.

24 Kjeldsen SE, Dahlof B, Devereux RB *et al.* Effects of losartan on cardiovascular morbidity and mortality in patients with isolated systolic hypertension and left ventricular hypertrophy: a Losartan Intervention For Endpoint Reduction (LIFE) study. *JAMA,* 2002; **288**(12): 1491–1498.

25 Azizi M and Menard J. Combined blockade of the renin-angiotensin system with angiotensin-converting enzyme inhibitors and angiotensin II type 1 receptor antagonists. *Circulation,* 2004; **109**(21): 2492–2499.

26 Verma S and Strauss M. Angiotensin receptor blockers and myocardial infarction. *BMJ,* 2004; **329**: 1248–1249.

27 McDonald MA, Simpson SH, Ezekowitz JA *et al.* Angiotensin receptor blockers and risk of myocardial infarction: systematic review. *BMJ,* 2005; **331**: 873.

Chapter 14

Atrial fibrillation

Atrial fibrillation (AF) is more common in older than younger people. It occurs in less than 2% of those below the age of 65 and in 5.9% of those over 65 years.[1] The prevalence rises to between 7% and 14% of the population over the age of 80, although these figures may underestimate the true prevalence of AF as unsustained episodes (paroxysmal AF (PAF)) are likely to have been missed.

AF can be provoked by almost any cardiac abnormality. Those who have had a previous MI, or have left ventricular impairment or atrial enlargement are at an increased risk of its development. Only around 15% occurs in people with structurally normal hearts ('lone' AF).[2]

The major adverse consequence of AF is the six-fold increased risk of stroke (the rate is even higher in those with AF secondary to mitral valve disease).[2] This is due to the formation and subsequent embolisation of thrombus – most typically from the left atrial appendage. On average the annual risk of stroke in people with AF but no antiplatelet or anticoagulation medication is around 5%, but this varies according to other risk factors. From the Stroke Prevention in AF II trial, the following clinical characteristics were associated with a higher risk of stroke: history of previous stroke or transient ischaemic attack (TIA); systolic blood pressure (BP) above 160 mmHg; left ventricular dysfunction; and age over 75 years.[3] Rating scales to estimate risk have been developed: one of these is CHADS2.[4] In this scheme one point is given for each of **C**ongestive cardiac failure history, **H**ypertension, **A**ge over 75 years and **D**iabetes, and a history of **S**troke scores **2** points (spelling CHADS2) – giving a score of 0–6. The estimated stroke rates for different scores are shown in Table 14.1.

Table 14.1   Estimated stroke rates for CHADS2 scores

CHADS2 score	0	1	2	3	4	5	6
Estimated stroke rate per 100 patient-years (for patients on neither warfarin nor antiplatelet agents)	1.9	2.8	4.0	5.9	8.5	12.5	18.2

Overall, around 15% of strokes are associated with AF, but this proportion is elevated in older patients, being around 36% in those over the age of 80.[5] Recurrent episodes of PAF appear to carry a similar thrombo-embolic risk to sustained AF.[3] However, the relevance of very infrequent, brief episodes, such as a single short run of AF detected on a 24-hour electrocardiograph (ECG), is unclear.

When evaluating a patient with AF it is important to look for reversible secondary causes. These include thyrotoxicosis and excessive alcohol intake. Twenty-four hour ECG recordings may detect previously unknown PAF or may be useful for judging rate control over a prolonged period. Echocardiography may provide information regarding left ventricular function, left atrial size, and valvular lesions but is unlikely to give additional information that would influence the decision regarding the suitability of an elderly patient for warfarinisation.[6]

Prevention of thrombo-embolic complications

Warfarin

Warfarin antagonises the effect of vitamin K in the process of production of its dependent clotting factors within the liver (factors VII, IX, X, prothrombin, and proteins C and S) (see Figure 5.9). This reduces the risk of forming blood clots within the left atrium due to blood stasis during AF. The overall efficacy of warfarin is in the order of around a 65% reduction in relative risk of stroke.[3,7] When real-life practice has been compared to the results of such trials, similar outcomes have been observed.[8] Of course, the absolute risk reduction depends on the individual's baseline risk of stroke, that is, those at highest risk benefit the most. Patients under the age of 65 years who have no history of vascular disease or diabetes are at a very low risk of thrombo-embolism and the benefits do not outweigh the risks of warfarinisation.[7]

The main side effect of warfarin is an elevated bleeding tendency. Contraindications to anticoagulation include recent bleeding, multiple falls (>2 in the past year), inability to consistently take the prescribed dose, uncontrolled hypertension and excessive alcohol intake.[6] Taking these factors into account, around half of older patients with AF would be suitable candidates for warfarin.[6]

Despite the evidence of benefit of warfarin in those with AF, only around 30% of such patients who do not have contraindications are receiving this therapy.[9] This is usually due to a perceived low risk of embolus or high risk of haemorrhage within particular patients. Having previously had a patient who sustained a serious bleeding complication appears to reduce the probability of a physician prescribing warfarin.[10]

The anticoagulant response to warfarin is increased with advanced age.[11] This difference is still apparent after correction for confounding variables such as body weight, medication interactions and comorbidity. Part of this difference may be due to dietary change. Vitamin K, which opposes the effect of warfarin, is found in leafy green vegetables. Therefore a diet containing less of these may make the effects of warfarin more pronounced.

Loading

The old regimen of 10 mg on three consecutive days resulted in over a third of patients being over-coagulated on the fourth day.[12] An early loading regimen that commenced with 10 mg but then varied according to international normalised ratio (INR) on day two was described by Fennerty et al.[12] This has largely been replaced in the elderly by regimens commencing with a 5 mg dose, which cause lower incidences of over-coagulation.[13] The initial dose may be further reduced in the presence of other factors increasing sensitivity to warfarin, such as liver disease or medication interactions.[14]

Complications

Complications of therapy are mainly due to increased bleeding. Overall, major bleeds occur at a rate of 2–7% per year[3,15] and fatal ones at a rate of 1% per year.[15,16] The risk rises proportionally with increasing INR values.[17] The bleeding risk is also elevated in this first few months of therapy and in those with unstable INRs.[16] Patients who have had one bleed are at a higher risk of additional events within the following year.[16] Age itself, when adjusted for confounding variables, does not appear to be a significant risk factor for overall rates of bleeding complications.[16,18,19] On the other hand, a doubling of risk for subdural haemorrhage with each additional decade has been reported.[18] Other risk factors for bleeding whilst on warfarin therapy include recent haemorrhage, binge drinking of alcohol, renal impairment, liver disease, non-steroidal anti-inflammatory drug (NSAID) use, and having a diagnosis of cancer.[14]

Intracranial bleeds occur at a rate of 0.3% to 1% per year in patients on warfarin, depending on baseline risk factors (such as hypertension and previous stroke).[20] Around 70% of intracranial bleeding occurring in people on warfarin is due to intracerebral haemorrhage (ICH) and most of the rest is due to subdural haematomas.[20] ICH in this population carries a 60% mortality rate. The size of the bleed often increases over a 24-hour period, making urgent reversal of the coagulation impairment imperative. This is best achieved with prothrombin complex concentrate infusion. ICH is further discussed on p 116.

In a study of 228 very old patients (mean age 81, range 76–94 years) on warfarin over a mean follow-up of 28 months, an annual incidence of 10% for major bleeding and 1% for fatal haemorrhage was detected.[21] Two intracranial bleeds occurred (0.4% per year) and these were both fatal. There was an associated 2.6% ischaemic stroke rate per year. The most common site of major bleeding was gastrointestinal (30%). Forty-two per cent of major bleeds occurred with INRs above the target range (>3), and 60% of fatal bleeds occurred with a very high INR (>5). The majority of the adverse bleeding events resulted in complete recovery. This suggests that the benefits of warfarin are still apparent in this age group, but emphasises the importance of INR control.

Even elderly patients in a controlled environment may also be at risk of unstable warfarin dosing. There is a high incidence of errors in the management of INRs within nursing homes,[22] with an increased chance of sub-therapeutic INRs or overcoagulation.[23]

Aspirin

Aspirin is less effective than warfarin in reducing the risk of thrombo-embolism in AF. The results of clinical trials have been conflicting. The Stroke Prevention in AF I study found a 42% relative risk reduction with the daily use of 325 mg of aspirin compared to placebo (absolute risks 3.6% vs 6.3% per year).[24] Another study failed to demonstrate a significant benefit in reducing thrombo-embolic complications with 75 mg of aspirin compared to placebo in 672 people.[25] An analysis of multiple trials concluded that aspirin resulted in approximately a 20% reduction in stroke risk.[3] Despite this demonstrated benefit, less than half of patients in AF who are ineligible for warfarin are on antiplatelet therapy.[26]

Clopidogrel

The combination of aspirin (75–100 mg) and clopidogrel (75 mg) has been compared to warfarin (INR 2–3) for the prevention of thrombo-embolic events in patients with AF.[27] In 6706 patients (mean age 70 years) with AF and a least one other risk factor for stroke who were randomised, it was found that both the risk of stroke (RR 1.44; 95% CI 1.18–1.76) and the risk of bleeding complications (RR 1.21; 95% CI 1.08–1.35) were higher in the aspirin and clopidogrel arm (the mean follow-up was 1.28 years). Therefore, warfarin appears to be the preferable option.

A further component of this study that compares aspirin alone to aspirin plus clopidogrel in this patient group is ongoing at the time of writing.

Cardioversion

Reversion of AF back into sinus rhythm is often possible with either DC cardioversion or medications (e.g. flecainide).[2] It is usually not performed in elderly people with reasonable rate control due to the high chance of relapse to AF following the procedure. A longer duration of AF and the presence of left atrial enlargement also make the procedure less likely to be effective.[28] When studies compared outcomes in patients randomly assigned to either a strategy of sinus rhythm restoration or rate control alone, attempts at rhythm control did not appear to offer any long-term benefit.[29]

Rate control

Pacemakers

When AF is associated with episodes of very fast and very slow heart rate (the tachycardia–bradycardia syndrome), it is best treated with a combination of pacemaker insertion and the use of rate-slowing drugs. Pacemakers should also be considered in the presence of prolonged and symptomatic pauses (e.g. >3 seconds).

Beta-blockers

Beta-blockers may be used to slow ventricular rate and may prevent episodes of arrhythmia in those with PAF.[30]

Sotalol is a beta-blocker that also has some class III anti-arrhythmic activity. In trials it has not proven to be more effective than standard beta-blockers.[30] It is associated with a stronger pro-arrhythmogenic tendency, especially in those with underlying heart disease. It is, therefore, best avoided in the elderly.

Digoxin

Digoxin does not result in an increased rate of reversion to sinus rhythm,[31] nor does it control the rate of AF during exertion,[14] or during episodes of AF in those with PAF.[31] It has a smaller rate limiting effect than most alternative agents. In a randomised controlled trial that compared intravenous digoxin to placebo, digoxin did not cause cardioversion but did result in a small, significant reduction in heart rate apparent after two hours (heart rate 105 per minute vs 117 per minute with placebo).[32]

Amiodarone

Amiodarone is a highly lipophilic compound and a large loading dose is required to maintain plasma drug levels. It is traditionally described as a Vaughan–Williams class III agent but also has some class I and II activity. It has been demonstrated to have the capacity to convert AF to sinus rhythm (SR), can maintain SR in PAF and can control rate in sustained AF.[33] In comparison to sotalol and various class I drugs it has been found to be superior in maintaining SR.[34] It also appears to be more effective than beta-blockers in preventing the onset of AF in high-risk patients.[35]

Along with the potential to induce life-threatening arrhythmias, there are a number of severe adverse reactions associated with amiodarone use – *see* Table 14.2.[36] The most common of these is hypothyroidism, which can be treated simply by hormone replacement. Hyperthyroidism is less common but far harder to treat.[37] Pulmonary infiltrates may occur more commonly after prolonged drug exposure.

Table 14.2 Annual incidence (%) of severe adverse reactions to amiodarone

Reaction	Annual incidence(%)
Hypothyroidism	5.9
Pulmonary infiltrates	1.1
Hyperthyroidism	0.9
Hepatic dysfunction	0.6
Peripheral neuropathy	0.3

Calcium channel antagonists

Diltiazem and verapamil may have a role in the slowing of heart rate in some patients who are intolerant to, or inadequately controlled by, alternative agents. They are best avoided in those with heart failure. Verapamil cannot be used in combination with beta-blockers.

References

1 Feinberg WM, Blackshear JL, Laupacis A *et al.* Prevalence, age distribution, and gender of patients with atrial fibrillation: analysis and implications. *Arch Intern Med,* 1995; **155**: 469–473.

2 Peters NS, Schilling RJ, Kanagaratnam P *et al.* Atrial fibrillation: strategies to control, combat, and cure. *Lancet,* 2002; **359**: 593–603.

3 Hart RG, Halperin JL, Pearce LA *et al.* Lessons from the Stroke Prevention in Atrial Fibrillation trials. *Ann Intern Med,* 2003; **138**(10): 831–838.

4   Gage BF, Waterman AD, Shannon W *et al.* Validation of clinical classification schemes for predicting stroke: results from the national registry of atrial fibrillation. *JAMA,* 2001; **285**(22): 2864–2870.

5   Wolf PA, Abbott RD and Kannel WB. Atrial fibrillation: a major contributor to stroke in the elderly: the Framingham study. *Arch Intern Med,* 1987; **147**: 1561–1564.

6   Sudlow M, Thompson R, Thwaites B *et al.* Prevalence of atrial fibrillation and eligibility for anticoagulants in the community. *Lancet,* 1998; **352**: 1167–1171.

7   Atrial Fibrillation Investigators *et al.* Risk factors for stroke and efficacy of antithrombotic therapy in atrial fibrillation: analysis of pooled data from five randomized controlled trials. *Arch Intern Med,* 1994; **154**: 1449–1457.

8   Kalra L, Yu G, Perez I *et al.* Prospective cohort study to determine if trial efficacy of anticoagulation for stroke prevention in atrial fibrillation translates into clinical effectiveness. *BMJ,* 2000; **320**: 1236–1239.

9   Bungard TJ, Ghali WA, Teo KK *et al.* Why do patients with atrial fibrillation not receive warfarin? *Arch Intern Med,* 2000; **160**: 41–46.

10 Choudhry NK, Anderson GM, Laupacis A *et al.* Impact of adverse events on prescribing warfarin in patients with atrial fibrillation: matched pair analysis. *BMJ,* 2006; **332**: 141–143.

11 Gurwitz JH, Avorn J, Ross-Degnan D *et al.* Aging and the anticoagulant response to warfarin therapy. *Ann Int Med,* 1992; **116**: 901–904.

12 Fennerty A, Dolben J, Thomas P *et al.* Flexible induction dose regimen for warfarin and prediction of maintenance dose. *BMJ,* 1984; **288**: 1268–1270.

13 Harrison L, Johnston M, Massicotte MP *et al.* Comparison of 5-mg and 10-mg loading doses in initiation of warfarin therapy. *Ann Intern Med,* 1997; **126**(2): 133–136.

14 Gage BF, Fihn SD and White RH. Warfarin therapy for an octogenarian who has atrial fibrillation. *Ann Intern Med,* 2001; **134**(6): 465–474.

15 Landefeld CS and Goldman L. Major bleeding in outpatients treated with warfarin: incidence and prediction by factors known at the start of outpatient therapy. *Am J Med,* 1989; **87**: 144–152.

16 Fihn SD, McDonell M, Martin D *et al.* Risk factors for complications of chronic anticoagulation: a multicenter study. *Ann Intern Med,* 1993; **118**: 511–520.

17 Landefeld CS, Rosenblatt MW and Goldman L. Bleeding in outpatients treated with warfarin: relation to the prothrombin time and important remediable lesions. *Am J Med,* 1989; **87**: 153–159.

18 Hylek EM and Singer DE. Risk factors for intracranial hemorrhage in outpatients taking warfarin. *Ann Intern Med,* 1994; **120**(11): 897–902.

19 Fihn SD, Callahan CM, Martin DC *et al.* The risk for and severity of bleeding complications in elderly patients treated with warfarin. *Ann Intern Med,* 1996; **124**(11): 970–979.

20 Hart RG, Boop BS and Anderson DC. Oral anticoagulants and intracranial haemorrhage: facts and hypotheses. *Stroke,* 1995; **26**(8): 1471–1477.

21 Johnson CE, Lim WK and Workman BS. People aged over 75 in atrial fibrillation on warfarin: the rate of major haemorrhage and stroke in more than 500 patient-years of follow-up. *JAGS,* 2005; **53**: 655–659.

22 Gurwitz JH, Field TS, Avorn J, *et al.* Incidence and preventability of adverse drug events in nursing homes. *Am J Med,* 2000; **109**: 87–94.

23 Gurwitz JH, Monette J, Rochon PA *et al.* Atrial fibrillation and stroke prevention with warfarin in the long-term care setting. *Arch Intern Med,* 1997; **157**: 978–984.

24 Stroke Prevention in Atrial Fibrillation Investigators. Stroke Prevention in Atrial Fibrillation Study: final results. *Circulation,* 1991; **84**: 527–539.

25 Petersen P, Boysen G, Godtfredsen J *et al.* Placebo-controlled, randomised trial of warfarin and aspirin for prevention of thromboembolic complications in chronic atrial fibrillation. *Lancet,* 1989; **1**: 175–179.

26 Antithrombotic Trialists' Collaboration. Collaborative meta-analysis of randomised trials of antiplatelet therapy for prevention of death, myocardial infarction, and stroke in high risk patients. *BMJ,* 2002; **324**: 71–86.

27 The ACTIVE Writing Group. Clopidogrel plus aspirin versus oral anticoagulation for atrial fibrillation in the Atrial fibrillation Clopidogrel Trial with Irbesartan for prevention of Vascular Events (ACTIVE W): a randomised controlled trial. *Lancet,* 2006; **367**(9526): 1903–1912.

28 Channer KS. Current management of symptomatic atrial fibrillation. *Drugs,* 2001; **61**(10): 1425–1437.

29 Page RL. Newly diagnosed atrial fibrillation. *NEJM,* 2004; **351**(23): 2408–2416.

30 Steeds RP, Birchall AS, Smith A *et al.* An open label, randomised, crossover study comparing sotalol and atenolol in the treatment of symptomatic paroxysmal atrial fibrillation. *Heart,* 1999; **82**(2): 170–175.

31 Robles de Medina EO and Algra A. Digoxin in the treatment of paroxysmal atrial fibrillation. *Lancet,* 1999; **354**: 882–883.

32 The Digitalis in Acute Atrial Fibrillation (DAAF) Trial Group. Intravenous digoxin in acute atrial fibrillation: results of a randomized, placebo-controlled multicentre trial of 239 patients. *Eur Heart J,* 1997; **18**: 649–654.

33 Connolly SJ. Evidence-based analysis of amiodarone efficacy and safety. *Circulation,* 1999; **100**: 2025–2034.

34 The AFFIRM First Antiarrhythmic Drug Study Investigators. Maintenance of sinus rhythm in patients with atrial fibrillation: an AFFIRM study of the first antiarrhythmic drug. *J Am Coll Cardiol,* 2003; **42**: 20–29.

35 Solomon AJ, Greenberg MD, Kilborn MJ *et al.* Amiodarone versus a beta-blocker to prevent atrial fibrillation after cardiovascular surgery. *Am Heart J,* 2001; **142**(5): 811–815.

36 Amiodarone Trials Meta-analysis Investigators. Effect of prophylactic amiodarone on mortality after acute myocardial infarction and in congestive heart failure: meta-analysis of individual data from 6500 patients in randomised trials. *Lancet,* 1997; **350**: 1417–1424.

37 Newman CM, Price A, Davies DW *et al.* Amiodarone and the thyroid: a practical guide to the management of thyroid dysfunction induced by amiodarone therapy. *Heart,* 1998; **79**: 121–127.

Immobility

Chapter 15

Rehabilitation

The terminology used in rehabilitation is undergoing change. 'Impairments' are the physical problems caused by illness, such as weakness secondary to a stroke. Traditionally, these caused 'disabilities' such as a reduced ability to mobilise, which led to 'handicap' – the loss of ability to perform functions such as gardening, dancing or playing golf. In an attempt to use more positive terminology the World Health Organization (WHO) has advised that the latter two terms be changed to 'activities' and 'participation'.

Rehabilitation is performed by teams of people. These usually include doctors, nurses, physiotherapists, social workers and occupational therapists. Other specialties may also be involved, for example speech and language therapy, and dietetics. In some centres the traditional distinctions between professions are becoming blurred with individuals taking on multiple roles.

The aim of rehabilitation is to reduce the impact of physical illness. This will mean different things to different individuals. Ideally, the physical disability will be lessened. If this cannot be done, then new techniques or strategies may be learned to circumvent the problems. This may include adaptation of the person's living environment. Common sense and lateral thinking are often more important than scientific knowledge to solve problems for an individual patient.

Given this individualised nature of aims, it is right that patients should be involved in the setting of appropriate and realistic goals with the help of medical personnel. Goals may be divided into an overall, long-term aim and a series of more easily achieved short-term ones. The acronym 'SMART' has been proposed to help set suitable goals:

S   specific
M   measurable
A   achievable
R   relevant
T   time-limited

For example, having a goal of walking the length of the ward within one minute is both specific and measurable. If this goal could realistically be attained within four weeks, then it may be defined as both achievable and time-limited. If it would make going home a possibility then it is clearly relevant to the individual. It may be broken down into a series of smaller stages, for example standing unaided, walking several steps, walking several metres, and so on. This can make it easier to monitor the patient's progress towards the longer-term goal and help maintain morale.

Performing clinical trials in the field of rehabilitation is fraught with problems. There have been few large-scale controlled trials in any aspect of it. For this reason the evidence basis behind practice is often weak, but there is some proof of benefit.[1]

Stroke

Stroke is a major cause of disability in the adult population. After six months, around one-third of survivors are dependent on others for their activities of daily living.[2] Attempts at rehabilitation may be hindered by associated cognitive deficits, especially receptive dysphasia, making in harder for the patient to comply with interventions. There may also be components of apraxia, visuospatial impairment, or neglect (*see* Chapter 5), which should be specifically looked for in these patients. When such problems are detected, rehabilitation therapy sessions and ward environments should be adapted to lessen disability and promote recovery.[3]

Following a stroke, patients usually have some degree of recovery, and this improvement process can continue for periods of over a year. However, it is hard to predict in which patients and to what degree significant improvements will occur. The recovery process is thought to initially be due to the return of normal neuronal functioning around the infarcted area, but in the longer term it is dependent on the formation of new inter-neuronal connections, similar to the normal process of learning new information.[4]

Inpatient rehabilitation is usual for those patients who are unable to safely return home. Its duration varies according to patient response. Typically a period of six to eight weeks will demonstrate the likely long-term functional need of the patient, enabling future care plans to be formulated. Early hospital discharge is sometimes appropriate with the continuation of rehabilitation in the community through specialised teams. The minimal functional requirement for most patients to manage this is to be able to independently transfer from bed to chair. Discharge often requires the provision, and education in the use of, equipment and the implementation of home adaptations (e.g. the provision of rails). Barriers to early discharge include the lack of wheelchair access or downstairs bathroom facilities (for downstairs living) in the home of the patient.

A study compared additional educational sessions for carers of stroke patients just prior to discharge to standard care.[5] These sessions included both factual and practical aspects involving topics such as handling, transfers, continence and communication. The carers attended between three and five sessions of around 40 minutes' duration. They found improved psychosocial scores in both patients and carers after one year within the treatment group, although there was no resultant improvement in mortality, disability scores or institutionalisation rates.

Correct patient positioning is important to prevent contractures, spasticity and pressure ulcers. Shoulder pain (but not subluxation) is common in people who have had a stroke. Prevention involves correct patient positioning, the use of supports and careful handling of hemiplegic limbs by staff.[3]

The initial aims of rehabilitation are usually modest, such as enabling a patient to transfer from bed to chair rather than to walk independently. For those with hemiplegia, one-handed techniques of self-care can be taught in the immediate phase. Once the affected limb has regained sufficient power to overcome gravity it may be incorporated into the performance of functional tasks. The best evidence for a benefit of physiotherapy after a stroke is for task-orientated exercise training, especially if intensive and performed in the early phase.[6] Team members other than the physiotherapist should then encourage the patient to incorporate the techniques into their usual daily routine.[3] An ankle–foot orthosis (AFO) may prevent footdrop hindering attempts at walking.[7] Foot inversion whilst walking can be prevented by a lateral ankle support.

Trials have demonstrated a small benefit of speech and language therapy for the treatment of dysphasia.[4] Patients with expressive dysphasia may be helped by the provision of communication aids. These include simple boards containing pictures or letters to which the patient points. More complex computerised speech-generation devices are also available.

Spasticity

'Spasticity' is a term for inappropriate increases in muscular tone. Not only can this cause reduced function of the affected area but also it may result in contracture formation and pain. Additionally, it may make dressing and personal hygiene more difficult (e.g. adequate cleaning of the palmar skin fold of a hand closed by spasticity). Appropriate joint positioning, movement and exercise, and splints or orthoses can reduce its development. It may be made worse by intercurrent illness, stress/anxiety or medication effects.[8]

Various oral antispasmodic agents have been tried for spasticity. Benzodiazepines have some efficacy but are rarely used due to associated side effects. Baclofen is a gamma-aminobutyric acid (GABA) agonist. It has a short half-life of around four hours. Side effects include sedation, confusion and muscle weakness. Tizanidine appears to be as effective as baclofen but causes less muscle weakness.[8,9] Its mechanism of action is not well understood but probably involves a norepinephrine alpha-2 agonist action within the spinal cord. It may take up to one week to have its maximal effect.[10] Observed side effects include somnolence (62%), dizziness (32%), dry mouth (21%) and hypotension (13%).[11] Abnormalities on liver function tests and occasional hallucinations have been reported.[9]

Non-oral techniques include phenol nerve blocks and botulinium toxin injections. This latter agent blocks the release of acetylcholine at nerve synapses. The toxin is injected directly into the target muscle. The effects last for around three months. It is very expensive and may be associated with a 'flu-like illness immediately after injections. When used in stroke patients to treat wrist and finger spasticity, 62% of the treatment group compared to 27% of the placebo arm reported at least some degree of improvement in severity of disability.[12]

Phenol nerve blocks involve the percutaneous injection of phenol into the target nerve. If a nerve that has mixed motor and sensory components is blocked, an area of dysaesthesia may develop.[8] The duration of effect is variable.

Swallowing

There are four phases described in the process of swallowing.

- *Oral preparation*: chewing and mixing with saliva.
- *Oral phase*: the bolus of food is moved backwards in the mouth by the tongue.
- *Pharyngeal phase*: there is closure of the velopharynx (to block off the nasal cavity) and the larynx (by an upward and anterior movement). There is pharyngeal

peristalsis to aid the transit. The food passes the cricopharyngeal muscle to enter the oesophagus.

- *Oesophageal phase*: transport to the stomach.

A simple bedside evaluation can be obtained by observing a patient swallowing a teaspoon of water and then asking the patient to give a cough or speak whilst listening for the moist sound of fluid in the airways or coughing/choking. More descriptive information can be obtained by the use of a videofluoroscopy test. This uses a swallowed radio-opaque substance under X-ray screening to watch the movement of food matter. In this way, a suitable food consistency for patients may also be identified during the test. The presence of a gag reflex is a poor predictor of swallowing ability. It is also absent in a number of normal individuals and can be unpleasant to elicit. For all of these reasons it has no place in the assessment of swallowing.

Parkinson's disease

Various swallowing problems have been associated with Parkinson's disease (PD). They include abnormal tongue control or festination, delayed swallowing reflex and impaired pharyngeal peristalsis.[13] Aspiration may occur without preceding reports of dysphagia. Swallowing improvements do not closely correlate with other motor benefits observed with levodopa. Techniques may be used that allow mechanical modification of the swallow process.

Stroke

Around 50% of patients have been found to have swallowing abnormalities by clinical testing immediately after admission to hospital because of a stroke, and this figure is around 60% when videofluoroscopy testing is used.[14] Screening for swallowing disorders is recommended in all patients following a stroke, and those with impairments should have specialist input.[3] Patients who have difficulty with swallowing on admission should be initially made nil by mouth and started on intravenous fluids. The use of thickened fluids, puréed/soft foods, and techniques such as using a chin tuck during swallowing can reduce the risk of aspiration in vulnerable patients. Around 90% of stroke survivors will return to a normal diet by six months.[14] The management of those patients who are unable to take sufficient oral nutrition is discussed on p 121.

Mobility aids

A range of mobility aids has been developed. They typically aim to improve a patient's gait pattern by allowing the support of some body weight through the arms rather than the legs. This may protect a painful, weakened or unstable joint. Balance and confidence may also benefit. The choice of which aid is most appropriate is usually based on individual patient preferences, ability and lifestyle, plus environmental factors within their discharge destination. Patients may decline, or never use, aids that they feel stigmatise them as disabled.

Sticks

The use of a walking stick provides a wider, and therefore more stable, base. For this purpose two sticks are better than one. For patients with an antalgic gait (e.g. due to unilateral hip pain) using a single stick there is controversy as to which hand should hold the stick – ipsilateral or contralateral to the painful side. Contralateral usage is less disruptive to the normal gait pattern (the patient tends not to lean over the stick) and provides a wider, more stable, base. But it does not allow as much weight to be transmitted through the stick (and so not through the painful limb) as ipsilateral use.

Sticks with three or four feet (tri- or tetrapods) are also available. These have wider bases, which can increase stability when walking on the flat. The disadvantage is having a larger stick that can be clumsy in narrow spaces such as doorways, plus they are less stable on uneven surfaces and unsuitable for use on stairs.

Crutches

Crutches are usually only for short-term use. They come in three main varieties. Axillary crutches are fitted under the arm. Elbow crutches have retaining cuffs around the forearm. This gives the advantage of making them easier to use on stairs and allows easier door opening by the user. Gutter crutches have supports that allow weight to be transferred through the forearms rather than the hands. They are for use by patients with reduced grip strength.

Frames

Frames have wider bases than either sticks or crutches and so provide the most stable base. The standard 'Zimmer' frame has four feet. The patient lifts the frame forwards and then walks into it. This creates an unnatural stop–start gait pattern. Gutter or pulpit frames provide support for the patient's forearms, which makes them more suitable for those with weakened grips.

An alternative is to have a frame with two wheels replacing the two front feet – a 'rollator' frame. This allows the frame to be pushed forwards over even surfaces, which produces a more natural gait. It also does not have to be lifted, which can help the very frail. Disadvantages include a mild reduction in stability and they tend to be less manoeuvrable in tight spaces.

Three- and four-wheeled frames without feet are suitable for patients requiring less support but requiring help with balance. They promote a more natural, unbroken gait pattern than standard frames. They may come with brakes, shopping baskets and seats (for resting between walking) attached. Larger wheels make it easier to get over outdoor obstacles. They may be foldable to allow easier transport and storage. Such frames may be too bulky for indoor use.

No frames are suitable for use on stairs and patients should not attempt to carry them up and down. Having a frame for upstairs and another for downstairs is an option. The correct height for a frame is such that a patient's elbows are flexed at approximately $15°$ when holding the handgrips at rest.

Wheelchairs

Wheelchairs come in a wide variety according to their planned usage. Factors that need to be considered include indoor, outdoor or mixed use, and self-propelled, pushed or motorised. A folding chair may be necessary for transportation in a car. Chairs with removable armrests allow sideways transfers. Cushioning and support can usually be tailored to the individual patient.

Early discharge teams

In some circumstances, specialised teams (including nurses, physiotherapists and occupational therapists) are able to provide rehabilitation to patients within their own homes. This may have the advantage of freeing up hospital beds and allowing patients to be in a preferred environment. The disadvantage may be a reduced access to therapists – typically three times a week or less, rather than daily. Available evidence suggests that they can improve patients' overall well-being without having a negative impact on functional outcomes.[15]

Day hospital

There is little trial evidence to support the efficacy of day hospital care.[16] An advantage for patients is the ability to see various disciplines in one visit, for example physiotherapy and occupational therapy.

Further reading

Barnes MP and Ward AB. *Textbook of Rehabilitation Medicine*. Oxford: Oxford University Press, 2000.

References

1 Rice-Oxley M. Effectiveness of brain injury rehabilitation. *Clin Rehabil*, 1999; **13** (Suppl. 1): 7–24.
2 Warlow CP. Epidemiology of stroke. *Lancet*, 1998; **352** (Suppl. III): 1–4.
3 Intercollegiate Stroke Working Party. National Clinical Guidelines for Stroke, second ed. (Available at: www.rcplondon.ac.uk/pubs/books/stroke/stroke_guidelines_2ed.pdf)
4 Dobkin BH. Rehabilitation after stroke. *NEJM*, 2005; **352**(16): 1677–1684.
5 Kalra L, Evans A, Perez I *et al.* Training care givers of stroke patients: randomised controlled trial. *BMJ*, 2004; **328**: 1099–1101.
6 Van Peppen RPS, Kwakkel G, Wood-Dauphinee S *et al.* The impact of physical therapy on functional outcomes after stroke: what's the evidence? *Clin Rehabil*, 2004; **18**: 833–862.
7 de Wit DCM, Buurke JH, Nijlant JMM *et al.* The effect of an ankle-foot orthosis on walking ability in chronic stroke patients: a randomized controlled trial. *Clin Rehabil*, 2004; **18**: 550–557.
8 Barnes MP. Management of spasticity. *Age Ageing*, 1998; **27**: 239–245.
9 Wallace JD. Summary of combined clinical analysis of controlled clinical trials with tizanidine. *Neurology*, 1994; **44** (Suppl. 9): S60–69.
10 The United Kingdom Tizanidine Trial Group. A double-blind, placebo-controlled trial of tizanidine in the treatment of spasticity caused by multiple sclerosis. *Neurology*, 1994; **44** (Suppl. 9): S70–78.

11 Gelber DA, Good DC, Dromerick A *et al.* Open-label dose-titration safety and efficacy study of tizanidine hydrochloride in the treatment of spasticity associated with chronic stroke. *Stroke,* 2001; **32**: 1841–1846.

12 Brashear A, Gordon MF, Elovic E *et al.* Intramuscular injection of botulinium toxin for the treatment of wrist and finger spasticity after a stroke. *NEJM,* 2002; **347**(6): 395–400.

13 Bushmann M, Dobmeyer SM, Leeker L *et al.* Swallowing abnormalities and their responses to treatment in Parkinson's disease. *Neurology,* 1989; **39**: 1309–1314.

14 Mann G, Dip PG, Hankey GJ *et al.* Swallowing function after stroke: prognosis and prognostic factors at 6 months. *Stroke,* 1999; **30**(4): 744–748.

15 Cunliffe AL, Gladman JRF, Husbands SL *et al.* Sooner and healthier: a randomised controlled trial and interview study of an early discharge rehabilitation service for older people. *Age Ageing,* 2004; **33**(3): 246–252.

16 Black DA. The geriatric day hospital. *Age Ageing,* 2005; **34**: 427–429.

Chapter 16

Skin ulceration

Pressure ulcers

Pressure ulcers (PU) are also known as 'pressure sores', 'bedsores' or 'decubitus ulcers'. They develop in areas where pressure on the skin overlying a bony prominence restricts capillary blood flow, resulting in tissue hypoxia then necrosis and breakdown. Classic sites are over the sacrum, ischial tuberosities and heels (*see* Figure 16.1). This process is worsened by a reduction in the natural padding provided by subcutaneous fat associated with poor nutrition and other factors such as moisture levels, shear forces and superimposed infections. They are also more commonly seen in patients who have delirium.[1]

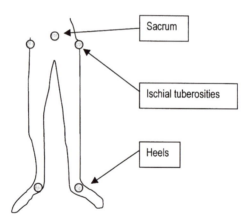

Sacrum

Ischial tuberosities

Heels

Figure 16.1   Common sites of pressure ulcers.

The pathogenesis has been subdivided into four stages but progression of the lesions does not always follow this linear pattern.[2] It is outlined below.

- Stage 1: Superficial skin changes (e.g. erythema, bogginess, increased tempera-ture).
- Stage 2: Shallow ulcer due to loss of epidermis and/or dermis.
- Stage 3: Full thickness skin loss with necrosis of subcutaneous fat.
- Stage 4: Involvement of bone, tendon or muscle.

Assessment

The site and stage of pressure damage should be recorded for all patients entering a geriatric unit. Assessment and monitoring of progression may be aided by the use of photographs. Swabs taken from wounds will always identify bacterial growth – often multiple organisms. This is probably only clinically significant when there is evidence of infection such as surrounding erythema, the characteristic odour of anaerobic organisms (usually *Bacteroides* species) or suspected osteomyelitis. Bone beneath deep ulcers is at risk of osteomyelitis. Changes seen on X-rays or bone scanning can help this diagnosis but bone culture is preferable.[3] This is best achieved during surgery but is sometimes possible via wound aspiration. An elevated white cell count (WCC) and inflammatory markers (e.g. erythrocyte sedimentation rate (ESR) or C-reactive protein (CRP)) may accompany infection. Newer techniques of labelled leucocyte scanning and magnetic resonance imaging (MRI) may aid the diagnosis of osteomyelitis.[4]

Prevention

Screening tools

Various screening tools have been developed to identify those patients most at risk and thus try to target intervention strategies. Among those commonly used are the Waterlow[5] and Braden[6] scores. In the Waterlow scale a score of 15 or more indicates high risk of decubitus ulcer development, in the Braden scale a score of 18 or less signifies increased risk. However, a recent study has questioned their actual predictive value.[7] It seems that, to date, an ideal tool has not been developed and, in addition, clinical judgement is still required to identify those at risk.

Patient turning

The more frequently the patient is turned the better. Ulcer formation has been known to occur after time intervals as short as two hours. A more practical target on general wards is more likely to be four-hourly turning. This should begin from the time of admission.

Pressure-relieving devices

Mattresses are subdivided into static and dynamic designs. Static devices are simply air-filled or made of foam. Dynamic devices are filled with air at alternating pressures. Specialised foam mattresses have been found to be superior to standard hospital mattresses in the prevention of PU.[8] In a study comparing the use of a foam mattress and a four-hourly turning regimen to an alternating pressure air mattress without turning in patients at high risk of PU, no difference in the incidence of ulceration was noted (15.6% vs 15.3%; $n = 447$; median age 82 years).[9] In an intensive therapy unit (ITU) setting, air-filled beds have been shown to be superior to standard ITU beds in reducing PU incidence.[10]

Treatment

Analgesia

PU can be associated with significant pain. When it occurs, analgesia is an important part of therapy.

Dressings

Non-gauze dressings are preferred, as they require less frequent changes (usually every three to four days) and are associated with mildly improved healing rates.[11] A wide range of dressings is available with differing clinical indications.[12] Vacuum-assisted dressings have also been developed. These create a negative pressure gradient across a suitably sized piece of polyurethane foam fitted into the wound cavity. It is felt that this may reduce wound healing times by the more effective reduction of wound exudates, surrounding oedema and bacterial colonisation.[13]

Nutrition

Logic suggests that measures to correct malnutrition should aid PU healing. To date, there is no evidence from clinical trials of a benefit from replacing vitamins or minerals to treat PU in the absence of a known deficiency.[14]

Larval therapy

Larval therapy is an old technique of debridement that has been reintroduced recently. Sterile fly maggots are now commercially available. The larvae are placed onto the wound and covered in a dressing. Their use has been evaluated in both PU and leg ulcers with high rates (88%) of complete debridement.[15] In an unrandomised, retrospective study, the use of larvae for chronic pressure ulcers was associated with more rapid healing than conventional therapy.[16] The main side effect noted was pain (4–24%). Potential barriers include psychological and aesthetic aspects. Randomised controlled trials are required to confirm these findings.

Surgery

Surgical intervention is usually only recommended for grade 3 or 4 ulcers in patients suitable to undergo an operation. Debridement is believed to improve wound healing by removing the necrotic tissue that has harmful effects on the wound. It has the added benefits of potentially unmasking underlying abscesses and allowing samples to be taken for culture, for example bone to diagnose osteomyelitis. Skin repair techniques include direct closure, skin grafts and the use of skin flaps.[3] They are associated with high recurrence and adverse-event rates in elderly, immobile patients and, therefore, appropriate patient selection is important.

Leg ulcers

Although leg ulcers are multi-factorial in their origin, they often are associated with reduced mobility and may even be caused by pressure ulceration, hence their inclusion within this section. They are estimated to have a prevalence of 1–2% in the over 65s.[17] The vast majority are caused by venous insufficiency, arterial, diabetic and mixed aetiologies.

Venous insufficiency

In around 70% of people with leg ulcers the mechanism includes increased venous blood pressure caused by incompetent venous valves, inadequate blood pumping due to reduced mobility, or occluded veins following venous thrombosis.[18] Venous incompetence may affect up to 10% of the population.[19] Venous ulcers are most commonly found around the malleoli. Clinical examination may reveal signs of venous insufficiency: oedema and trophic skin changes (e.g. lipodermatosclerosis and hyperpigmentation). Lipodermatosclerosis is caused by fibrotic changes in the dermis and subcutaneous tissues and results in toughening of the skin that can lead to an 'inverted champagne bottle' appearance.[19] The hyperpigmentation is due to the leakage and subsequent breakdown of blood cells. This may stimulate melanin deposition causing a brown colouration.[19] Treatment usually involves compression bandaging. As there is a risk of an arterial component, an ankle–brachial pressure index (ABPI) should be performed prior to bandaging. This test compares the standard blood pressure (BP) measured at the arm to the pressure at the ankle. The lower the figure, the more likely that arterial insufficiency is a factor. A value of 0.8 or above should be obtained if compression bandaging is to be applied.

Treatment

Pressure bandaging has been shown to increase healing rates compared to no compression in clinical trials.[20] The amount of pressure that should be exerted by the treating bandages has been an area of uncertainty. A trial comparing elasticated (higher pressure) with unelasticated (lower pressure) bandages in 112 people with venous leg ulcers failed to demonstrate any significant difference in efficacy or adverse events.[18] Approximately 60% of ulcers had healed at six months in both groups. Large ulcers heal more slowly than small ones.

Simple measures to treat ulceration and prevent recurrence include leg elevation, improved mobility and nutrition, and reductions in obesity.[21] Antibiotics are necessary only when the lesions become infected. Likely organisms are *Staphylococcus aureus, Pseudomonas aeruginosa* and beta-haemolytic streptococci.[19] Surgical debridement may be appropriate in certain circumstances. This is most often undertaken when there are signs of infection.[22] Removal of the dead tissue is thought to increase the chance of wound granulation and reduce infection risk. Removed tissues can be sent for culture. For large ulcers that fail to heal, skin grafting has been tried. There is some evidence that, in combination with compression bandaging, this can improve healing rates.[23]

Arterial ulcers

Large vessel ischaemia is associated with signs of arterial insufficiency, i.e. pallor, reduced temperature, prolonged capillary refill time and absent pulses. These signs may be absent if small vessel disease is the cause of the ulceration. Assessment should include identifying vascular risk factors. An ABPI should be performed; it is usually below 0.5 in cases of arterial insufficiency. Vascular surgery may be indicated to restore adequate blood flow. Secondary vascular prevention medication should be commenced (e.g. antiplatelets and statins). Smoking-cessation and diabetic control may also be appropriate.

Diabetic ulcers

Peripheral neuropathy and arterial insufficiency may be present alone or in combination in diabetic foot ulcers. Prevention is aided by careful footwear selection, tight glucose control and revascularisation where appropriate. Surgical debridement and eradication of infection, including osteomyelitis, are necessary once an ulcer has developed.

Other aetiologies

Pressure ulcers may develop on the leg, especially over the heel. Less common causes of ulceration include vasculitis and malignancy. Vasculitis may initially present as an area of cutaneous purpura. It is associated with unexplained raised inflammatory markers, black necrosis and irregular borders to the ulcers. Malignancies causing ulceration are most likely to be squamous cell or basal cell carcinomas. They usually occur on sun-exposed skin areas. Rarely, other skin conditions can present as ulcers in the elderly, for example pyoderma gangrenosum associated with inflammatory bowel disease.

Further reading

Mekkes JR, Loots MAM, Van der Wal AC *et al.* Causes, investigation and treatment of leg ulceration. *Br J Derm*, 2003; **148**: 388–401.

References

1 American Psychiatric Association. Practice guideline for the treatment of patients with delirium. *Am J Psychiatry*, 1999; **156**(5 Suppl.): 1–20.
2 Parish LC and Witkowski JA. Controversies about the decubitus ulcer. *Dermatol Clin*, 2004; **22**: 87–91.
3 Sorensen JL, Jorgensen B and Gottrup F. Surgical treatment of pressure ulcers. *Am J Surg*, 2004; **188** (Suppl.1A): 42–51.
4 Mekkes JR, Loots MAM, Van der Wal AC *et al.* Causes, investigation and treatment of leg ulceration. *Br J Derm*, 2003; **148**: 388–401.
5 Waterlow J. A risk assessment card. *Nurs Times*, 1985; **81**(48): 49–55.
6 Braden BJ and Bergstrom N. Predictive validity of the Braden scale for pressure sore risk in a nursing home population. *Res Nurs Health*, 1994; **17**: 459–470.
7 Schoonhoven L, Haalboom JRE, Bousema MT *et al.* Prospective cohort study of routine use of risk assessment scales for prediction of pressure ulcers. *BMJ*, 2002; **325**: 797–800.
8 Cullum N, McInnes E, Bell-Syer SEM *et al.* Support surfaces for pressure ulcer prevention. Cochrane Database Syst Rev 2004, Issue 3. Art. No.: CD001735. DOI: 10.1002/14651858. CD001735.pub2.
9 Vanderwee K, Grypdonck MHF and Defloor T. Effectiveness of an alternating pressure air mattress for the prevention of pressure ulcers. *Age Ageing*, 2005; **34**: 261–267.
10 Inman KJ, Sibbald WJ, Rutledge FS *et al.* Clinical utility and cost-effectiveness of an air suspension bed in the prevent of pressure ulcers. *JAMA*, 1993; **269**(9): 1139–1143.
11 Xakellis GC and Chrischilles EA. Hydrocolloid versus saline-gauze dressings in treating pressure ulcers: a cost-effectiveness analysis. *Arch Phys Med Rehabil*, 1992; **73**: 463–469.
12 Lyder CH. Pressure ulcer prevention and management. *JAMA*, 2003; **289**(2): 223–226.
13 Baxter H and Ballard K. Vacuum-assisted closure. *Nursing Times*, 2001; **97**(35): 51–52.

14 Langer G, Schloemer G, Knerr A *et al.* Nutritional interventions for preventing and treating pressure ulcers. Cochrane Database Syst Rev 2003, Issue 4. Art. No.: CD003216. DOI: 10.1002/14651858.CD003216.

15 Mumcuoglu KY, Ingber A, Gilead L *et al.* Maggot therapy for the treatment of intractable wounds. *Int J Derm*, 1999; **38**(8): 623–627.

16 Sherman RA. Maggot versus conservative therapy for the treatment of pressure ulcers. *Wound Rep Regen*, 2002; **10**(4): 208–214.

17 Callam MJ, Ruckley CV, Harper DR *et al.* Chronic ulceration of the leg: extent of the problem and provision of care. *BMJ*, 1985; **290**: 1855–1856.

18 Meyer FJ, Burnand KG, Lagattolla NRF *et al.* Randomized clinical trial comparing the efficacy of two bandaging regimens in the treatment of venous leg ulcers. *Br J Surg*, 2002; **89**: 40–44.

19 Grey JE, Enoch S and Harding KG. Venous and arterial leg ulcers. *BMJ*, 2006; **332**: 347–350.

20 Cullum N, Nelson EA, Fletcher AW *et al.* Compression for venous leg ulcers. Cochrane Database Syst Rev 2001, Issue 2. Art. No.: CD000265. DOI: 10.1002/14651858.CD000265.

21 Simon DA, Dix FP, McCollum CN. Management of venous leg ulcers. *BMJ,* 2004; **328**: 1358–1362.

22 Brem H, Kirsner RS and Falanga V. Protocol for the successful treatment of venous ulcers. *Am J Surg*, 2004; **188** (Suppl.): 1S–8S.

23 Jones JE and Nelson EA. Skin grafting for venous leg ulcers. Cochrane Database Syst Rev 2000, Issue 2. Art. No.: CD001737. DOI: 10.1002/14651858.CD001737.pub2.

Therapeutics

Chapter 17

Therapeutics

Medical research does not always answer physicians' dilemmas. Subgroups of patients, such as the elderly, are often not adequately represented in trials to be sure that results are also applicable to them. Trials may even specifically exclude this age group,[1] so evidence-based medicine may not support some common prescribing practices in the elderly. The other side to this is that by not prescribing certain treatments, elderly people may be unfairly denied therapies that work at least as well within their age group. There is evidence to suggest that many older people are not on treatments that are of proven benefit, such as aspirin for ischaemic heart disease and angiotensin-converting enzyme (ACE) inhibitors in heart failure.[2] Therefore, the geriatrician has to tread a careful path between the potential negative effects of both polypharmacy and unreasonable under-treatment.

There is a further difficulty that confronts all physicians. The design and reporting of many drug trials is influenced by the drug company that will benefit from subsequent marketing. The potential conflict of interest is quite obvious. Perhaps more disturbingly, a number of authors of clinical guidelines are in receipt of grants from, or hold shares, in pharmaceutical companies.[3]

Inappropriate medication use

A number of medications have been adjudged to be inappropriate for use in the majority of older people due to inefficacy, unacceptable side effects or the availability of more suitable alternatives. An example is the use of sedative hypnotics, which appear to be associated with a small increase in sleep duration (mean 25 minutes) with a number needed to treat (NNT) of 13, but have many adverse effects (e.g. cognitive impairment and falls) with a number needed to harm of just six.[4]

Benzodiazepines have few indications for use in the elderly, yet they are the most commonly prescribed of the psychotropic drugs in these people. A study found that 30% of the over 85s are on such agents.[5] They are associated with an increased risk of falls (see p 185), cognitive impairment[4] and fracture-related mortality.[5] If their use is absolutely necessary then drugs with shorter half-lives and lower lipid solubility are probably safer (e.g. lorazepam or oxazepam).[6] Other drugs often deemed inappropriate include those with anticholinergic properties.[6,7] These are discussed further on p 148 and in Tables 2.1 and 3.2. Non-steroidal anti-inflammatory drugs (NSAIDs) are also associated with high rates of side effects in the elderly and are usually best avoided.[6]

Despite these recommendations, there is evidence that elderly people are commonly prescribed such agents. One study found that 24% of people of 65 years or older were on at least one drug that was deemed unsuitable according to expert guidelines and 20% of these people were on two or more.[8] This appears to be worse among nursing home residents, where 40% have been found to be on inappropriate drugs.[9] This value represented 7% of all prescriptions in this group. In the UK around 25% of nursing home residents are on antipsychotic medications, and around 85% of these prescriptions are inappropriate according to expert guidelines.[10,11] Many of these people are on higher than recommended doses or even multiple agents.

Pharmacokinetics

Generally speaking, elderly patients absorb medications similarly to younger individuals. The main differences in the pharmacokinetics occur with drug distribution and elimination. The concentration of albumin in the blood does not change significantly with ageing in the absence of severe illness. Therefore, protein binding is not usually altered. But the body composition does change as people age. Older individuals have a higher proportion of body fat compared to water than the young. Body fat changes from 18% to 36% in men and from 33% to 45% in women, as they grow old.[12] At the same time body water reduces by 10% to 15%.[12] This affects the volume of distribution (Vd) of drugs. It is increased for lipophilic drugs and reduced for hydrophilic ones. As the half-life of a drug is proportional to its Vd divided by clearance, a larger Vd can increase a drug's half-life. Examples of drugs with longer half-lives in the elderly for this reason include benzodiazepines and barbiturates.[6] Similarly, a reduced clearance may have an additional effect.

The two main mechanisms of drug elimination are metabolism in the liver and excretion via the kidneys. Both of these are impaired in older age. The reduced hepatic metabolic capacity may be related to several processes, including reduced blood flow or enzyme activity. However, an age-related reduction in liver mass appears to be the most important factor.[13] The liver mass has been found to reduce by 20–50% by the time people reach 80 years of age.[12]

The glomerular filtration rate (GFR) also progressively declines with advancing age. This factor is taken into account in calculations to estimate GFR such as the Cockcroft–Gault formula:[14]

$$\frac{(140 - \text{age})(\text{body weight in kg}) \text{ (multiply by 0.85 for females)}}{72 \text{ (serum creatinine (mg/dl))}}$$

This is associated with a reduced renal mass and blood flow with advancing age.[12] Digoxin is an example of a drug with a reduced renal clearance and increased risk of toxicity in the elderly.[6]

Additionally, there may be changes in the sensitivity of target organs to certain concentrations of drugs compared to younger counterparts (pharmacodynamics). This causes either increased or decreased drug efficacies at similar plasma concentrations compared to younger people. One example is the apparent increased sensitivity of older people to psychoactive medications.[12]

So, the elderly are prone to variation in drug peak concentrations and half-lives. Altering the size of drug doses or their frequency can compensate for this.

Adverse drug reactions

Adverse drug reactions may account for around 12% of admissions to hospital in the over-70s.[15] These may be unrelated to drug doses (idiosyncratic) but most are dose-dependent. For this reason it is generally preferable to use the lowest possible effective dose of a drug. Some adverse reactions may develop after a prolonged exposure, for example tardive dyskinesia with neuroleptic agents (*see* p 81). Therefore medications should be reviewed and withdrawn, when possible, at periodic intervals.

Adverse drug reactions appear to occur commonly in the elderly,[12] especially among those in nursing homes.[16] This probably reflects the fact that elderly people are on many different agents simultaneously. Studies have found that the use of three or more medications significantly increases the chance of an adverse reaction.[15,17] Of the adverse events that are potentially preventable, more than half are related to the use of psychoactive medications, with antipsychotics being the most common offenders.[16]

Polypharmacy

Polypharmacy is a term used to describe a large number of medications given to a patient. Precise definitions vary but it is often taken as being on four or more regular medications. As people age they accumulate diagnoses and, consequently, medications. Many conditions require two or more agents to control them, for example osteoporosis, heart failure, hypertension and ischaemic heart disease. A study found that a sample of people over the age of 72 (mean age 81 years) were on a mean number of 2.2 medications (range 0–15).[18] In a random sample of community-dwelling people over the age of 65, 19% of men and 23% of women regularly took five or more prescription drugs.[19] When a group of nursing home residents (mean age 84 years) was assessed, they were receiving an average number of 4.8 regular medications each.[20] A sample of people aged 65 years or over who resided in residential care or assisted living settings averaged 5.8 regular medications per person.[7]

Polypharmacy may become exacerbated by the addition of more drugs to treat adverse effects of current agents, for example the addition of a diuretic agent to reduce the leg oedema caused by a calcium channel-blocker. This process is what is called the 'prescribing cascade'.[21] To try and prevent this cycle, new symptoms should always be evaluated as possible drug adverse effects.

It is not uncommon to find the co-prescription of agents that have directly opposing mechanisms of action, for example beta-blockers and salbutamol or furosemide and fludrocortisone. Also, a recent trend of prescribing anticholinergic agents with cholinesterase inhibitors appears to have developed. This may be true for as many as 35% of those on cholinesterase inhibitors.[22] This may sometimes be caused by the commencement of anticholinergic agents to treat urinary incontinence precipitated by the cholinesterase inhibitors.[23]

The use of multiple agents increases the risks of side effects and interactions; also, patients' adherence to their medication regimen reduces as the number of drugs increases. A regular review of medications and their ongoing justification and safety should be undertaken whenever possible. Agents without clear benefit should be withdrawn. This often occurs at the time of hospital admission, when the results of medication adjustments can be closely monitored.

Medication concordance

The old term 'compliance' is being replaced by the term 'concordance' to describe a patient's adherence to prescribed therapies. This is based on the philosophy that doctors and patients are entering into an alliance and good communication between these parties is essential to its proper functioning. The patient should not merely comply with instructions but should agree with the reasoning and be a willing participant in any treatment. An alternative term is 'medication adherence'.

Estimates of concordance rates depend on what definition is applied. The value falls among patients who are being treated for illnesses of long compared to short duration and figures between 40% and 80% have been found in clinical trials of chronic conditions.[24] There is also a reduction with increasing medication regimen complexity. Patients on once-daily medications will take them around 80% of the time, whereas those on four times daily dosing will take only 50% of their medication.[24] Other factors that have been associated with reduced concordance include the presence of psychiatric disorders (e.g. depression and dementia), medications for conditions that cause no symptoms (e.g. hypertension) and the side effects of drugs.[24]

The identification of patients who are not taking their medications is not always easy. Sometimes drug levels (e.g. phenytoin), physiological parameters (e.g. blood pressure) or pill counts provide a clue. Usually patient self-reporting is relied upon. It is important not to be confrontational when enquiring about concordance, as this will tend to cause patients to over-report their taking of medications. Accepting that all patients will lapse from time to time, questions should focus on how often this occurs.

Patient education on the value of their various drugs may improve the situation but is unlikely to solve the problem altogether. A logical first step is to try to reduce the number of medications and limit the number of times they are to be taken each day. For example, a once-daily formulation could be used in place of one taken twice daily. Medication aids, as discussed below, may be beneficial in selected patients.

Medication aids

Various devices and methods of drug packaging have been designed to try and improve the concordance of elderly patients with their medications. They include multi-compartment and blister packs. They usually have individual slots for tablets to be taken in the morning, lunch, afternoon, and night time and span over a one-week period. Accepted wisdom is that they are of benefit; however, this is not evidence-based. Trials that have utilised them have not shown clear benefits in improved medication concordance.[25] That said, large-sized trials assessing their use in the frail elderly have not been performed. They are often started without adequate patient assessment and as many as half of these patients may do as well without them.[26] They may disassociate the patient from their medications as they become all mixed together. They are also only suitable for some drugs. Liquids or inhaled medications cannot be dispensed this way. Other medications, such as bisphosphonates or levodopa, may need to be taken at specific times or in specific ways.

References

1 Gurwitz JH. Polypharmacy: a new paradigm for quality drug therapy in the elderly? *Arch Int Med*, 2004; **164**: 1957–1959.

2 Sloane PD, Gruber-Baldini AL, Zimmerman S *et al.* Medication undertreatment in assisted living settings. *Arch Int Med*, 2004; **164**: 2031–2037.

3 Taylor R and Giles J. Cash interests taint drug advice. *Nature*, 2005; **437**: 1070–1071.

4 Glass J, Lanctot KL, Herrmann N *et al.* Sedative hypnotics in older people with insomnia: meta-analysis of risks and benefits. *BMJ*, 2005; **331**: 1169–1173.

5 Vinkers DJ, Gussekloo J, van der Mast RC *et al.* Benzodiazepine use and risk of mortality in individuals aged 85 years or over. *JAMA*, 2003; **290**(22): 2942–2943.

6 Chutka DS, Takahashi PY and Hoel RW. Inappropriate medications for elderly patients. *Mayo Clin Proc*, 2004; **79**: 122–139.

7 Sloane PD, Zimmerman S, Brown LC *et al.* Inappropriate medication prescribing in residential care/assisted living facilities. *JAGS*, 2002; **50**: 1001–1011.

8 Wilcox SM, Himmelstein DU and Woolhandler S. Inappropriate drug prescribing for the community-dwelling elderly. *JAMA*, 1994; **272**(4): 292–296.

9 Beers MH, Ouslander JG, Fingold SF *et al.* Inappropriate medication prescribing in skilled-nursing facilities. *Ann Int Med*, 1992; **117**(8): 684–689.

10 McGrath AM and Jackson GA. Survey of neuroleptic prescribing in residents of nursing homes in Glasgow. *BMJ*, 1996; **312**: 611–612.

11 Oborne CA, Hooper R, Chi Li K *et al.* An indicator of appropriate neuroleptic prescribing in nursing homes. *Age Ageing*, 2002; **31**: 435–439.

12 Vestal RE. Aging and pharmacology. *Cancer*, 1997; **80**: 1302–1310.

13 Wynne HA, Cope LH, James OFW *et al.* The effect of age and frailty upon acetanilide clearance in man. *Age Ageing*, 1989; **18**: 415–418.

14 Friedman JR, Norman DC and Yoshikawa TT. Correlation of estimated renal function parameters versus 24-hour creatinine clearance in ambulatory elderly. *JAGS*, 1989; **37**: 145–149.

15 Mannesse CK, Derkx FHM, de Ridder MAJ *et al.* Contribution of adverse drug reactions to hospital admission of older patients. *Age Ageing*, 2000; **29**: 35–39.

16 Gurwitz JH, Field TS, Avorn J *et al.* Incidence and preventability of adverse drug events in nursing homes. *Am J Med*, 2000; **109**: 87–94.

17 von Renteln-Kruse W, Thiesemann N, Thiesemann R *et al.* Does frailty predispose to adverse drug reactions in older patients? *Age Ageing*, 2000; **29**: 461–462.

18 Agostini JV, Han L and Tinetti ME. The relationships between number of medications and weight loss or impaired balance in older adults. *JAGS*, 2004; **52**(10): 1719–1723.

19 Kaufman DW, Kelly JP, Rosenberg L *et al.* Recent patterns of medication use in the ambulatory adult population of the United States: the Sloane Survey. *JAMA*, 2002; **287**(3): 337–344.

20 Roberts MS, King M, Stokes JA *et al.* Medication prescribing and administration in nursing homes. *Age Ageing*, 1998; **27**: 385–392.

21 Rochon PA and Gurwitz JH. Optimising drug treatment for elderly people: the prescribing cascade. *BMJ*, 1997; **315**: 1096–1099.

22 Carnaham RM, Lund BC, Perry PJ *et al.* The concurrent use of anticholinergics and cholinesterase inhibitors: rare event or common practice? *JAGS*, 2004; **52**: 2082–2087.

23 Gill SS, Mamdani M, Naglie G *et al.* A prescribing cascade involving cholinesterase inhibitors and anticholinergic drugs. *Arch Int Med*, 2005; **165**: 808–813.

24 Osterberg L and Blaschkle T. Adherence to medication. *NEJM*, 2005; **353**(5): 487–497.

25 Huang H, Maguire MG, Miller ER *et al.* Impact of pill organizers and blister packs on adherence to pill taking in two vitamin supplementation trials. *Am J Epidemiol*, 2000; **152**: 780–787.

26 Raynor DK and Nunney JM. Medicine compliance aids are a partial solution, not panacea. *BMJ*, 2002; **324**: 1338.

End of life

Chapter 18

Palliative care

Palliative care is the treatment of advanced, incurable disease. This includes planning for death and may extend to bereavement support. Its main aims are excellent symptom control coupled with excellent communication with patients and their carers to maximise quality of life. Its purpose is neither to shorten life, nor to prolong the dying process. A thorough review of all aspects of the specialty is beyond the scope of this book. Here a brief review of the management of some of the specific problems of palliative care is presented. For those in search of further information, a useful, free online resource is available at: www.helpthehospices. org.uk/elearning/index.htm.

Traditionally the focus for this specialty has been on cancer care, but more recently this has extended into other conditions, such as heart failure and Parkinson's disease. There are many similarities with standard geriatric management, including the involvement of team members from different disciplines, the implementation of goal setting and the use of intermediary care facilities (day centre, respite and rehabilitation units). Currently, around two-thirds of deaths in the UK occur within standard hospitals[1] and the majority of these are geriatric patients. The care of dying patients should be inherent to our practice. Palliative care services augment this role by providing expert assistance with difficult symptom control and additional resources, such as community teams, enabling patients to die at home.

Many barriers to effective management of dying patients within hospitals exist. These include the fundamental hospital culture of investigating until a definitive diagnosis has been made, and persevering with interventions even when they are likely to be futile.[1] In the past, healthcare professionals, often in conjunction with families' wishes, have avoided revealing the true facts during discussions with the terminally ill. However, studies suggest that openness and honesty are the best strategies in the longer term.[2] It is, of course, unethical to withhold or give dishonest information to patients when asked.

A 'good' death

Recognising that a patient is dying and communicating this to them and their relatives is a key step towards achieving optimal care.[1] Doing this allows appropriate planning to be made – both medical and social. Following this, several processes should take place. These include the discontinuation of unnecessary medications (e.g. statins for long-term cardiovascular risk reduction) and investigations (e.g. blood tests and vital signs). A plan of care that respects religious and spiritual needs can also be formulated in conjunction with the patient and their relatives. Issues regarding nutrition or hydration and resuscitation can be discussed (*see* later). Good mouth care is an important component, and can also be a process in which family members can be involved. All of this should occur in conjunction with optimal symptom control.

Pain

'Pain' is a broad term for an unpleasant sensation that may have many different causations and mechanisms. The various subgroups respond to differing degrees to treatment modalities, for example bone pain, neuropathic pain and the pain of muscular spasm do not always improve with opiate therapy. A patient may have many different pains with different causes, and a careful history to elucidate all of the components is required. Emotional factors such as anger, depression or anxiety may also be involved.[3] Dying in pain is a significant fear for many patients. Yet it has commonly been found that relatives judge their loved one to be in discomfort in their final days of life despite palliative care input.[4]

Regular medication to prevent pain is far superior to allowing a patient to suffer pain prior to receiving 'as required' medication. 'Breakthrough' analgesia is additional medication that is given on top of the background analgesia at times when pain intensity increases. A common method of dose titration is to start with a low dose of four-hourly short-acting agents (such as morphine liquid) plus breakthrough doses.[3] After a period on this regimen, the total medication used can be converted to an equivalent dose of a regular longer-acting drug plus breakthrough short-acting doses. The assessment of symptoms is then repeated and doses titrated until pain control is achieved.

Analgesic agents are often used in combination. They are increased in a step-wise fashion as outlined in the World Health Organization (WHO) analgesic ladder (*see* Figure 18.1) until pain control is achieved.[5] Adjuvant agents may be used in some circumstances. These include steroids for raised intracranial pressure and nerve compression, bisphosphonates for bone pain and antidepressants or anticonvulsants for neuropathic pain (*see below*).[3]

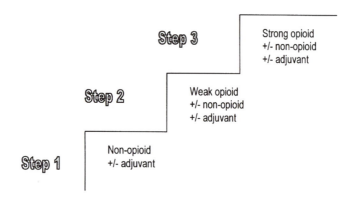

Figure 18.1 The World Health Organization (WHO) analgesic ladder: reach the maximum dose of each agent before moving to the next step.

Opiates act at receptors at the terminal end of pain fibres within the dorsal columns of the spinal cord. The medium strengthen opiate agent tramadol also has non-opiate, mainly serotinergically mediated, properties. Non-steroidal anti-inflammatory drugs (NSAIDs) act by preventing the formation of prostaglandins at sites of inflammation. The mechanism of action of paracetamol is poorly understood.

Opiates

Standard-release morphine is usually started at low doses (2.5 mg to 5 mg) given four-hourly and 'breakthrough' doses are also given as required. According to the requirements for additional medication, the regular doses can be adjusted. Once a stable dose has been reached, it can be converted to the equivalent amount as a slow-release formulation (e.g. MST).

There is no pharmacological logic in combining weak and strong opioid agents. Side effects include sedation, nausea/vomiting and constipation. The nausea and vomiting may settle after several days of therapy, but anti-emetics may be initially required. There is some evidence that different opiates may cause differing degrees of constipation. In a non-randomised study, transdermal fentanyl use was associated with lesser requirement for aperients than oral morphine.[6] When constipation is opiate-induced, there is some evidence from studies in younger people that orally taken inhibitors of opiate receptors (e.g. naloxone) that have poor systemic absorption may be beneficial without significantly affecting pain control.[7,8] Tolerance and addiction are not seen in the context of acute pain. Toxicity can cause delirium and myoclonic jerks.[3] Warning signs of toxicity include pinpoint pupils and oversedation.[9] The risk is increased in those with renal impairment and smaller, less frequent doses are usually required in such patients.

Subcutaneous administration is suitable for patients unable to take oral morphine. Diamorphine has the advantage of being extremely soluble in a small volume of liquid and is therefore ideal for use with a subcutaneous infusion pump. The required dose is estimated by dividing the total daily morphine dose by three.[9] Four-hourly breakthrough doses should also be prescribed.

Transdermal fentanyl is an alternative for those unable to take oral medication. The patches are changed very 72 hours. The disadvantage of this approach is that it takes up to 24 hours to reach a steady plasma drug level.[9] The available doses of the patches are also limited, making titration more difficult.

Neuropathic pain

Neuropathic pain is caused by damage to nerves causing abnormal function. Figure 18.2 outlines the key differences between nocioceptive and this type of pain. It may be attributed to a wide range of aetiologies and may be either peripheral (e.g. trigeminal neuralgia) or central (e.g. post-stroke pain). The pain may be provoked by a stimulus or may occur spontaneously. Stimuli causing pain may be normally non-noxious (allodynia) or may be an exaggerated response to a mildly noxious stimulus (hyperalgesia). The history may elucidate the particular characteristics of neuropathic pain, which is often described by terms such as 'burning', 'shooting' and 'tingling'. The underlying cause may be identified (e.g. history of diabetes or shingles). The distribution of pain will guide towards the causative structures. Examination may reveal a region of altered sensation (either increased or reduced) in the region of the pain. Other neurological signs may suggest the underlying mechanism (e.g. stroke or Parkinson's disease).

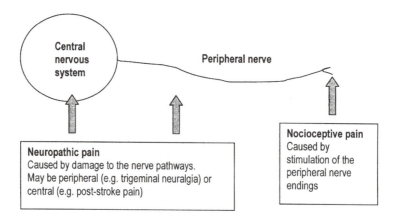

Figure 18.2 Sites of causation of nociceptive and neuropathic pain.

Treatment

Control of the symptoms of neuropathic pain can be difficult and may take some time to achieve. An adequate trial of therapy will take at least two weeks once a therapeutic dose is attained. Pharmacological management must be linked with patient education and reassurance. Non-pharmacological strategies may also play a role. Given the diverse nature of neuropathic pain and the multiple possible treatment combinations, the best management strategy for all situations is not well established. What works well in one patient may be ineffective in another. The approaches most likely to be beneficial are listed in Table 18.1.

Table 18.1 Techniques for controlling neuropathic pain

Method	Comments
Tricyclic antidepressants (TCA)	Usually as a low dose given at night (*see* p 51)
Anticonvulsants (e.g. gabapentin and carbamazepine)	Action probably due to glutamate inhibition within the central nervous system (CNS)
Lidocaine gel or patches	May have a role in peripherally caused pains
Opiates	Not usually very effective alone for this type of pain; may be used in combination with other agents
Tramadol	Has some additional serotinergic-type action similar to TCA
Ketamine	Originally an anaesthetic agent. *N*-methyl-D-aspartate (NMDA) blocking action; used in low doses for pain control, under specialist supervision
Spinal analgesia	For severe pains unresponsive to less invasive measures; patients may be able to be managed in the community with spinal catheters connected to syringe-driver infusions for periods of several months
Nerve blocks	When a single causative, peripheral nerve can be identified
Transcutaneous electrical nerve stimulation (TENS)	Not effective in all patients, but non-invasive and with few side effects

More than one modality may be needed to control symptoms. It may be reasonable to start with either a tricyclic antidepressant (TCA) or anticonvulsant initially, and proceed to both agents in combination as a second-line strategy. If this fails, the addition of further agents or spinal analgesia may be considered. A recent trial suggested that the combination of gabapentin and morphine might be superior to either agent alone.[10]

The assessment of response to treatment may be helped by using a standard 0–10 scale (0 = no pain, 10 = worst pain ever experienced). Specific scales for the assessment of neuropathic pain have also been developed.[11]

Nausea and vomiting

Nausea and vomiting are common symptoms encountered in palliative care caused by a variety of mechanisms. Components of the vomiting pathway and the most important associated receptors are shown in Figure 18.3. Anti-emetic drugs should be targeted towards the most likely receptor group involved in symptom genesis. Listed below are some example drugs with actions at the associated receptor type:

- histamine – cyclizine
- acetlycholine – hyoscine
- serotonin – ondansetron
- dopamine – haloperidol, metoclopramide and domperidone (peripheral action only).

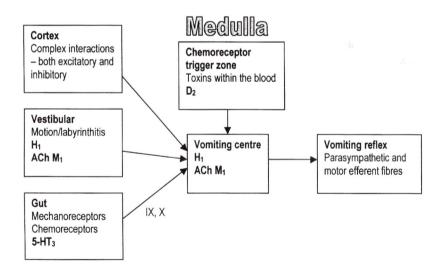

Figure 18.3 Pathways involved in the vomiting reflex. H_1 = histamine type 1 receptor; ACh M_1 = acetylcholine muscarinic receptor type 1; 5-HT_3 = serotonin type 3 receptor; D_2 = dopamine type 2 receptor; IX = glossopharyngeal nerve; X = vagus nerve.

Artificial nutrition and hydration

The terminal stages of illness are often accompanied by a reduced oral intake. This often leads carers to be concerned about associated suffering due to hunger or thirst. When 32 patients (mean age 75 years, most with advanced cancer) in a palliative care setting, who were able to express themselves, were given food only when asked for, 63% experienced no hunger despite only a small oral intake of nutrition.[12] Thirty-four per cent experienced only initial hunger and only one patient had hunger up to the time of death. It, therefore, seems likely that comfort can be achieved in the dying despite minimal oral intake.

The General Medical Council guidance on good practice in withholding and withdrawing treatment (including artificial nutrition and hydration) is available on their website (www.gmc-uk.org/guidance/library/W_&_W.pdf).

Links to ethical information for those outside the UK are contained in Box 1.3.

Death rattle

'Death rattle' is a term coined for the gurgling sounds caused by air passing over secretions within the oropharynx in patients in a terminal phase of their condition. It occurs in around 50% of the dying, with a mean duration of around two days.[13] It is not clear whether this causes patients any distress but it is a source of concern for attending relatives.[4] The best treatment may simply be reassurance for the family members. When it is felt necessary, several therapeutic options are available. Non-pharmacological measures that may help include more upright positioning of the patient and the use of suctioning. Anticholinergic drugs that act at muscarinic receptors have been shown to be effective. These include hyoscine hydrobromide and butylbromide, and glycopyrronium.

Available evidence suggests a similar efficacy for all of these agents. A significant reduction in death rattle is observed in around 80% of treated patients.[13] When these medications are given intravenously (IV) they have a more rapid onset but shorter duration of action than intramuscular (IM) dosing. A 24-hour subcutaneous infusion is probably preferable in most patients. Hyoscine is also available as a transdermal patch. Table 18.2 compares some of the characteristics of these agents.

Table 18.2 Comparison of characteristics of some anticholinergic agents. Doses as listed in the *BNF* No. 52, September 2006

Agent	Single dose duration (hours)	Suitable dose for 24-hour subcutaneous infusion	Heart rate	Confusion
Hyoscine butylbromide	1	20–60 mg	↑	+
Hyoscine hydrobromide	6	0.6–2.4 mg	↓	–
Glycopyrronium	6	0.6–1.2 mg	↓	–

Hyoscine butylbromide is able to cross the blood–brain barrier and may cause confusion. Glycopyrronium and hyoscine hydrobromide may cause bradycardia, whereas hyoscine butylbromide may cause tachycardia. All of these agents may induce urinary retention.

Cardiopulmonary resuscitation

The outcomes of cardiopulmonary resuscitation (CPR) attempts in general are poor.[14] When considering elderly populations, these become even less impressive. An analysis of 503 patients over the age of 70, who had sustained a cardiac arrest, found that only 3.8% survived to discharge.[15] The outcome was worse in the subgroup who sustained an arrest in the community (0.8%) compared to those who arrested in hospital (6.5%). However, two other studies found contrasting results in people aged over 70 years: none of 77 patients who sustained an arrest within a hospital survived,[16] and yet 10% of 140 patients who sustained an arrest in the community did survive to discharge.[17] In comparison to people who arrest in their own home, those who reside in nursing homes have worse outcomes. A study found that 11% of community-dwelling people over the age of 65 survived to discharge compared to only 2% of those from nursing homes.[18] The outcomes of cardiac arrests within a long-term care facility, which had a resident advanced cardiac life support (ACLS) trained team has also been evaluated.[19] Despite an initial 20% response to CPR, none of 57 residents survived to hospital discharge.

The initial rhythm is associated with the probability of a successful outcome. Those in ventricular fibrillation (VF) or ventricular tachycardia (VT) generally do better than those in asystole or pulseless electrical activity (PEA). We may also expect that complications such as fractured ribs and cerebral hypoxic damage may be more pronounced in this age group due to more prevalent comorbidities such as osteoporosis and dementia. In those who do survive resuscitation, a significant number will be left with a neurological impairment that limits function.

The majority of patients, when asked, appear to express an interest in being involved in the decision-making process regarding the receipt of CPR.[20] For CPR to occur it is clear that patients should be informed of the process and likely outcomes as their decisions may be influenced by unrealistic expectations. A large number of patients appear to gain their knowledge of CPR from watching television programmes, where outcomes are generally overly optimistic.[20] Around 70% of older patients rate themselves as having little or no knowledge of the procedure involved.[20] A study found that 41% of 287 elderly patients (mean age 77, range 60–99 years) initially expressed a wish to receive CPR in the event of a cardiac arrest.[21] This figure fell to 22% once the subjects were informed of only a 10–17% estimated chance of survival to discharge after such an event. Of course, it may have been even lower if the 3.8% survival chance figure, as stated above, had been quoted.

In summary, a lot of time in hospitals is spent discussing CPR decisions yet the outcome in elderly people is poor (0–10%). The public is, generally, unaware of this. If patients and relatives are to be involved in such decisions, it is right that they should be informed of the chances of success and the potential harms that it could cause.

Further reading

Twycross R. *Introducing Palliative Care*, 3rd ed. Oxford: Radcliffe Medical Press, 1999.

Watson M, Lucas C, Hoy A *et al. Oxford Handbook of Palliative Care*. Oxford: Oxford University Press, 2005.

Dworkin RH, Backonja M, Rowbotham MC *et al.* Advances in neuropathic pain: diagnosis, mechanisms, and treatment recommendations. *Arch Neurol,* 2003; **60**: 1524–1534.

References

1   Ellershaw J and Ward C. Care of the dying patient: the last hours or days of life. *BMJ,* 2003; **326**: 30–34.
2   Fallowfield LJ, Jenkins VA and Beveridge HA. Truth may hurt but deceit hurts more: communication in palliative care. *Palliative Med*, 2002; **16**: 297–303.
3   O'Neill B and Fallon M. ABC of palliative care: principles of palliative care and pain control. *BMJ*, 1997; **315**: 801–804.
4   Hallenbeck J. Palliative care in the final days of life: "They were expecting it at any time." *JAMA*, 2005; **293**(18): 2265–2271.
5   World Health Organization. *WHO Guidelines: cancer pain relief,* 2nd ed. Geneva: WHO, 1996.
6   Radbruch L, Sabatowski R, Loick G *et al.* Constipation and the use of laxatives: a comparison between transdermal fentanyl and oral morphine. *Palliative Med,* 2000; **14**: 111–119.
7   Yuan C, Foss JF, O'Connor M *et al.* Methylnaltrexone for reversal of constipation due to chronic methadone use: a randomized controlled trial. *JAMA,* 2000; **283**(3): 367–372.
8   Meissner W, Schmidt U, Hartmann M *et al.* Oral naloxone reverses opioid-associated constipation. *Pain,* 2000; **84**: 105–109.
9   Quigley C. The role of opioids in cancer pain. *BMJ,* 2005; **331**: 825–829.
10 Gilron MD, Bailey JM, Tu D *et al.* Morphine, gabapentin, or their combination for neuropathic pain. *NEJM,* 2005; **352**(13): 1324–1334.
11 Galer BS and Jensen MP. Development and preliminary validation of a pain measure specific to neuropathic pain: the Neuropathic Pain Scale. *Neurology,* 1997; **48**: 332–338.
12 McCann RM, Hall WJ and Groth-Juncker A. Comfort care for terminally ill patients: the appropriate use of nutrition and hydration. *JAMA,* 1994; **272**(16): 1263–1266.
13 Bennett M, Lucas V, Brennan M *et al.* Using anti-muscarinic drugs in the management of death rattle: evidence-based guidelines for palliative care. *Palliative Med,* 2002; **16**: 369–374.
14 Bedell SE, Delbanco TL, Cook EF *et al.* Survival after cardiopulmonary resuscitation in the hospital. *NEJM,* 1983; **309**(10): 569–576.
15 Murphy DJ, Murray AM, Robinson BE *et al.* Outcomes of cardiopulmonary resuscitation in the elderly. *Ann Int Med,* 1989; **111**: 199–205.
16 Taffet GE, Teasdale TA and Luchi RJ. In-hospital cardiopulmonary resuscitation. *JAMA,* 1988; **260**(14): 2069–2072.
17 Longstreth WT, Cobb LA, Fahrenbruch CE *et al.* Does age affect outcomes of out-of-hospital cardiopulmonary resuscitation? *JAMA,* 1990; **264**: 2109–2110.
18 Applebaum GE, King JE and Finucane TE. The outcomes of CPR initiated in nursing homes. *JAGS,* 1990; **38**: 197–200.
19 Awoke S, Mouton CP and Parrott M. Outcomes of skilled cardiopulmonary resuscitation in a long-term-care facility: futile therapy? *JAGS,* 1992; **40**: 593–595.
20 Godkin MD and Toth EL. Cardiopulmonary resuscitation and older adults' expectations. *Gerontologist,* 1994; **34**(6): 797–802.
21 Murphy DJ, Burrows D, Santilli S *et al.* The influence of the probability of survival on patients' preferences regarding cardiopulmonary resuscitation. *NEJM,* 1994; **330**: 545–549.

Rating scales

Abbreviated mental test

The Abbreviated Mental Test (AMT) is a quick to use 10-point scale for screening for cognitive impairment. It predominantly assesses short- and long-term memory, attention and orientation. A score of less than 8 is usually taken to imply a significant cognitive deficit,[1] such as delirium or dementia, the cause of which can only be determined by more detailed evaluation.

Alzheimer's disease assessment scale – cognitive sub-scale

The Alzheimer's Disease Assessment Scale – cognitive subscale (ADAS-cog)[2] is a score to assess severity of cognitive dysfunction in Alzheimer's disease (AD). It gives values for a variety of clinical features, including language, recall, praxis and orientation, which are then added up. The total score is between 0 and 70. A higher score suggests a more severely impaired patient.

Barthel index

The Barthel index[3] is a rating scale used to assess recovery with rehabilitation. Scores are given for various daily activities, including continence, self-care, mobility and transfers. The value ranges from 0 to 100, with a higher score suggesting greater functionality and independence. Scores achieved by the time of discharge appear to reflect eventual destination. Those scoring less than 10 commonly require nursing home placement.[4]

Confusion Assessment Method

The Confusion Assessment Method[5] is a screening test for the detection of delirium. For a positive result the patient must have evidence of both items 1 and 2, plus either 3 or 4 as listed below:

1 acute confusion with a fluctuating pattern
2 inattention
3 disorganised speech
4 altered level of consciousness.

Geriatric Depression Scale

The Geriatric Depression Scale (GDS) was initially developed as a 30-question form[6] but more recently as a 15-question version of yes/no answers. It can be self- or carer-administered. A cut-off score of 5 or more is suggestive of depression. Depending on cut-off used, sensitivities and specificities of 82–100% and 72–82%, respectively, have been demonstrated.[7]

The five-item GDS is an abbreviated version of the GDS that appears to be as effective as the standard GDS, yet is administered in less time.[8] The five questions are as follows:

- Are you basically satisfied with your life?
- Do you often get bored?
- Do you often feel helpless?
- Do you prefer to stay at home rather than going out and doing new things?
- Do you feel pretty worthless the way you are now?

A score of 2 or more is suggestive of depression.

Hospital Anxiety and Depression Scale

The Hospital Anxiety and Depression Scale (HAD) is a screening tool for anxiety and depression. The patients fill in the questionnaire themselves. There are 14 questions, seven of which look for signs of anxiety and seven for depression. Each is given a score between 0 and 3, leading to maximum scores of 21 for each aspect. A higher score suggests more significant impairment. A score of 11 or above is usually taken to indicate a significant disorder.[9]

Hoehn and Yahr

The Hoehn and Yahr[10] is a rating scale used to assess the severity of Parkinson's disease (PD). There are five stages as outlined below:

I   Unilateral disease.
II   Bilateral disease.
III   Postural instability.
IV   Advanced disease with severe disability but still able to walk.
V   Confined to wheelchair or bed.

More recently, a modified version of this has been developed.[11]

- Stage 0.0   No signs of PD.
- Stage 1.0   Unilateral disease.
- Stage 1.5   Unilateral and axial disease.
- Stage 2.0   Bilateral disease.
- Stage 2.5   Mild bilateral disease and recovery on the pull test.
- Stage 3.0   Postural instability.
- Stage 4.0   Advanced disease with severe disability but still able to walk.
- Stage 5.0   Confined to wheelchair or bed.

Mini Mental State Examination

The Mini Mental State Examination (MMSE)[12] is a 30-point assessment scale used in the diagnosis and monitoring of cognitive impairment. The higher the score, the better the cerebral function. A score of 25 or below is usually used to indicate significant impairment. Its clinical utility is limited and it may well not detect impairment due to frontal lobe dysfunction in the early stages of frontotemporal dementia (FTD). A score of 30 does not automatically mean no impairment (ceiling effect) and a score of 0 does not mean no brain function (floor effect). Its value may be hard to interpret in the presence of illiteracy, dysphasia or visual loss, or in people who do not speak English. When used to monitor dementia, a rate of decline of around three points per year is commonly seen. It also appears to have a role in the diagnosis and monitoring of patients with delirium.[13]

Neuropsychiatric inventory

The Neuropsychiatric Inventory (NPI)[14] is a score to assess behavioural problems in dementia. It assesses 10 domains (delusions, hallucinations, agitation/aggression, depression/dysphoria, anxiety, elation/euphoria, apathy/indifference, disinhibition, irritability/lability and aberrant motor behaviour). Each domain is scored out of 12 (by multiplying a severity (0–3) and frequency (0–4) value together). The total score is the sum of these domain scores, which will be between 0 and 120. A higher score suggests a worse behavioural disturbance.

Unified Parkinson's Disease Rating Scale

The Unified Parkinson's Disease Rating Scale (UPDRS)[15] is an assessment tool for use with patients with PD. The total score is between 0 and 199. A higher score suggests a more severe impairment. It has four main parts (the maximum scores for the individual sections are shown in brackets):

- I   Mentation, behaviour and mood (16)
- II   Activities of daily living (52)
- III Motor (108)
- IV Complications of therapy (23).

References

1 Jitapunkul S, Pillay I and Ebrahim S. The abbreviated mental test: its use and validity. *Age Ageing*, 1991; **20**: 332–336.
2 Doraiswamy PM, Bieber F, Kaiser L *et al.* The Alzheimer's disease assessment scale: patterns and predictors of baseline cognitive performance in multicenter Alzheimer's disease trials. *Neurology*, 1997; **48**: 1511–1517.
3 Mahoney F and Barthel D. Functional evaluation: Barthel index. *Md State Med J*, 1965; **14**: 61–65.
4 Stone SP, Ali B, Auberleek I *et al.* The Barthel index in clinical practice: use on a rehabilitation ward for elderly people. *J Royal Coll Phys*, 1994; **28**(5): 419–423.

5   Inouye SK, van Dyck CH, Alessi CA *et al.* Clarifying confusion: the confusion assessment method. A new method for detection of delirium. *Ann Intern Med,* 1990; **113**(12): 941–948.

6   Brink TL, Yesavage JA, Lum O *et al.* Screening tests for geriatric depression. *Clin Gerontol,* 1982; 1: 37–43.

7   Watson LC and Pignone MP. Screening accuracy for late-life depression in primary care: a systematic review. *J Fam Prac,* 2003; **52**(12): 956–964.

8   Hoyl TM, Alessi CA, Harker JO *et al.* Development and testing of a five-item version of the Geriatric Depression Scale. *JAGS,* 1999; **47**: 873–878.

9   Zigmond AS and Snaith RP. The Hospital Anxiety and Depression Scale. *Acta Psychiatr Scand,* 1983; **67**: 361–370.

10 Hoehn MM and Yahr MD. Parkinsonism: onset, progression and mortality. *Neurology,* 1967; 17: 427–442.

11 Lang AE and Fahn S. Assessment of Parkinson's disease. In: Munsat TL, *Quantification of Neurologic Deficit.* Stoneham: Butterworth-Heineman, 1989.

12 Folstein MF, Folstein SE and McHugh PR. 'Mini-mental state'. A practical method for grading the cognitive state of patients for the physician. *J Psychiatr Res,* 1975; **12**: 189–198.

13 O'Keeffe ST, Mulkerrin EC, Nayeem K *et al.* Use of serial mini-mental state examinations to diagnose and monitor delirium in elderly hospital patients. *JAGS,* 2005; **53**: 867–870.

14 Cummings JL, Mega M, Gray K *et al.* The Neuropsychiatric Inventory: comprehensive assessment of psychopathology in dementia. *Neurology,* 1994; **44**: 2308–2314.

15 Fahn S, Elton RL and UPDRS Development Committee. Unified Parkinson's Disease Rating Scale. In: Fahn S, Marsden CD, Calne DB *et al., Recent Developments in Parkinson's Disease,* Vol 2. Florham Park, NJ: MacMillan Healthcare Information, 1987: 153–163.

Abbreviations

ABC	Antecedents, behaviour and consequences
ABG	Arterial blood gas
ABPI	Ankle–brachial pressure index
ACA	Anterior cerebral artery
ACE	Angiotensin-converting enzyme
ACEi	Angiotensin-converting enzyme inhibitor
ACh	Acetylcholine
ACLS	Advanced cardiac life support
AD	Alzheimer's disease
ADAS-cog	Alzheimer's Disease Assessment Scale – cognitive sub-scale
AF	Atrial fibrillation
AFO	Ankle–foot orthosis
ALP	Alkaline phosphatase
AMT	Abbreviated mental test
ANP	Atrial natriuretic peptide
ARB	Angiotensin type II receptor blockers
ARD	Alcohol-related dementia
AVM	Arteriovenous malformation
BADLS	Bristol Activities of Daily Living Scale
bd	Twice daily
BMD	Bone mineral density
BMI	Body mass index
BMT	Behavioural management techniques
BNP	Brain natriuretic peptide
BP	Blood pressure
BPH	Benign prostatic hyperplasia
BPPV	Benign paroxysmal positional vertigo
BPSD	Behavioural and psychological symptoms of dementia
BT	Behavioural treatment
CAA	Cerebral amyloid angiopathy
CADASIL	Cerebral autosomal dominant arteriopathy with subcortical infarcts and leukoencephalopathy
CAM	Confusion assessment method
CBD	Corticobasal degeneration
CCF	Congestive cardiac failure
CE	Carotid endarterectomy
CI	Confidence interval
CICSS	Cardio-inhibitory carotid sinus syndrome
CJD	Creutzfeldt–Jakob disease

CK	Creatine kinase
CNP	C-type natriuretic peptide
CNS	Central nervous system
COMT	Catechol-o-methyltransferase
COMTi	Catechol-o-methytransferase inhibitor
CPR	Cardiopulmonary resuscitation
CR	Controlled-release
CRP	C-reactive protein
CSF	Cerebrospinal fluid
CSH	Carotid sinus hypersensitivity
CSM	Carotid sinus massage
CSS	Carotid sinus syndrome
CT	Computerised tomography
CVA	Cerebrovascular accident
DBS	Deep brain stimulation
DEXA	Dual-energy X-ray absorptiometry
DHT	Dihydrotestosterone
DI	Dual incontinence
DIC	Disseminated intravascular coagulation
DLB	Dementia with Lewy bodies
DVT	Deep vein thrombosis
ECG	Electrocardiograph
ECT	Electroconvulsive therapy
EEG	Electroencephalography
ELD	External lumbar drainage
EPS	Electrophysiological studies
ESR	Erythrocyte sedimentation rate
ET	Essential tremor
FBC	Full blood count
FFP	Fresh frozen plasma
FI	Faecal incontinence
FTD	Frontotemporal dementia
GABA	Gamma-aminobutyric acid
GCA	Giant cell arteritis
GCS	Glasgow Coma Scale
GDNF	Glial cell derived neurotrophic factor
GDS	Geriatric depression score
GFR	Glomerular filtration rate
GnRH	Gonadotrophin-releasing hormone
GPi	Globus pallidus interna
GTN	Glyceryl trinitrate
HAD	Hospital Anxiety and Depression Scale
HIV	Human immunodeficiency virus
HR	Hazard ratio

| HRT | Hormone replacement therapy |
| HUT | Head-up tilt |

ICD	Implantable cardioverter-defibrillator
ICH	Intracranial haemorrhage
IM	Intramuscular
INR	International normalised ratio
ISH	Isolated systolic hypertension
ITU	Intensive therapy unit
IV	Intravenous

| JVP | Jugular venous pressure |

LACI	Lacunar circulation infarct
LACS	Lacunar circulation stroke
LH	Luteinising hormone

MAOI	Monoamine oxidase inhibitor
MCA	Middle cerebral artery
MDMA	Methylenedioxymethamphetamine
MELAS	Mitochondrial encephalomyopathy, lactic acidosis and stroke-like episodes
MI	Myocardial infarct
MMSE	Mini Mental State Examination
MND	Motor neuron disease
MRI	Magnetic resonance imaging
MSA	Multiple system atrophy
MSU	Mid-stream urine

NG	Nasogastric
NHS	National Health Service
NICE	National Institute for Clinical Excellence
NMDA	N-methyl-D-aspartate
NMS	Neuroleptic malignant syndrome
NNT	Number needed to treat
NPH	Normal pressure hydrocephalus
NPI	Neuropsychiatric inventory
NSAID	Non-steroidal anti-inflammatory drug

OH	Orthostatic hypotension
OR	Odds ratio
OSA	Obstructive sleep apnoea

PACI	Partial anterior circulation infarct
PACS	Partial anterior circulation stroke
PAF	Paroxysmal atrial fibrillation
PCA	Posterior cerebral artery
PCC	Prothrombin complex concentrate
PD	Parkinson's disease

PDD	Parkinson's disease dementia
PE	Pulmonary embolism
PEA	Pulseless electrical activity
PEG	Percutaneous endoscopic gastrostomy
PET	Positron emission tomography
PFO	Patent foramen ovale
PMC	Pseudomembranous colitis
POCI	Posterior circulation infarct
POCS	Posterior circulation stroke
POTS	Paroxysmal orthostatic tachycardia syndrome
PPI	Proton pump inhibitor
PR	Per rectum
PSA	Prostate specific antigen
PSP	Progressive supranuclear palsy
PTH	Parathyroid hormone
PU	Pressure ulcers
RCT	Randomised controlled trial
RR	Risk ratio
Rt-PA	Recombinant tissue plasminogen activator
SAH	Subarachnoid haemorrhage
SC	Subcutaneous
SD	Standard deviation
SHBG	Sex hormone binding globulin
SIADH	Syndrome of inappropriate antidiuretic hormone
SLE	Systemic lupus erythematosus
SR	Sinus rhythm
SSRI	Selective serotonin reuptake inhibitor
STN	Subthalamic nucleus
TACI	Total anterior circulation infarct
TACS	Total anterior circulation stroke
TCA	Tricyclic antidepressant
TD	Tardive dyskinesia
tds	Three times daily
TENS	Transcutaneous electrical nerve stimulation
TGA	Transient global amnesia
TIA	Transient ischaemic attack
TOE	Transoesophageal echocardiography
TSH	Thyroid stimulating hormone
TURP	Trans-urethral resection of prostate
UI	Urinary incontinence
UMN	Upper motor neuron
UPDRS	Unified Parkinson's Disease Rating Scale
UTI	Urinary tract infection
UV	Ultra violet

VaD	Vascular dementia
Vd	Volume of distribution
VDCSS	Vasodepressor carotid sinus syndrome
VDRL	Venereal disease research laboratory test
VF	Ventricular fibrillation
VP	Vascular Parkinsonism
VT	Ventricular tachycardia
VVS	Vasovagal syndrome (or syncope)
WHO	World Health Organization

Index